Blood Cells

A PRACTICAL GUIDE

Barbara J Bain MB BS MRC Path FRCP
*Senior Lecturer in Haematology and Consultant Haematologist,
St Mary's Hospital, London, UK*

J. B. Lippincott Company PHILADELPHIA
Gower Medical Publishing LONDON · NEW YORK

Distributed in USA and Canada by:
J.B. Lippincott Company
East Washington Square
Philadelphia, PA 19105
USA

Distributed in UK and Continental Europe by:
Harper & Row Ltd
Middlesex House
34–42 Cleveland Street
London W1P 5FB
UK

**Distributed in Philippines/Guam, Middle East,
Latin America and Africa by:**
Harper & Row International
East Washington Square
Philadelphia, PA 19105
USA

Distributed in Australia and New Zealand by:
Harper & Row (Australasia) Pty Ltd
P.O. Box 226
Artarmon, N.S.W. 2064
Australia

Distributed in Japan by:
Igaku Shoin Ltd
Tokyo International
P.O. Box 5063
Tokyo
Japan

**Distributed in Southeast Asia, Hong Kong,
India and Pakistan by:**
Harper & Row Publishers (Asia) Pte Ltd
37 Jalan Pemimpin 02–01
Singapore 2057

Project editors:
Leslie Smillie
Marion Jowett

Design:
Michel Laake
Mark Willey

Line artists:
Marion Tasker
Mark Willey
Michael Rabess
Sue Allison

Library of Congress Catalog Number: 88–81403

British Library Cataloguing in Publication Data:
Bain, Barbara J. (Barbara Jane)
    Blood Cells.
    1. Man. Blood. Cells
    i. Title
    612'.11

ISBN: 0–397–44558–X (Lippincott/Gower)

Originated in Hong Kong by Mandarin Offset.

Typesetting by IC Dawkins (typesetters) Ltd., London.

Text set in Aldus; captions and figures set in Futura.

Printed in Hong Kong by Imago Publishing Ltd.

Preface

I have written this book with both the practising haematologist and the trainee in mind. My aim has been to provide a guide to the morphology of blood cells which is both sufficiently straightforward to be intelligible to the trainee and also sufficiently comprehensive to be a reference source for the qualified haematologist. Since in modern haematological practice blood films are rarely assessed other than in relation to blood counts I have also sought to explain the principles underlying the performance of the blood count and the approach the haematologist might take to the interpretation of the data produced. This has necessarily involved a consideration of the range of normality. I have not discussed bone marrow morphology other than to the very limited extent necessary to put in context the abnormalities which may be noted in the peripheral blood but I have indicated when a bone marrow examination or other specialized tests are indicated. The morphological descriptions relate particularly to Romanowsky-stained blood films, but important cytochemical tests applicable to the peripheral blood have also been discussed.

My hope is that this book will give the medically trained haematologist a fuller understanding of the scientific basis of an important segment of laboratory haematology and at the same time will give the scientifically trained laboratory worker a deeper understanding of the purpose and clinical relevance of the tests being performed. If I succeed in sending the reader back to the microscope with renewed interest and enthusiasm I shall be satisfied.

B.J.B.

Acknowledgements

I should like to thank the following people who have helped in various ways: Dr S. Abdalla, Dr I. Bunce, Mr A. Dean, Dr D. Gill, Dr N. Parker, Dr M. Pippard, Dr M. Taylor, Dr M. Walker, Professor S. Wickramasinghe and Mr J. Williams for lending blood films for photography; Professor J. Stewart for the photograph of the Chédiak–Higashi syndrome; Dr D. Coleman for the photograph of the Ph[1] chromosome and Mr J. Griffiths for the printout of the Ortho ELT 800 WCS automated counter. My thanks are also due to a number of people who read and criticized sections of the text and in particular to Dr J. Matthews and Mr A. Dean who assiduously read the entire manuscript.

Contents

1. Blood sampling and film preparation

OBTAINING A BLOOD SPECIMEN

The identity of the patient requiring venepuncture should be carefully checked prior to obtaining a blood specimen. Patients should either sit or lie comfortably and should be reassured that the procedure causes only moderate discomfort; they should not be told that venepuncture is painless since this is not so. It is preferable for apprehensive patients to lie down. Chairs used for seating patients requiring venepuncture should have arm rests, both for convenience and to prevent a faint patient from falling from the chair. (The author has personally observed a skull fracture sustained when a patient fainted at the conclusion of a venepuncture and fell forward onto a hard floor.) If venepunctures are being performed on children or on patients unable to cooperate fully then the arm for venepuncture should be gently but firmly immobilized by an assistant.

PERIPHERAL VENOUS BLOOD

In an adult, peripheral venous blood is most readily obtained from a vein in the antecubital fossa (Fig.1.1), using either a needle and a plastic syringe or a needle and an evacuated tube. Of the veins in the antecubital region the median cubital vein is preferred, since it is usually large and well anchored in tissues, but the cephalic and basilic veins are also often satisfactory. Other forearm veins can be used, although they are often more mobile and therefore more difficult to penetrate. Veins on the dorsum of the wrist and hand often have a poorer flow and performing venepuncture at these sites is more likely to lead to bruising. This is also true of the anterior surface of the wrist where, in addition, venepuncture tends to be more painful. When a vein is identified it is palpated to ensure that it is patent. If a vein is not visible (in dark-skinned people

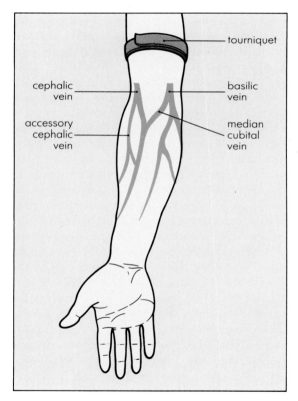

Fig.1.1 *The veins of the antecubital fossa which are most suitable for venepuncture.*

and in some overweight people) then palpation is required to make one identifiable. If veins appear very small, warming of the arm to produce vasodilation is helpful, as is tapping the vein and asking the patient to clench and unclench the fist several times.

The arm should be positioned on the arm rest so that the selected vein is under some tension and its mobility is reduced. The skin should be cleansed with 70% ethanol or 0.5% chlorhexidine, and allowed to dry. A tourniquet is applied to the arm sufficiently tightly to distend the vein but not in such a manner as to cause discomfort. Alternatively a sphygmomanometer cuff may be applied and inflated to diastolic presure, but a tourniquet is usually quicker and simpler. The tourniquet should preferably be left on the arm only long enough to allow penetration of the vein. If it is necessary to leave the tourniquet applied in order to get an adequate flow of blood, it should be applied for no more than a minute if possible. However, the degree of haemoconcentration caused by a tourniquet applied in this manner, even for 10 minutes, is not great; the increase in haemoglobin (Hb) concentration and red cell count (RBC) is about 3 percent at 2 and at 10 minutes.[5]

A 19 or 20 gauge needle is suitable for an adult and a smaller gauge (21 or 23) for a child or an adult with small veins. The needle, attached to the syringe, is inserted into the vein with the bevel upwards. This may be done with a single movement or in two separate movements for the skin and the vein, depending on personal preference and on how superficial the vein is. With one hand steadying the barrel of the syringe so that the needle is not accidentally withdrawn from the vein, blood is drawn into the syringe using minimum possible negative pressure. Care needs to be taken that an attempt is not made to aspirate more rapidly than blood is entering the vein, or the wall of the vein may be drawn against the bevel of the needle and cut off the flow of blood. If the tourniquet has not already been released this must be done prior to withdrawal of the needle. Following needle withdrawal direct pressure is applied to the puncture with a sterile dry gauze square, the arm being held straight and, if preferred, somewhat elevated. Adhesive plaster should not be applied until pressure has been applied for long enough for haemostasis to be achieved.

The needle should be removed from the syringe prior to expelling the blood, great care being taken to avoid self-injury with the needle. It is generally regarded as safer to put the needle directly into a special receptacle for sharp objects without resheathing it. (Hepatitis B virus can readily be transmitted by a needle-prick injury, as may other infections. The transmissibility of the human immunodeficiency virus (HIV) by needle-prick injury is much less than that of hepatitis B virus, but a risk does exist.)

Following removal of the needle the blood specimen is expelled gently from the syringe into a bottle containing anticoagulant. Forceful ejection of the blood may cause lysis. The blood is mixed with the anticoagulant by inverting the bottle four or five times. Shaking should be avoided. The anticoagulant of choice is a salt of ethylenediaminetetraacetic acid (EDTA) also known as sequestrene. In the United Kingdom dry K_2EDTA to give a final concentration of 1.5 mg/ml is favoured, whereas in North America liquid K_3EDTA to give a final concentration of 1.5 mg/ml is most often used. The preference for an anticoagulant in solution in North America is because mixing of the blood specimen is easier and clotted specimens are therefore less likely. Na_2EDTA may also be employed, but it is less soluble than are the potassium salts. It should be noted that some haematological parameters are altered by dilution if EDTA in solution is used, and if too little blood is taken into a tube then dilution may be appreciable. Measurements of some parameters differ according to the specific salt of EDTA which is used (see page 17). Excess EDTA also has deleterious effects on cell morphology in stained blood films (see page 86) and alters the microhaematocrit.

Following gentle mixing of the blood specimen and the anticoagulant the tubes should be labelled with the patient's name, other identifying details and the time of venepuncture. Bottles should not be labelled in advance away from the patient's bedside as this increases the chances of putting a blood sample into a mislabelled bottle. Recording the time of venepuncture is important both to allow the clinician to relate the laboratory result to the condition of the patient at the time, and also to allow the laboratory to check that there was no undue delay between venepuncture and performing the test.

When blood is taken into an evacuated tube the technique of venepuncture is basically similar. A double-ended needle is screwed into a holder which allows it to be manipulated for insertion into the vein. After insertion the evacuated tube is inserted into the holder and its rubber cap is penetrated by the needle, breaking the vacuum and causing blood to be aspirated into the tube. If veins are small an appropriately small vacuum tube should be used as excess vacuum may cause the vein to collapse. Evacuated tubes are very convenient if multiple samples are to be taken, since selected evacuated tubes can be applied in turn. Only sterile vacuum tubes should be used for obtaining blood specimens.

If a large specimen is required and an evacuated tube

system is not in use, blood can be collected through a 'butterfly', that is, through a needle fused to a small flexible tube (Fig. 1.2). The tubing can be easily pinched off to allow several syringes in turn to be attached.

'CAPILLARY' BLOOD

It is often advisable to obtain blood by skin puncture rather than venepuncture in babies and infants, and in adults with poor veins.

'Capillary' or, more probably, arteriolar blood may be obtained from a freely flowing stab wound made with a sterile lancet on the plantar surface of a warmed and cleansed heel (babies less than three months of age and infants), the plantar aspect of the big toe (infants) or a finger, thumb or ear lobe (older children and adults). The correct site for puncture of a heel is shown in Fig. 1.3. The lateral or posterior aspect of the heel should not be used in a baby as the underlying bone is much closer to the skin surface than it is on the plantar aspect. In older patients a finger (excluding the fifth finger) or the thumb is preferred to an ear lobe since bleeding from the ear lobe may be prolonged in a patient with a haemostatic defect and pressure is difficult to apply. The palmar surface of the distal phalanx is the preferred site on a digit since the underlying bone is closer to the skin surface on other aspects. Skin punctures should ideally be more than 1.5 mm deep in order that the lancet passes through the dermal–subcutaneous junction, where the concentration of blood vessels is greatest, and a free flow of blood occurs. Lancets used for heel puncture in babies must not exceed 2.4 mm in depth since this is the depth below the skin of the calcaneal bone. Osteomyelitis of the calcaneus has resulted from inadvertent puncture of the bone.[2] Previous puncture sites should be avoided to lessen the risk of infection.

Capillary samples should be obtained from warm tissues so that a free flow of blood is more easily obtained. If the area is cool then it should be warmed with a wet cloth no hotter than 42°C. The skin should then be cleansed with 70% isopropanol and dried with a sterile gauze square (since traces of alcohol may lead to haemolysis of the specimen). The first drop of blood may be diluted with tissue fluid and should be wiped away with a sterile gauze square. Flow of blood may be promoted by gentle pressure, but a massaging or pumping action should not be employed since this may lead to tissue fluid being mixed with the blood.

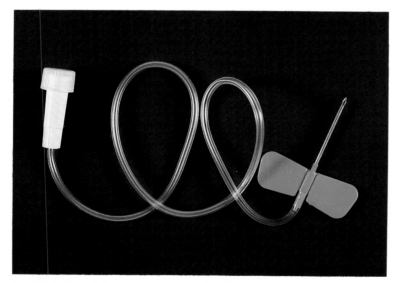

Fig.1.2 A 'butterfly' infusion set suitable for obtaining a blood sample. Following insertion of the needle into the vein the cap is removed and a syringe attached.

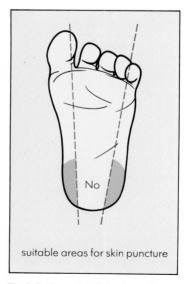

suitable areas for skin puncture

Fig.1.3 The sole of the foot of an infant showing the areas which are suitable for skin puncture.

Capillary blood may be collected into reusable glass pipettes or into glass capillary tubes. Capillary tubes containing EDTA may be used, but tubes containing heparin should not be used for full blood count (FBC) specimens since cellular morphology and staining characteristics are altered. Disposable pipettes complete with diluent, suitable for both automated and manual counts, are commercially available.

Platelet counts performed on capillary blood are often lower than on venous blood.[1] Other haematological parameters may also vary with the site of sampling (see Chapter 6).

CORD BLOOD

Blood samples may be obtained from the umbilical cord immediately after birth. Cord blood is best obtained from the cord vessel by means of a syringe and needle. Expressing blood from the cut end of the cord may introduce Wharton's jelly into the blood sample with subsequent red cell agglutination. Laboratory results on cord blood are not necessarily identical to those obtained on capillary or venous specimens from the neonate (see Chapter 6).

OTHER SITES

It may sometimes be necessary to obtain blood from ankle veins, from the femoral vein or from indwelling cannulae in various sites. If the blood is obtained from a cannula the first sample obtained may be diluted by infusion fluid or contaminated by heparin and should be discarded. In infants, blood may be obtained from scalp veins and jugular veins.

MAKING A BLOOD FILM

A blood film may be made from non-anticoagulated (native) blood, obtained either from a vein or a capillary, or from EDTA-anticoagulated blood. Chelation of calcium by EDTA hinders platelet aggregation so that platelets are evenly spread and their numbers can be assessed more easily (Fig. 1.4). Films prepared from capillary blood usually show prominent platelet aggregation (Fig. 1.5) and films from non-anti-coagulated venous blood often show small aggregates (Fig. 1.6). Films prepared from non-anticoagulated venous or capillary blood are free of artefacts due to storage or the effects of the anticoagulant. Many laboratories use such films as a matter of normal practice, and they are obligatory for investigating abnormalities such as red cell crenation or white cell or platelet aggregation, which may be induced by EDTA (see page 32). Conversely, the use of a blood film prepared from EDTA-anticoagulated blood after arrival of the blood specimen in the laboratory has the advantage that some of the abnormalities which may

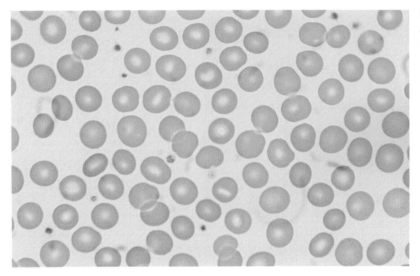

Fig. 1.4 *A blood film from EDTA-anticoagulated blood showing the even distribution of platelets. ×960.*

effect the validity of results obtained from automated instruments are more likely to be detected, for example the formation of fibrin strands, platelet aggregates, or red cell agglutinates consequent on the presence of a cold agglutinin.

MANUAL SPREADING OF A BLOOD FILM ON A GLASS SLIDE (WEDGE-SPREAD FILM)

Glass slides must be clean and free of grease. A spreader is also required and must be narrower than the slide; if the slide is to have a coverslip mounted, the spreader must also be narrower than the coverslip so that cells at the edges of the film are beneath the coverslip and may be easily examined microscopically. A spreader may be readily prepared by breaking the corner off a glass slide after marking it with a diamond pen; this provides a smooth-edged spreader which is large enough to be manipulated easily. This technique provides superior spreaders to those made by cutting transverse pieces from a slide with a diamond pen; the latter technique leaves at least one rough edge which may damage the fingers.

A drop of native or well mixed anticoagulated blood is placed near one end of the slide; anticoagulated blood is applied with a capillary tube which is then discarded. The spreader is applied at an angle of 25–30 degrees, in front of the drop of blood and is *drawn back into it*.

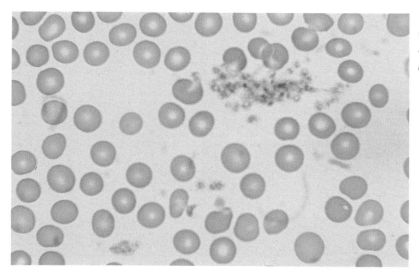

Fig.1.5 *A blood film from non-anticoagulated capillary blood showing the aggregation of platelets which usually occurs.* ×960.

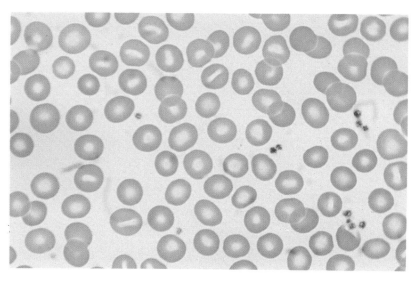

Fig.1.6 *A blood film from non-anticoagulated venous blood showing the minor degree of platelet aggregation which usually occurs.* ×960.

Once the blood has run along the edge of the spreader, the spreader is advanced with a smooth steady motion so that a thin film of blood is spread over the slide (Fig. 1.7). If the angle of the spreader is too obtuse or the speed of spreading is too fast, the film will be too short. An experienced operator learns to recognize blood with

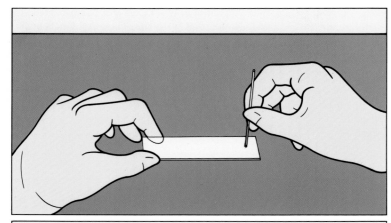

Fig. 1.7 *The making of a wedge-spread blood film:*
(a) *a drop of blood is applied near one end of the slide, using a capillary tube.*

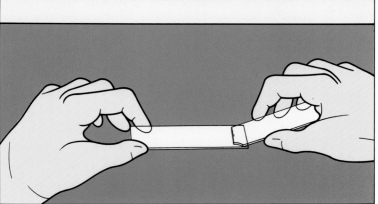

(b) *the spreader is drawn back into the drop of blood and is held there until some blood has spread across its width.*

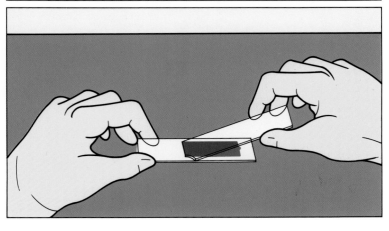

(c) *the spreader, at an angle of about 25 degrees, is pushed steadily along the slide to produce a thin, even film of blood.*

a higher than normal haematocrit, which is more viscous and requires a more acute angle to make a satisfactory film, and, conversely, blood with a lower than normal haematocrit, which requires a more obtuse angle. The film is dried rapidly; if the laboratory atmosphere is humid then it may be necessary to use a fan or a hot-air drier such as a hair drier.

Figure 1.8 shows a well-made blood film plus examples of poor films resulting from faulty technique.

The slide is labelled with the date and the patient's name or with an identifying number. Labelling may be done by writing on the thicker part of the film with a pencil or by using a marker which is not soluble in methanol. A diamond pen can also be used, but this is slower. If preferred, slides frosted at one end so that they can readily be labelled with a pencil can be used, though they tend to be marginally more expensive.

It is important that the spreader is wiped thoroughly with a dry tissue or gauze square after each use since it is possible to transfer abnormal cells from one blood film to another by the use of an inadequately cleaned spreader (Fig.1.9).

Unless otherwise stated, this book deals with morphology as observed in wedge-spread films. Most of the photographs are of wedge-spread films which have been prepared manually from recently collected EDTA-anticoagulated blood.

AUTOMATED SPREADING OF A BLOOD FILM ON A GLASS SLIDE
Wedge-spread films may also be prepared using a mechanical spreader. Mechanical spreaders may give more consistent results than manual wedge-spreading.

COVERSLIP FILMS
Slides may also be prepared by placing a drop of blood on a coverslip, adding a second coverslip, and allowing the blood to spread between the two by capillary action. The two coverslips are then separated by pulling them in opposite directions. Coverslip films are difficult to

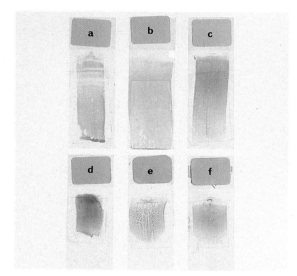

Fig.1.8 *Unsatisfactory and satisfactory blood films: (a) uneven pressure has produced ridges; (b) too broad and too long — the edges and tail of the film cannot be examined adequately; (c) too long, and streaked by an uneven spreader; (d) too thick and short due to wrong angle or speed of spreading; (e) fat globules on a greasy slide interrupt the distribution of the blood cells; (f) satisfactory.*

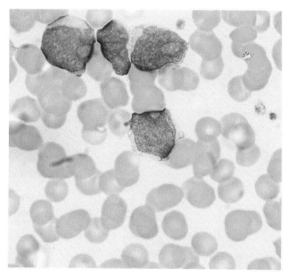

Fig.1.9 *Blast cells from a patient with leukaemia have been inadvertently transferred to the blood film of another patient by the use of an inadequately cleaned spreader. ×960.*

handle until they have been stained and themselves mounted on slides. They do not lend themselves to automated staining. The distribution of white cells may be more even than in wedge-spread films, but red cell morphology is often less satisfactory.

FILMS PREPARED BY CENTRIFUGATION

A film of blood one cell thick may be spread on a glass slide by centrifugation at an appropriate speed in a specially designed centrifuge. These preparations have the advantage that cells of different types are distributed similarly throughout the film and fragile cells (such as the lymphocytes of chronic lymphocytic leukaemia) are not smeared or smudged. Films prepared by this method are required for some automated differential counting machines, but they are also suitable for microscopic examination.

FILMS FROM BLOOD WITH A VERY HIGH HAEMATOCRIT

The increased viscosity of very polycythaemic blood (for example of blood with a Hb concentration greater than 20 g/dl or with a haematocrit greater than 0.60) may make it difficult to spread a film which is sufficiently thin for cellular morphology to be assessed, even when the spreader is applied at a more acute angle. In these circumstances it is useful to add a drop of AB plasma or saline to a drop of blood; a suitably thin film can then be made.

BUFFY-COAT FILMS

In order to inspect large numbers of nucleated cells it is sometimes useful to centrifuge a blood specimen and make a blood film in the normal way from the buffy coat which has been mixed with an equal volume of autologous EDTA–plasma. This technique can be used when a manual differential count is required on a specimen with a very low white cell count. It is also useful for the detection of bacteria or abnormal cells present at low frequency (for example, blast cells, hairy cells, ring sideroblasts or megaloblasts).

THICK FILMS

Thick films are required for examination for malarial parasites and certain other parasites, the red cells being lysed before the film is examined. Parasites are much more concentrated in a thick film than in a thin film. To make a thick film several drops of native or EDTA-anti-coagulated blood are placed in the centre of a slide and spread with a capillary tube into a pool of blood of such thickness that typescript or a watch face can just be read through the blood. The blood film is not fixed but, following drying, is placed directly into an aqueous stain (see below) so that lysis of the red cells occurs (Fig.1.10); this allows the organisms to be seen more clearly. Placing the film in an incubator at 37°C for 10 minutes both accelerates drying and renders the blood film less likely to lift off the slide during staining.

FIXATION, STAINING AND MOUNTING
FIXATION

Following air drying, thin films are fixed in absolute methanol for 10–20 minutes. Poor fixation and characteristic artefactual changes occur if the methanol has more than a few percent of water (Fig.1.11); this renders interpretation of morphology, particularly red cell morphology, impossible. In warm humid climates it may be necessary to change methanol solutions several times a day. Similar artefactual changes may be produced by condensation on slides. In a humid atmosphere slides should be fixed as soon as they are adequately dry.

STAINING

There is little consistency between laboratories in the precise stain used to prepare a blood film for microscopic examination, but the multitude of stains in use are all based on the Romanowsky stain, developed by the Russian protozoologist in the late nineteenth century.[6] Romanowsky used a mixture of old methylene blue and eosin to stain the nucleus of a malarial parasite purple and the cytoplasm blue. Subsequently Giemsa modified the stain, combining methylene azure and eosin. The stain most commonly used in the United Kingdom is a combination of Giemsa's stain with May–Grünwald stain; it is therefore designated May–Grünwald–Giemsa (MGG) stain. The stain most commonly used in North America is Wright's stain, which contains methylene blue and eosin; the methylene blue has been heated, or 'polychromed', to produce analogues of methylene blue.

It has recently been demonstrated using chromatography that dyes prepared by traditional organic chemistry methods are not pure, dyes sold under the same designation containing a variable mixture of five to ten dyes.[4] Variation between different batches prepared by the same manufacturer also occurs.

The essential components of a Romanowsky-type stain are: a basic or cationic dye, such as azure B, which conveys a blue-violet or blue colour to nucleic acids (DNA and RNA) and to nucleoprotein, to the granules of basophils and, weakly, to the granules of neutrophils; and an acidic or anionic dye, such as eosin, which conveys a red or orange colour to haemoglobin and the eosinophil granules. A stain containing azure B and eosin provides a satisfactory Romanowsky stain,[6] as does a mixture of azure B, methylene blue and eosin.[4]

Traditionally, cytoplasm which stains blue and granules which stain deep purple have both been designated 'basophilic' and granules which stain violet or pinkish-purple have been designated 'azurophilic'. In fact all these hues are achieved by uptake of a single basic dye such as azure B or azure A. 'Acidophilic' and 'eosinophilic' both refer to uptake of the acidic dye eosin, although 'acidophilic' has often been used to describe cell components staining pink, and 'eosinophilic' to describe cell components staining orange. The range of colours which a Romanowsky stain should produce are shown in Fig.1.12.

Satisfactory and consistent staining can be achieved using good quality commercial stains (see appendix). Pure azure B and eosin Y, as used in the ICSH (International Committee for Standardization in Haematology) reference method for the Romanowsky stain,[3] are now commercially available. A mixture of these dyes gives a very satisfactory result but such pure dyes are too expensive for routine use.

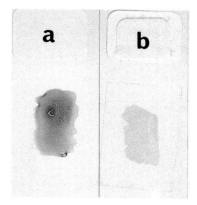

Fig.1.10 *Thick films for examination for malarial parasites: (a) unstained film; (b) film stained without fixation, causing lysis of the red cells.*

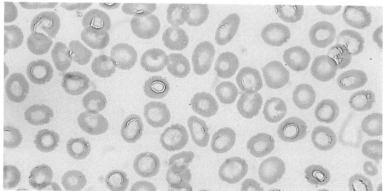

Fig.1.11 *Artefactual changes produced by five percent of water in methanol used for fixation. ×960.*

Fig.1.12 *Characteristic staining of different cell components by Romanowsky stains.*

Cell component staining	Colour
chromatin (including Howell–Jolly bodies)	purple
promyelocyte granules and Auer rods	purplish-red
cytoplasm of lymphocytes	blue
cytoplasm of monocytes	blue-grey
cytoplasm rich in RNA (i.e. 'basophilic cytoplasm')	deep blue
Döhle bodies	blue-grey
neutrophil-specific granules, 'azurophilic' granules of lymphocytes, granulomere of platelets	light purple or pink
granules of basophils	deep purple
granules of eosinophils	orange
red cells	pink

Staining must be performed at the correct pH. If the pH is too low, basophilic components do not stain well. Leucocytes are generally pale with eosinophil granules a brilliant vermilion. If the pH is too high, uptake of the basic dye may be excessive so that there is general over-staining, it becomes difficult to distinguish between normal and polychromatic red cells, eosinophil granules are blue or dark grey, and the granules of normal neutrophils are heavily stained, simulating toxic granulation.

Destaining a May–Grünwald–Giemsa-stained blood film may be done by flooding the slide with methanol, washing in water, and then repeating the sequence until all the stain has gone. This may be useful if only a single blood film is available and a further stain (for example an iron stain) is required.

Unless otherwise stated all descriptions of morphology and the staining characteristics of cells in this book refer to MGG-stained blood films.

Staining films for detection of malarial parasites

The detection and identification of malarial parasites is facilitated if blood films are stained with Giemsa stain at pH 7.2. At this pH cells which have been parasitized by either *Plasmodium vivax* or *Plasmodium ovale* have different tinctorial qualities from non-parasitized cells and are easily identified (see Chapter 3). The following method also gives good staining of inclusions in parasitized red cells. A standard methanol-fixed wedge-spread thin film and an unfixed thick film are air dried (or for greater speed are dried with a hot-air blower or in an incubator at 37°C) and are placed on a rack over a sink. The slides are flooded with freshly prepared unfiltered Giemsa stain in buffered distilled water (Sorensen's buffer, pH 7.2). Best results are obtained with 5% Giemsa stain for 20 minutes, but if greater speed is required 10% Giemsa stain for 10 minutes can be used. At the end of the staining period the stain is washed from the slides with running tap water. It is preferable not to pick up the slide and tip off the stain since this may leave stain deposits on the slide. Thick films must be washed very gently or the film of blood may be washed from the slide; it may be necessary to allow water to remain on the slide for some minutes to complete lysis and wash away the haemoglobin. Thin films can be washed with more vigour than thick films. Giemsa staining at pH 7.2 is also suitable for staining for other protozoan parasites, such as trypanosomes, and for microfilariae.

MOUNTING

If films are to be stored, mounting gives them the best protection against dust and scratching. As stated above, the coverslip should be sufficiently wide to cover the edges of the blood film. A neutral mountant which is miscible with xylene is required.

As an alternative to mounting, blood films may be sprayed with a polystyrene or acrylic resin.

Films which are not to be stored may be mounted temporarily by placing a coverslip on top of a drop of oil or xylene; alternatively, a thin film of oil may be smeared over the blood film to allow examination under low power before adding a drop of oil for examination under high power.

STORAGE OF SLIDES

Ideal patient care and continuing education of haematologists dictate that blood films should be stored as long as is practicable, preferably for some years. The most economical way to store slides is in metal racks in stacking drawers. Labels showing the date, test number and patient's name should be applied in such a way that they can be read while slides are in storage. Slides which have been freshly mounted should be kept in cardboard trays or stacked in racks separated from each other by wire loops until the mountant has hardened and dried. When the mountant is no longer sticky, slides may be stacked closely together for maximum economy of space.

References

1. Brecher G, Schneiderman M & Cronkite EP (1953) The reproducibility of the platelet count. *American Journal of Clinical Pathology*, **23**, 15–26.
2. Hammond KB (1980) Blood specimen collection from infants by skin puncture. *Laboratory Medicine*, **11**, 9–12.
3. ICSH (1984) ICSH reference method for staining blood and bone marrow film by azure B and eosin Y. *British Journal of Haematology*, **57**, 707–710.
4. Marshall PN, Bentley SA & Lewis SM (1975) A standardized Romanowsky stain prepared from pure dyes. *Journal of Clinical Pathology*, **28**, 920–923.
5. Mull JD & Murphy WR (1963) Effects of tourniquet-induced stasis on blood determinations. *American Journal of Clinical Pathology*, **39**, 134–136.
6. Wittekind D (1979) On the nature of the Romanowsky dyes and the Romanowsky–Giemsa effect. *Clinical and Laboratory Haematology*, **1**, 247–262.

2. Principles of performing a blood count

The tests included in a routine blood count have changed with time. Twenty years ago, using labour-intensive manual techniques, most laboratories estimated only haemoglobin concentration (Hb), packed cell volume (PCV) and white cell count (WBC) on a regular basis. Hb was measured by a method depending on optical density and PCV by centrifugation of a blood sample; white cells were counted micro-scopically in a diluted blood sample in a haemocyto-meter, a counting chamber of known volume. From the haemoglobin concentration and the PCV, the mean corpuscular haemoglobin concentration (MCHC) was calculated.

$$MCHC = \frac{Hb\ concentration\ (g/dl)}{PCV\ (l/l)}$$

For example, if $Hb = 12.3\ g/dl$

$$and\ PCV = 0.33,$$

$$then\ MCHC = \frac{12.3}{0.33} = 37.3\ g/dl.$$

Measurement of the red cell count (RBC) was required for calculation of the mean cell volume (MCV). Since counting of red cells in a haemocytometer was very time-consuming, an RBC was only made when there was a clear clinical indication for the calculation of the MCV.

$$MCV = \frac{PCV\ (l/l) \times 1000}{RBC\ (cells/l) \times 10^{-12}}$$

For example, if $PCV = 0.33$

$$and\ RBC = 4.1 \times 10^{12}/l,$$

$$then\ MCV = \frac{0.33 \times 1000}{4.1} = 80.5\ fl.$$

Availability of the RBC also allowed calculation of the mean corpuscular haemoglobin (MCH):

$$MCH = \frac{Hb\ concentration\ (g/dl) \times 10}{RBC\ (cells/l) \times 10^{-12}}$$

For example, if $Hb = 12.3\ g/dl$

$$and\ RBC = 4.1 \times 10^{12}/l,$$

$$then\ MCH = \frac{12.3 \times 10}{4.1} = 30\ pg.$$

With manual techniques there were thus three measured parameters (Hb, PCV and RBC) and three calculated parameters (MCHC, MCV and MCH). With the introduction of semiautomated and automated haematological counters the measurement of Hb, RBC and WBC became rapid and precise. These instruments generally measured Hb by a modification of traditional methods but introduced novel methods of counting cells by means of the light they scattered or the alteration in electrical impedance they caused. Some instruments were designed to measure the PCV (from which the MCV could be calculated, as with the manual techniques) and others to measure the MCV (from which the PCV could be calculated, given knowledge of the RBC). MCH and MCHC could be calculated as before. The WBC and six red cell parameters were thus readily and rapidly available and haematologists soon found new uses for the RBC and MCV.

Platelets were initially counted in a haemocytometer, using light or phase-contrast microscopy. As this manual technique was very time-consuming the test was performed only when there was a clear clinical indication. The first advance in making platelet counts more readily available was the introduction of automated counting of platelets in platelet-rich plasma, the method being dependent on the alteration of electrical impedance caused by the platelets. More recently several methods have been devised to count platelets in a sample of whole blood. As was the case for the more readily available red cell parameters, new clinical needs for the now readily available platelet count were soon found.

Current automated blood counters now usually produce, as a minimum, a WBC, six red cell parameters and a platelet count. Other newer parameters, not yet of such clear clinical relevance, are also being produced (see page 27). Manual methods remain important for the calibration of automated instruments and as reference methods.

BASIC TECHNIQUES
HAEMOGLOBIN CONCENTRATION

To measure the concentration of haemoglobin, a known volume of carefully mixed whole blood is added to a diluent which lyses red cells to produce a haemoglobin solution; lysis occurs because of the hypotonicity of the diluent, but may be accelerated by the inclusion in the diluent of a non-ionic detergent to act as a lytic agent.

The concentration of haemoglobin is then determined from the light absorbance (optical density) of the solution of haemoglobin or its derivative at a selected wavelength.

Cyanmethaemoglobin methods

The International Committee for Standardization in Haematology (ICSH) has recommended the use of a method in which haemoglobin is converted to cyanmethaemoglobin (haemiglobincyanide).[11] This method has three significant advantages. First haemoglobin, methaemoglobin and carboxyhaemoglobin are all converted to cyanmethaemoglobin and are therefore included in the measurement; of the forms of haemoglobin likely to be present in blood, only sulphaemoglobin — usually present in negligible amounts — is not converted to cyanmethaemoglobin, although carboxyhaemoglobin is more slowly converted than the other forms. Secondly, stable secondary cyanmethaemoglobin standards which have been compared with the WHO International Standard are readily available for calibration. Thirdly, cyanmethaemoglobin has an absorbance band at 540 nm which is broad and relatively flat (Fig. 2.1), and thus measurements can be made either on a narrow-band spectrophotometer or on a filter photometer or colorimeter which reads over a wide band of wavelengths.

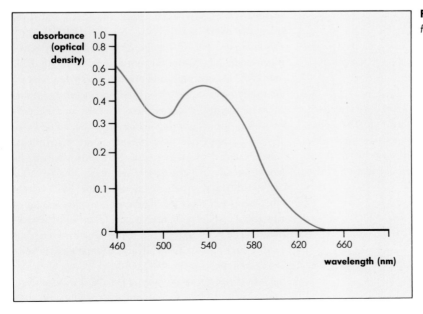

Fig. 2.1 *Absorbance spectrum for cyanmethaemoglobin.*

The reference method requires the addition of a diluent which contains: potassium cyanide and potassium ferricyanide, to effect the conversion to cyanmethaemoglobin; dihydrogen potassium phosphate, to lower the pH, accelerate the reaction, and allow the reading of light absorbance at 3 minutes rather than 10–15 minutes; and a non-ionic detergent, to accelerate cell lysis and lessen the turbidity due to precipitation of lipoproteins (and to a lesser extent red cell stroma) which is otherwise a consequence of the lower pH achieved by the dihydrogen potassium phosphate.[28] The absorbance of light by the solution is measured at 540 nm in a spectrophotometer. At this wavelength the light absorbance of the diluent itself is zero; either water or, preferably, the diluent can be used as the blank. No standard is required, since the haemoglobin concentration can be calculated from the absorbance, given that the molecular weight and the millimolar extinction coefficient of haemoglobin are known. However, the wavelength of light produced by the instrument must be verified and the absorbance scale calibrated. A reference solution of cyanmethaemoglobin can be used for calibration.

In routine practice, haemoglobin concentration is usually measured by means of a photometer or colorimeter in which light of approximately 540 nm is produced by the use of a yellow-green filter such as the Ilford 625. The light passing through the solution is detected by a photoelectric cell and the instrument scale shows either light absorbance or transmittance. Comparison of the instrument reading with that for a reference solution allows calculation of the haemoglobin concentration; this is most conveniently done using a standard curve or a conversion table. Alternatively the photometer may be calibrated to produce a direct readout in haemoglobin concentration units; a reference cyanmethaemoglobin solution is suitable for verifying the accuracy of instruments of this type.

Certain characteristics of pathological blood samples may lead to inaccuracy in a cyanmethaemoglobin estimation of haemoglobin. The presence of sulphaemoglobin will lead to slight underestimation of the total haemoglobin: a concentration of 15 g/dl will be measured as 14.8 g/dl if 5 percent of the haemoglobin is present as sulphaemoglobin.[28] The slow conversion of carboxyhaemoglobin to methaemoglobin leads to overestimation of the haemoglobin concentration if the test is read at 3 minutes, since carboxyhaemoglobin absorbs more light at 540 nm than does cyanmethaemoglobin;

the maximum possible error which could be caused if 20 percent of the haemoglobin were in the form of carboxyhaemoglobin, a degree of abnormality which may be found in heavy smokers, would be 6 percent overestimation.[28]

Spectrophotometers and photometers are both sensitive to the effects of turbidity, which may be caused by a high WBC, high levels of lipids or plasma proteins, or non-lysed RBC. Increased turbidity causes a factitiously elevated measure of haemoglobin concentration. When the WBC is high, turbidity effects are circumvented by centrifugation or filtration of the solution prior to reading the absorbance. When turbidity is due to high levels of protein (either when a paraprotein is present or when there is severe chronic infection or inflammation), it can be cleared by the addition of either potassium carbonate or a drop of 25% ammonia. When turbidity is due to hyperlipidaemia, a blank may be prepared from the diluent and the patient's plasma or the lipid may be removed by diethyl ether extraction and centrifugation. The target cells of liver disease or red cells containing haemoglobin S or C may fail to lyse in the diluent and, again, increased turbidity produces a factitiously high reading of haemoglobin concentration. Occasionally this phenomenon is observed without there being any identifiable abnormality in the red cells to account for it. Making a 1:1 dilution in distilled water ensures complete lysis of osmotically resistant cells.

Other methods

In theory, if absorbance is measured at about 548.5 nm, at which wavelength deoxyhaemoglobin and oxyhaemoglobin have the same optical density and that of carboxyhaemoglobin is not much less, the haemoglobin concentration can be measured directly. Hb is calculated by comparison of absorbance with that of an artificial standard. However, a haemoglobinometer based on this principle was found in one quality control survey to give lower concentrations than the cyanmethaemoglobin method[15] and the method has now generally fallen into disuse.

Haemoglobin may also be measured as oxyhaemoglobin (in which case carboxyhaemoglobin, sulphaemoglobin and methaemoglobin will not be measured), or as haematin produced in acid or alkaline conditions. The acid haematin method is not recommended because of its inaccuracy. Sulphaemoglobin, methaemoglobin and carboxyhaemoglobin are insoluble in acid solution and the presence of an increased concentration of protein or lipid causes an artefactual increase of Hb. In the alkaline haematin method lipids and abnormal proteins do not interfere if the blood sample and diluent are well and quickly mixed but this method will not accurately measure fetal haemoglobin and haemoglobin Barts, which are resistant to alkaline denaturation. Oxy-haemoglobin methods were found to give a lower concentration than cyanmethaemoglobin methods in one quality control survey and they are now little used.[15] All these methods require artificial standards. Haemoglobin can also be measured as azidmethaemo-globin, following the addition of sodium nitrate and sodium azide; this method is employed in one currently available portable haemoglobinometer. However, in general, haemoglobinometers now rarely employ methods other than those based on cyanmethaemo-globin conversion.

Most automated multiparameter haemotological counters also measure haemoglobin by a cyan-methaemoglobin method, though at varying wave-lengths and often at a shorter, but constant, time after mixture of the diluent and the aliquot of blood. Incomplete conversion to cyanmethaemoglobin does not necessarily lead to inaccuracy since the instruments should be calibrated with fresh blood, to which the correct value for haemoglobin concentration has been assigned, and this calibrant will also be incompletely converted. One exception to the general use of a modified cyanmethaemoglobin methodology is the Contraves Model 801 Autoanalyzer which integrates absorbance between 500 and 600 nm, the integral absorbance of oxyhaemoglobin, deoxyhaemoglobin and carboxyhaemoglobin being similar in this waveband; this method correlates well with an oxyhaemoglobin method but less well with a cyanmethaemoglobin method.[29]

The ICSH recommends that haemoglobin concentration be expressed either in g/l or in mmol/l with the monomer or tetramer being specified in the latter case. However, the use of g/dl remains wide-spread. It is likely that were Hb to be expressed in mmol/l there would be widespread confusion among those interpreting laboratory test results and it is to be hoped that laboratories will continue to use either g/l or g/dl. A Hb of 10 g/dl, or 100 g/l, is equivalent to a concentration of 1.55 mmol/l of the tetramer or 6.2 mmol/l of the monomer.

PACKED CELL VOLUME (HAEMATOCRIT)
The packed cell volume (PCV) or haematocrit (Hct) is the proportion of a column of centrifuged blood which is occupied by red cells; some of the measured column of red cells represents plasma trapped between red cells. The haematocrit was originally expressed as a percentage but is now commonly expressed as a decimal fraction representing l/l (litres/litre). The haematocrit, as introduced by Maxwell Wintrobe, required one ml of blood, graduated glass tubes with a constant internal bore (Fig. 2.2), a large centrifuge (g value achieved being about 2260) and a centrifugation time of either half an hour or an hour. This method, now sometimes designated the macrohaematocrit, is the basis of the international reference method for the PCV.[12] It was chosen because the results obtained are accurate and precise. In the reference method it is modified by the addition of $[^{131}I]$-albumin, to enable measurement of the plasma trapped within the red cell column. The reference method is important in assessing the accuracy of automated methods of measuring the PCV. Within the diagnostic laboratory, however, the macrohaemato-crit has largely fallen into disuse and has been replaced by the microhaematocrit or by one of the automated methods. Some haematologists prefer the term 'haematocrit' to 'packed cell volume' when referring to the results of automated measurements which do not generally involve packing of the cells but it is legitimate to regard the terms as interchangeable since both were originally used to describe the same test.

In the microhaematocrit a small volume of blood is taken into an ungraduated capillary tube (usually 75 × 1.5mm) and the end of the tube distant from the column of blood is sealed by heat or with modelling clay or a similar product. It is then centrifuged for 5 or 10 minutes, at a high g value (for example 10 000–12 000 g) in a small, specially designed centrifuge. The micro-haematocrit (Fig. 2.3) is less accurate and precise than the macrohaematocrit because it is more difficult to read levels in a smaller tube, the microhaematocrit tubes commonly taper or are of uneven bore, and it is impossible to get a flat bottom to the column of blood. Heat sealing gives a convex seal and use of a modelling clay-like substance gives a concave seal (Fig. 2.4); this has a minor effect on the final reading.[3] The ICSH has published a selected method for the microhaemato-crit:[14] it requires tubes with a uniform internal bore of approximately 1.2 mm and centrifugation is for 5 minutes at 10 000–15 000 g (if the blood is poly-cythaemic a further 3 minutes' centrifugation is advised[10]).

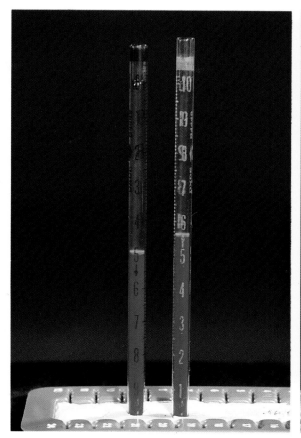

Fig. 2.2 *Measurement of the PCV by the macrohaematocrit technique; tests from two patients are shown.*

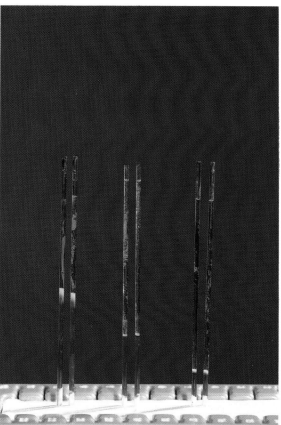

Fig. 2.3 *Measurement of the PCV by the microhaematocrit technique; paired tests from each of three patients are shown.*

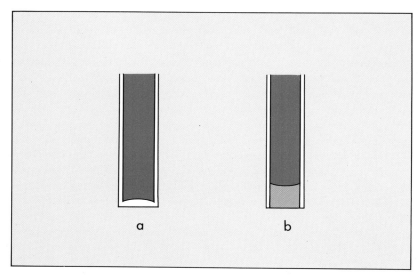

Fig. 2.4 *Diagrammatic representation of the end of a microhaematocrit tube showing the effect of sealing (a) with heat or (b) with a modelling clay equivalent.*

There is less plasma trapping at the higher *g* values achieved in the microhaematocrit than there is in the macrohaematocrit. As a consequence the measured PCV and the calculated MCV are lower and the calculated MCHC is higher. In the macrohaematocrit the red cell column in blood from healthy individuals includes 2–5 percent of trapped plasma, whereas in the microhaematocrit it includes in the order of 1–3 percent. Although the microhaematocrit is less accurate and precise than the macrohaematocrit, it is a more useful practical test for a diagnostic laboratory; its accuracy and precision can be increased by making a number of replicate estimations and averaging them, and this should be done when a microhaematocrit is being used to calibrate an automated instrument.

The macrohaematocrit requires venous blood whereas the microhaematocrit can be performed on either capillary or venous blood. If blood from a skin puncture is to be taken directly into a microhaematocrit tube, the interior of the tube must be coated with heparin (2 IU).

Plasma trapping correction

The calculation of the amount of trapped plasma using [131I]-albumin makes it possible to correct the microhaematocrit as well as the macrohaematocrit for trapped plasma, leading to a more accurate estimation of the true size of the red blood cell. Since this is clearly quite impractical for routine diagnostic tests, the custom has arisen of correcting the PCV for the amount of plasma which is believed to be there, on the basis of previous experimental work. This is more likely to be done when an automated instrument is calibrated than when a manual estimation of the haematocrit is performed. The MCV is necessarily corrected by the same percentage. This arbitrary application of a plasma trapping correction has some disadvantages and no clear advantages. The percentage of the red cell column occupied by trapped plasma varies between individuals and there is no agreement between different studies as to its average percentage in blood from healthy individuals: Garby and Vuille[9] found plasma trapping to average 1.3 percent (range 1.1–1.5 percent) after 10 minutes centrifugation at 10 000 *g*; Furth[8] found a mean value of 2 percent after 4 minutes centrifugation at approximately 10 000 *g*; Pearson and Guthrie[21] found a mean value of 1.53 percent (range approximately 1.2–1.8 percent) after 10 minutes centrifugation at a *g* value estimated at 12 500–14 400 at the level of the buffy coat; and England *et al*[7]. found a mean value of 3.2 percent (range approximately 1.7–4.2 percent) after 5 minutes centrifugation at 12 000 *g*. Estimates of the percentage of plasma trapped are lower when [131I]-fibrinogen is used in the estimation than when [131I]-albumin is used.[3] In view of the varying results obtained, the correction to be applied is arbitrary and is not necessarily correct for the specific bloods being used for calibration.

The use of a correction factor by some but not all laboratories and in some countries but not in others is the main reason that the introduction of correction of the PCV has caused problems. Laboratories which do not conform to current local practice will appear out of consensus in external quality control programmes. It can also be difficult to interpret published studies on the clinical significance of minor degrees of microcytosis and macrocytosis since authors commonly do not state whether a correction factor has been applied. For the same reasons it can be difficult to apply the various nomograms devised to assist in the differential diagnosis of iron deficiency and thalassaemia traits. Clinical decisions may be influenced by whether or not plasma trapping correction is applied (and by other apparently minor variations in method). In polycythaemic patients a precise knowledge of the PCV may be very important in indicating the adequacy of treatment, since above a certain level the whole blood viscosity rises exponentially with the PCV; guidelines suggested for control of the disease[22] may be invalidated if a different method is used (see pages 23 and 25) or if a different policy is adopted with reference to the use of a plasma trapping correction. In blood transfusion practice, if the PCV is used to assess a volunteer's suitability to donate blood, minor alterations in method can alter markedly the percentage of prospective donors whose donation is deferred.

Many British laboratories introduced a plasma trapping correction during late 1974 or early 1975 without realizing that they were doing so. This occurrence was consequent on the widespread practice of using the Coulter Electronics Quality Control material, 4C, as if it were a calibrant (a procedure *not* recommended by the manufacturer). Until 1974 the stated values for this product had no correction for plasma trapping. Subsequently, following publication of data suggesting that plasma trapping in the blood of healthy subjects was about 3 percent, [7] the measured PCV was reduced by 3 percent when assigning values to the PCV and the MCV on the product sheet. If this product is used to calibrate an instrument, then the measured PCV and MCV on patient samples will be 3 percent lower and the measured MCHC 3 percent higher than if such a correction is not applied. No such plasma trapping correction was introduced in most US laboratories and the US reference procedure, promulgated by the National Committee for Clinical Laboratory Standards, does not include a correction. The ICSH Committee on Cytometry also does not advise a plasma trapping correction when calibrating an automated instrument. Plasma trapping is more variable in pathological samples than in samples from healthy subjects so that such samples are likely to show a greater discrepancy between the micro- and automated haematocrits. Pathological samples such as those showing microcytosis should not be used for calibrating automated counters.

Factors affecting the microhaematocrit, including those altering the amount of trapped plasma, are shown in Fig. 2.5. These factors do not affect the automated PCV, except in those instruments where it is determined by centrifugation.

	Factors decreasing the microhaematocrit	Factors increasing the microhaematocrit
Consequent on an alteration of the amount of trapped plasma	longer period of centrifugation increased centrifugal force (i.e. increased radius of centrifuge or increased speed of centrifugation) elevated ESR dilution (e.g. EDTA in solution rather than dry EDTA)	polycythaemia microcytosis (e.g. iron deficiency or thalassaemia) sickle cell trait[7] sickle cell disease[7, 21] spherocytosis[8] reduced red cell flexibility, as when blood has been stored for a prolonged period
Consequent on cell shrinkage	excess EDTA[16, 23] K_3EDTA rather than K_2EDTA or Na_2EDTA	
Uncertain mechanisms	storage of blood at room temperature for greater than 24 hours[17] narrower tubes (0.5–0.6 mm rather than 1.1–1.2 mm)[26]	

Fig. 2.5 *Some factors affecting the microhaematocrit.*

A correction for plasma trapping should be applied if the microhaematocrit is used for blood volume measurements. Allowance should be made for the greater degree of plasma trapping with polycythaemic blood.[13] It is suggested that if the PCV is less than 0.50 after centrifugation for 5 minutes, 2 percent correction should be applied; if the PCV is greater than 0.50, a further 5 minutes centrifugation should be carried out and a 3 percent correction then be applied.

Other factors affecting the PCV

The microhaematocrit is also affected by cell shrinkage which may occur with excess EDTA or with certain salts of EDTA. If K_2EDTA is used as an anticoagulant a concentration of 1.2^{14} or 1.5^4 mg/ml is recommended. A concentration of more than 2 mg/ml causes cell shrinkage and therefore a lower PCV; if the taking of a small sample leads to a concentration as high as 16 mg/ml, the PCV is reduced by 6–16 percent.[23] Similarly, for Na_2EDTA, if 2 ml of blood is put into a tube intended to receive 7 ml, the PCV is lowered by 5 percent, and reducing the volume of blood to 1 ml causes a 10 percent error in the PCV.[16] Excess EDTA does not affect the automated PCV (with the exception of instruments using centrifugation) but it is important that specimens used for calibration should have the correct EDTA concentration, otherwise errors occurring in the microhaematocrit will be reflected in the automated haematocrit. The use of K_3EDTA rather than K_2EDTA, even in the recommended concentrations, causes shrinkage of the red cells so that PCV is lowered by about 3 percent.[19] As blood is commonly taken into K_3EDTA in the US[19] and into K_2EDTA in the UK there is likely to be a difference of about 3 percent between manual PCVs in the two countries; if the same procedures were used for calibration then a similar difference would be seen in automated PCVs and MCVs. In fact, the different policies as to correction for plasma trapping in the two countries may fortuitously remove the difference.

Other methods of measuring the PCV

It is also possible to calculate the PCV indirectly by adding trace quantities of $[^{131}I]$-albumin to blood and then measuring the radioactivity of both plasma and whole blood.[5] This method correlates well with a macrohaematocrit corrected for plasma trapping. It is not suitable for measuring the PCV for diagnostic purposes but is an interesting research technique.

Automated instruments may: include a centrifuge and measure the PCV in the traditional manner; estimate the PCV from the conductivity of blood (plasma being a much better conductor than red cells); sum the pulse heights produced by impedance or light-scattering methods; or multiply together the MCV and the RBC produced by impedance or light-scattering methods (see page 20). Instruments using the first two of these are no longer in current use. When the PCV was calculated from conductivity, factitiously low results were produced by excess EDTA and factitiously high results by hyperproteinaemia and marked leucocytosis; the relation of PCV to conductivity was non-linear outside a PCV range of 0.15–0.55.

THE RED CELL COUNT

The red cell count (RBC) was initially performed by counting red cells in a carefully diluted sample of blood in a counting chamber (haemocytometer) of known volume.[4] In this method the white cells are distinguished from red cells by their larger size, the presence of a nucleus and their somewhat irregular shape, and are excluded from the count. The ease of identification of red cells may be improved by the inclusion in the diluent of methyl violet, which stains leucocyte nuclei. Although this method was capable of producing satisfactory results if great care was exercised, it proved rather unreliable in routine use[1] and was also very time-consuming. For this reason the RBC and the parameters dependent on it (see below) were determined on only a minority of blood samples.

Attempts to automate the RBC commenced in the nineteenth century, early methods depending on a relation between turbidity of a suspension of red cells and the number of cells. A major advance occurred in the 1950s when a satisfactory cell counting instrument, based on impedance technology, was designed. This instrument and its successors made determining the RBC and the derived parameters practical, and their clinical usefulness was soon apparent. Early impedance counters and some current models (such as the Coulter Counter model ZM) count red cells in an accurately fixed and known volume of diluted blood so that, although accurate setting of thresholds is needed, they do not require calibration. Later generations of fully automated instruments do require calibration. After the development of impedance counters other instruments were designed which counted cells by light-scattering techniques. Automated red cell counts which are generated are usually non-linear with increasing cell concentration, consequent on the greater likelihood of two or more cells passing through the counting zone simultaneously (coincidence); a correction is required (coincidence correction). Instruments based on impedance technology and light-scattering usually count white cells together with red cells; as red cells are normally a hundred-fold more numerous, the inaccuracy introduced is not great. In a recent instrument dependent on light scattering at two angles (the Technicon H.1), red cells can be distinguished from white cells and counted separately.

Automated instruments count in the order of 20 000 to 50 000 red cells, so that precision is much greater than with a haemocytometer count based on 500 – 1000 cells.

DERIVED PARAMETERS (MCV, MCH, MCHC)

Given the three measured parameters (Hb, RBC and PCV) three other parameters can be calculated as detailed on page 11 . Because of plasma trapping the measured MCV may be an overestimate of the true MCV (see page 14) and the MCHC may be an underestimation of the true MCHC. (For the same reason the MCV may be higher and the MCHC lower when they are derived from a macrohaematocrit rather than a microhaematocrit.)

WHITE CELL COUNT (WBC)

Diluting a well-mixed sample of blood in a weak acid solution lyses the red cells, leaving the white cells to be counted in a counting chamber (haemocytometer) of known volume;[4] the nuclei of the white cells are visualized by the addition of a stain such as gentian violet to the diluting fluid. Nucleated red blood cells (NRBC) cannot be distinguished from white cells; if they are present it is necessary to count the ratio of NRBC to white cells on a stained blood film in order to correct the total nucleated cell count to a true WBC.

The WBC can also be determined by impedance or light-scattering technology (see pages 20 and 23 in which case, also, some or all of any NRBC are likely to be included in the WBC.

Automated instruments count in the order of 10 000– 20 000 white cells when the WBC is normal, compared with the 100–200 cells counted in a haemocytometer count; precision is therefore much greater.

PLATELET COUNT

Platelets may be counted in a counting chamber using either diluted whole blood (in which red cells can either be left intact or can be lysed) or platelet-rich plasma (prepared by sedimentation or centrifugation). If very large platelets are present a whole-blood method is preferred to the use of platelet-rich plasma in order to avoid any risk of large, heavy platelets being lost during the sedimentation or centrifugation process. Platelet-rich plasma may be preferred if the platelet count is low. When the method leaves red cells intact, large platelets can be distinguished from small red cells by the platelet shape, which can be oval rather than round, and by its irregular outline, with fine projections sometimes being visible. Use of ammonium oxalate as a diluent, with lysis of red cells, produces a higher and more accurate count than use of formol-citrate, with red cells remaining intact.[18]

Platelets may be visualized in the counting chamber by light or phase-contrast microscopy. When using light microscopy, brilliant cresyl blue can be added to the diluent; this stains platelets light blue and facilitates their identification. On light microscopy platelet identification is aided by their refractility. It is easier to identify platelets by phase-contrast microscopy and such counts are therefore generally more precise.

The first automated platelet counters, early models of Coulter counters, depended on impedance technology (see page 20) and required platelet-rich plasma. Coincidence correction was required. Platelets were counted between two thresholds so that any contaminating red cells and white cells were excluded from the count. Heavy red cell contamination was, however, noted to lead to a false low count.[2] Platelet-rich plasma could be prepared by sedimentation but the count was available more rapidly if centrifugation was employed, and a specially adapted centrifuge (the Thrombofuge) was designed for this purpose. The Thrombofuge sometimes failed to produce sufficient platelet-rich plasma in polycythaemic patients or when plasma viscosity was high. The need to prepare platelet-rich plasma also meant that accurate counts could not be performed when the platelets were particularly large, since some were lost during processing.

Instruments subsequently became available which counted platelets by light-scattering methods, and both they and later impedance instruments were able to count platelets in samples of whole blood. The introduction of laser technology improved separation of red cells and platelets in comparison with light-scattering methods using white light.

Automated platelet counts are much more precise than haemocytometer counts. The influence of method on the accuracy of the platelet count is discussed further in Chapter 5.

PRINCIPLES OF AUTOMATED HAEMATOLOGY COUNTERS

Members of the current generation of automated haematology counters aspirate and dilute a blood sample and determine eight parameters (WBC, RBC, Hb, PCV, MCV, MCH, MCHC, platelet count). Some also determine other parameters relating to platelets or red cells or perform an automated differential count (see Chapter 4). Apart from the measurement of haemoglobin, all parameters depend on the counting and sizing of particles, whether red cells, white cells or platelets. Particles may be counted and sized either by electrical impedance or by light scattering. Electrical impedance technology was devised and developed by Wallace Coulter in the late 1940s and 1950s, with such instruments subsequently produced by Coulter Electronics; after the expiry of the initial patent the principle was adopted by numerous other companies. Light-scattering methods have been employed by Ortho Instruments and Technicon International.

Automated instruments have at least two channels. In one channel a diluent is added and red cells are counted and sized. In another channel a lytic agent is added, together with the diluent, in order to reduce red cells to stroma, leaving the white cells intact for counting and also producing a solution for the measurement of haemoglobin concentration. In Ortho instruments two separate channels serve these functions. Instruments with a short time interval between aspirating and counting need a strong lytic agent; in some circumstances this may also lyse white cells to produce a falsely low WBC. Conversely, instruments having a slower passage of the sample through the instrument and using weaker lytic agents have, in some circumstances, produced false high 'white cell' counts due to non-lysed red cells being counted.

Automated differential counts are discussed on page 105 and newer white cell parameters on page 118; other aspects of automated counters are dealt with in the section which now follows.

COULTER COUNTERS AND OTHER INSTRUMENTS DEPENDING ON ELECTRICAL IMPEDANCE

Blood cells are extremely poor conductors of electricity. When single red cells in a conducting medium flow through a small aperture across which an electric current is applied (Figs 2.6 and 2.7), there is a measurable increase in the electrical impedance across the aperture, this increase being proportional to the volume of conducting medium displaced. Cells can thus be both counted and sized from the electrical pulses which they generate. Aperture impedance is determined by capacitance and inductance as well as by resistance. Various factors apart from cell volume also influence the amplitude, duration and form of the pulse, these being related to the disturbance of electrical lines of force as well as to displacement of the conducting medium. Cell shape is relevant as well as cell volume, so that cells of increased deformability which elongate in response to shear forces appear smaller than their actual size and rigid cells appear larger.[25] Furthermore, cells which pass through the aperture off-centre produce aberrant impulses and appear larger than their actual size. Cells which recirculate through the edge of the electrical field produce an aberrant impulse which is smaller than that normally produced by a red cell but may be similar to that of a platelet. Cells which pass through the aperture simultaneously, or almost so, are counted as a single cell; the inaccuracy introduced requires coincidence correction. In early single-channel Coulter counters coincidence correction required reference to a table, but in the later semi-automated counters such as the ZM, and in automated counters, such as the Coulter S and the S Plus series, coincidence correction is an automatic function of the instrument. The S Plus series has also introduced edit circuitry, that is, electronic circuitry which recognizes and rejects aberrant pulses; the artefactual increase in the pulse height produced by cells passing through the edge of the aperture is thus eliminated. Other instruments have used sheathed flow, which directs a cell to the centre of the aperture, to prevent this problem.

The measurement of MCV and RBC by Coulter counters allows the PCV to be calculated. Some other instruments based on electrical impedance integrate pulse heights to produce the PCV and calculate MCV from the PCV and RBC. Most impedance counters measure haemoglobin by a cyanmethaemoglobin method; for example, with the Coulter Counter S Plus IV the Hb is derived from the optical density at approximately 525 nm after a reaction time of 20–25 s. MCH is derived from the Hb concentration and the RBC. MCHC is derived from the Hb concentration, RBC and MCV.

White cells are also present in the red cell channel and they are counted and sized with the red cells. Since there are normally 50–100 red cells to each white cell, the inaccuracy introduced is not generally very great, but if there is a marked leucocytosis, with or without

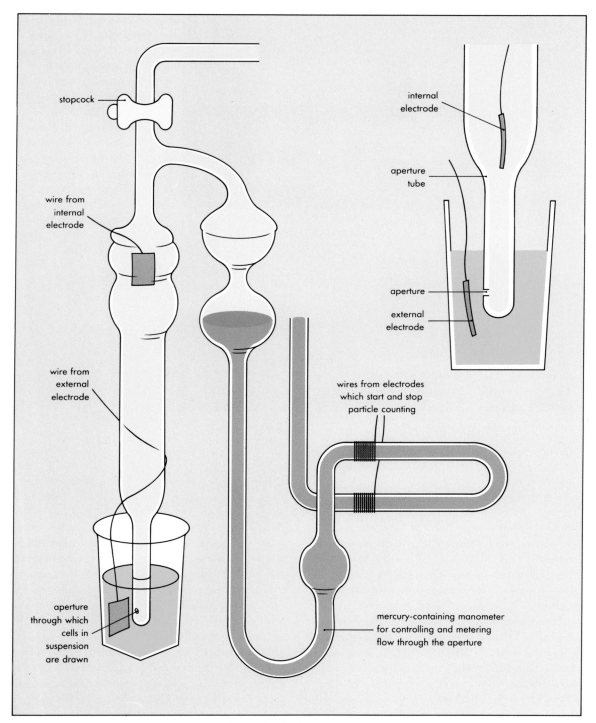

Fig. 2.6 *Semi-diagrammatic representation of part of a Coulter counter model FN showing the aperture tube and the manometer used for metering the volume of cell suspension counted. Inset: diagrammatic cross-section of the aperture tube of an impedance counter.*

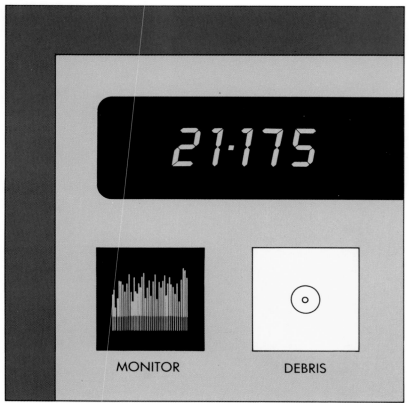

Fig. 2.7 *Numerical display and monitors of the Coulter counter model FN. The left-hand monitor is an oscilloscope showing voltage pulses generated by particles passing through the aperture, pulse height being proportional to cell size; that part of the pulse above the threshold appears brighter. The right-hand monitor is a projection of the actual aperture, allowing any debris to be visualized.*

anaemia, then not only is the 'RBC' elevated, but, since white cells are larger than red cells, a false macrocytosis is produced, and the RBC and PCV are falsely elevated. As turbidity can increase the apparent haemoglobin concentration, all six red cell parameters are likely to be inaccurate.

If red cells are selectively lysed then white cells can be counted and sized in the same channel as is used for determining the Hb; NRBC are usually counted with white cells so that the term 'total nucleated cell count' is more accurate then WBC. However, NRBC are somewhat smaller than WBC so that, depending on the threshold above which particles are counted as WBC, they will not necessarily all be included with the WBC.

If a method is devised for detecting overlapping of the pulses generated by large platelets with those generated by very microcytic red cells, thresholds can be set appropriately and pulse height analysis can be used to count platelets as well as red cells in a whole blood sample. Electronic circuitry to fit curves to the observed data may be used to extrapolate beyond the counting thresholds. Since red cells which recirculate into the edge of the electrical field produce a brief pulse of low amplitude, it is necessary to prevent red cell recirculation if platelets are to be counted accurately. This was achieved in Coulter counters of the S Plus series by the introduction of sweep flow behind the orifice, so that particles which traverse the orifice are swept away. Other manufacturers use other devices, such as sheathed flow, or a perforated plate behind the orifice so that particles attempting to recirculate strike the plate. Sheathed flow gives a good separation of red cell and platelet pulses.

Instruments based on impedance technology allow rapid, precise blood counts and have revolutionized the practice of haematology. Unfortunately not all parameters are determined accurately, particularly when dealing with pathological blood samples. As stated above, the pulse height produced by a particle of low conductivity passing through the sensing zone is related to cell shape as well as volume. A cell passing through the sensing zone produces an electrical shadow, that is, it produces a voltage pulse which suggests a particle of a certain size and shape. A normal red cell probably passes through in a fusiform or cigar shape,[25] producing an electrical shadow similar to its actual volume, whereas a sphere produces an electrical shadow approximately 1.5 times its actual volume.[25] The pulse height is related to electrical shadow rather than the actual volume, so that any rigid fixed cell will appear larger than its actual size.

Furthermore, cell deformability is a function of haemoglobin concentration within an individual cell. A hypochromic cell with a low MCHC elongates more than a normal cell and its electrical shadow is correspondingly less. Its MCV is therefore falsely low as is its PCV, whereas its MCHC is falsely elevated.[6] This factor operates with blood from healthy subjects, when the MCHC is within normal limits; it is an even more major factor when cells are markedly hypochromic. It is mainly for this reason that the low MCHC, a sensitive indicator of iron deficiency with manual methods, is a very insensitive indicator when a Coulter counter or similar instrument is used. Another factor contributing to the low MCHC seen in iron deficiency when manual methods are used is the increased trapping of plasma. This is not reproduced by automated counters, providing a second reason for the lower sensitivity to iron deficiency of the automated MCHC in comparison with the manual MCHC. The falsely low MCV and PCV of hypochromic cells with instruments based on impedance technology (and with most instruments based on light scattering; see page 16) has implications for the diagnosis of thalassaemia and for the control of therapy in polycythaemic patients.[22] The error is greater with Coulter counters of the S Plus series than with those of the S series.[6]

INSTRUMENTS DEPENDING ON LIGHT SCATTERING

Instruments which depend on light scattering to count and size cells may use white light, laser light or both. The underlying principles are similar. A cell passing through a focussed beam scatters the light, the intensity of scattering at a defined angle being related to the size of the cell. A light detector placed at an angle to the beam of incident light can thus be used both to count and to size the cell. An instrument may also have a detector placed forward of the flowing stream of cells, which can be used both to count cells and measure light absorbance.

Technicon Instruments

Technicon International have produced a series of automated haematology counters which use light scattering to count and, in later models, to size cells. The major instruments in the series are the Hemalog and Hemalog 8, the Hemalog D, the H 6000 and the H.1. The first such counters were continuous-flow instruments with air-bubble separation of successive samples.

A stream of cells in single file passes through a narrow beam of light. A photodetector cell is placed forward of the stream of cells at a small angle to the incoming light beam. A dark field stop in the light beam ensures that light reaches the photodetector cell only if it is diffracted by a cell passing through the beam. Since cells generally pass through the light beam singly, coincidence is not a major problem.

The first instrument in this series, the Hemalog, differed from its successor, the Hemalog 8, in that it had the capacity to perform some coagulation tests, and estimated the PCV both by centrifugation and by conductivity measurements. The Hemalog 8 was a five-channel instrument which did not perform coagulation tests and measured the PCV only by optically monitoring the interface of the red cells and the buffy coat during centrifugation of the blood in a J-tube. Otherwise the principles underlying the two instruments were similar. The MCV was computed from the RBC and the PCV. Haemoglobin was meausured by a cyanmethaemoglobin method with the colour development being accelerated by ultraviolet light. The MCH and MCHC were computed.

These two instruments were the first automated haematology counters to count platelets on a whole-blood sample and to produce a platelet count as an integral part of each full blood count. Platelets were counted in a channel in which red cells were lysed; the refractive index of the diluent matched that of the red cell stroma so that light was not scattered by the stroma. White cells were counted with the platelets, but the inaccuracy introduced was not great if the two classes of

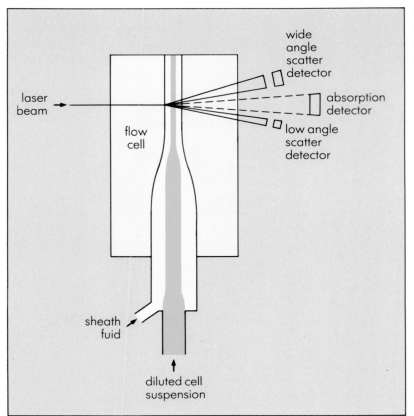

Fig. 2.8 *Diagrammatic representation of the cell detection and measuring system of the Technicon H.1 counter.*

wide angle scatter detector

absorption detector

laser beam

low angle scatter detector

flow cell

sheath fuid

diluted cell suspension

cells were present in their normal ratio. Conversely, if the platelet count was very high some platelets were counted as white cells. The Hemalog and Hemalog 8 were large instruments which were unsuitable for rapid analysis of urgent specimens. The MCV derived from the spun PCV was less precise than that produced by impedance counters.

The Hemalog 8 was later joined by the Hemalog D, another large, continuous-flow instrument producing a WBC and, by means of a combination of cell size and cytochemical reactions, a differential white cell count (see Chapter 4); it was possible to couple together the two instruments.

The next instrument in the series, the H 6000, combined the capabilities of the two preceeding instruments in a single, large continuous-flow instrument. Alterations were made in the method for identifying the different classes of leucocytes (see Chapter 4) and for measuring the PCV and the MCV Like the Hemalog D this instrument used sheathed flow so that the cells passed through the focussed light beam at the centre of the flow cell. This made it possible to size as well as count cells by the measurement of forward-angle light-scatter. Since such light-scatter is determined by particle shape and orientation as well as by size, an agent was introduced to cause isovolumetric sphering of red cells. With all cells being spherical the effects of both shape and orientation have been removed and light-scatter has become largely a function of cell size. The scattered light is converted to an electrical impulse and integration of such impulses followed by multiplication by a calibration factor allows calculation of the PCV. The MCV is then estimated by dividing the PCV by the RBC. Haemoglobin concentration is determined by a cyanmethaemoglobin method with measurement of light absorbance at about 550 nm.

Although conditions for determining cell size from light-scatter have been improved, some problems remain, since the refractive index of red cells is not

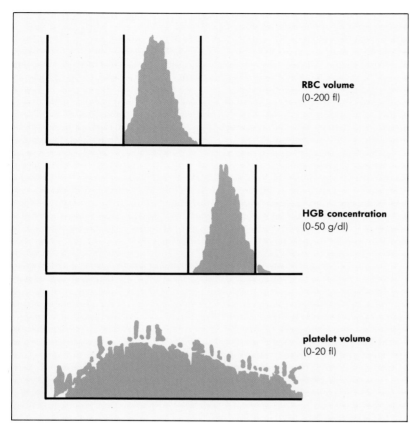

RBC volume
(0-200 fl)

HGB concentration
(0-50 g/dl)

platelet volume
(0-20 fl)

Fig. 2.9 *Histograms of distribution of size and haemoglobin content of red cells and size distribution of platelets produced by the Technicon H.1 counter.*

constant but is determined by their haemoglobin concentration. This varies between cells in the one sample and may vary greatly between samples. A consequence of this dependence of light-scatter on the refractive index is that there is an underestimation of the MCV when the cell is hypochromic, that is, when the MCHC is reduced. The net result is very similar to the underestimation of the MCV of hypochromic cells when the impedance method is employed. There is a false lowering of the PCV and a false elevation of the MCHC. The slope of the regression line of measured MCHC on 'true' MCHC is relatively flat, with a positive intercept, even for samples derived from healthy subjects.[6] The inaccuracy in the determination of the MCV, PCV and MCHC is similar to that in impedance systems and has the same implications for patient management. In macrocytic patients the MCV as measured by the H 6000 is not as high as that measured by impedance technology. The H 6000 is able to separate platelets and red cells on the basis of size and

thus can count and size both cell types in the one channel.

The most recent instrument introduced by Technicon is the H.1. It is more compact than its predecessors and accepts single samples rather than being a continuous-flow instrument. The H.1 continues to use the scattering of white light for counting and sizing white cells, but laser technology has been used to count and size red cells and platelets separately. Laser light scattered forward by red cells is measured at a narrow angle (2–3 degrees) and at a wider angle (5–15 degrees) (Fig. 2.8), and a comparison of the two allows a computation of the size and haemoglobin content of each individual cell. A histogram of the cell volumes (Fig. 2.9) is used to derive the mean cell volume (MCV), the coefficient of deviation of cell volumes (RDW) and the packed cell volume (PCV). Similarly, a histogram of haemoglobin concentrations of individual cells (Fig. 2.9) is used to measure the mean cell haemoglobin concentration — designated CHCM to distinguish it from MCHC derived by more traditional methods. The CHCM and the traditional MCHC are compared as an internal quality control mechanism; errors in the estimation of the haemoglobin concentration – for example, consequent on a very high white cell count — could cause a discrepancy between the MCHC and the CHCM.

The technology of the H.1 appears to produce accurate estimations of MCV, PCV and MCHC which agree well with reference methods.[20,27] and the inaccuracies observed with previous light-scattering technology appear to have been reduced. The only estimates noted to be inaccurate were those on very dense sickle cells; this was probably consequent on failure to convert irreversibly sickled cells into spheres.[20]

Ortho Instruments

Ortho Instruments have developed automated haematology counters using laser beam optics to count and size cells. Successive instruments in the Ortho series are the Hemac 630L, the ELT 8, ELT 800, ELT 15

and ELT 1500. Red cells and platelets passing through a laser beam are separated on the basis of size as determined by the optical detection of low-angle forward scatter of light (Fig. 2.10); both cell types are counted and red cells are sized. Thresholds separating red cells and platelets depend on transit times as well as light-scatter. Overlapping of the two populations, which may indicate microcytic red cells or giant platelets, is indicated. PCV is computed by integration of the amplitude of the red cell pulses and MCV is computed from the PCV and the RBC. White cells are counted in a second channel, following lysis of red cells. Haemoglobin is estimated in a third channel by a modified cyanmethaemoglobin method; in the ELT 800, for example, light absorbance is measured at approximately 540 nm after a reaction time of 20–25 seconds.[6] MCV, MCH and MCHC are calculated from the measured parameters. Laminar flow of a sheathed stream of a diluted sample ensures that cells generally pass through the laser beam in single file so that little coincidence occurs and coincidence correction is not necessary. Like the Technicon H 6000, the Ortho series

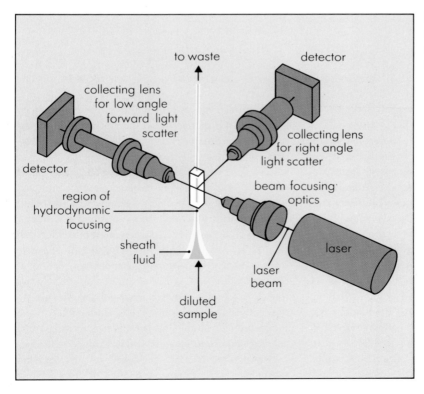

Fig. 2.10 *Diagrammatic representation of the cell detection and measuring system of the Ortho ELT 1500 counter.*

of instruments show less change in the MCV with increasing degrees of macrocytosis than is seen with impedance counters. As with impedance and light-scattering instruments the regression line of measured MCHC on reference MCHC is reltively flat.[6] The ELT 15 and ELT 1500 instruments have a capacity for a limited differential count and earlier models can be upgraded to include this capacity (see Chapter 4).

Newer red cell parameters

With the development of automated multiparameter haematology counters efforts have been made to automate the assessment of anisocytosis and to produce other new parameters relating to red cells.

In Coulter S Plus systems a histogram of red cell size distribution is produced and anisocytosis is assessed by the red cell distribution width (RDW), a measure of heterogeneity of cell size. Particles falling between 360 and 36 fl are classified as red cells and sized. Initially, in the Coulter S Plus Phase 1, the RDW was determined from the 20th and 80th percentiles of red cell size according to the formula:

$$\frac{20\text{th percentile of vol.} - 80\text{th percentile of vol.}}{20\text{th percentile of vol.} + 80\text{th percentile of vol.}} \times 100 \times 0.66$$

the factor of 0.66 being introduced to give an average value of approximately 10.[25] In later models the RDW was defined as the coefficient of variation (CV) of the RBC size distribution expressed as a percentage, with typical values being about 12–13. A typical set of histograms of size of white cell residues, red cells and platelets produced by a Coulter S Plus IV is shown in Fig. 2.11.

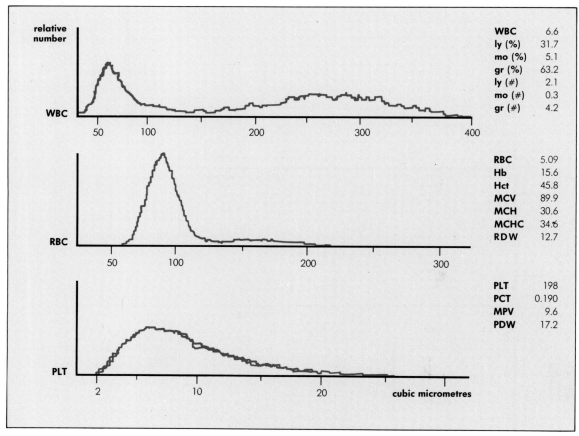

Fig. 2.11 *Typical histograms of size distribution of particles representing white cells, red cells and platelets produced by Coulter S Plus IV; for platelets both the instrument counts and the fitted curve derived from them are plotted.*

Another instrument using impedance technology, the E 5000 (TOA Medical Electronics Ltd, Kobe, Japan), also produces a measure of anisocytosis, but uses a different formula; with this instrument the RDW is defined as the size distribution in fl at 20 percent of the height from the base to the peak of the red cell histogram.

The Technicon H 6000 produces a histogram of the distribution of red cell size and indicates the degree of anisocytosis by the RDW, which is the CV of the red cell volume distribution. Later Ortho instruments produce histograms showing size distribution of white cells, red cells, and platelets (Fig. 2.12) together with an indication of morphological abnormality. A red cell morphology index (RCMI) of less than −2 or greater than +2 is said to indicate the presence of 10 percent or more of abnormal cells. The histograms produced by the impedance counters and light-scattering counters are similar but by no means the same. Histograms produced by the Coulter S Plus series of instruments have a tail of apparently larger cells (Fig. 2.11). This feature is seen to only a minor extent on the histograms produced by Ortho instruments (Fig. 2.12) while those produced by the H 6000 are symmetrical.

The Technicon H.1 measures the size and haemoglobin concentration of individual red cells and produces histograms of their distributions (Fig. 2.9).

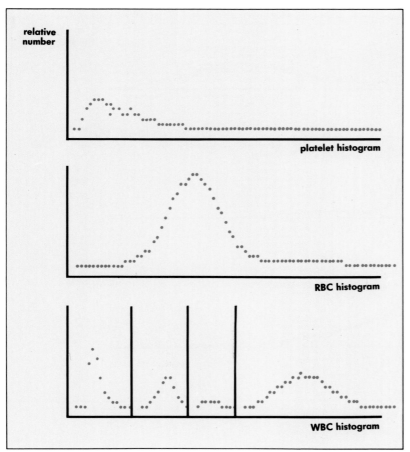

Fig. 2.12 *Typical Ortho ELT 800 WCS (white cell screen) histograms showing*
(a) *size distribution of platelets.*

(b) *size distribution of red cells.*

(c) *distribution of white cells into clusters according to light scatter at two angles; debris such as red cell stroma appears to the left of the histogram component representing lymphocytes.*

From the histogram of red cell size it is possible to give an indication of anisocytosis (depending on the red cell distribution width), and of microcytosis and macrocytosis (depending on the proportion of cells beyond present thresholds). The degree of abnormality is graded as + to ++ (for microcytrosis and macrocytosis) or + to +++ (for anisocytosis) rather than numerical values being given. From the histogram of red cell haemoglobin concentration it is similarly possible to assess anisochromasia (the degree of variation of haemoglobinization) (graded + to +++) and hypochromia and hyperchromia (graded + to ++). Indication of hyperchromia is a useful confirmation that spherocytes are present.

Comparison of the histograms of red cell volume and red cell haemoglobin concentration produced by the H.1 with the red cell size histograms of both the Coulter systems and the Technicon H 6000 shows that many samples which appeared to be dimorphic with regard to size are actually monomorphic with regard to size and dimorphic with regard to haemoglobin concentration. The apparent microcytes appear to be normocytic cells whose volume has been underestimated as a consequence of a low haemoglobin concentration affecting cell deformability and cell refractive index respectively.

Newer platelet parameters

Automated multiparameter haematology counters have the capacity to size as well as count platelets, using the same impedance or light-scattering technology as is used for sizing the red cells. This has allowed the estimation of platelet size (mean platelet volume, MPV) and an assessment of platelet size distributions and the degree of platelet anisocytosis (platelet distribution width, PDW). It is also possible to multiply the platelet count by the MPV to produce a plateletcrit, which is analogous to the PCV (haematocrit) of the red cells.

Calibration for platelet size is difficult. In impedance systems latex beads are customarily used. This creates two problems. First, there has not always been agreement as to the size assigned to latex beads; in 1983 there was an 8 percent increase in the size assigned to calibrant latex beads used by Coulter Electronics Ltd in the UK with a consequent 8 percent increase in the measured platelet size. This alteration did at least bring platelet size measurements in the UK into line with those in the USA. Secondly, although the shape assumed by platelets in any particular blood specimen as they pass through the counting and sizing aperture is unknown there is certainly no reason to assume that they have the same shape and electrical shadow as latex beads of identical volume. It must therefore be accepted that the size assigned to platelets is somewhat arbitrary. The size of platelets is also considerably affected by the conditions of blood collection and storage. When blood is taken into EDTA there is a rapid increase in platelet size as measured by impedance technology; this is probably consequent on progressive sphering of the platelets. Conversely, when light scattering technology is employed the size of platelets in EDTA-anticoagulated blood appears to decrease on storage.[24]

References

1. Biggs R & MacMillan RL (1948) The error in the red cell count. *Journal of Clinical Pathology*, **1**, 288–291.
2. Brown B (1980) *Hematology: principles and procedures.* Lea and Febiger, Philadelphia.
3. Crosland-Taylor PJ (1982) The micro PCV. In van Assendelft OW & England JM (Eds) *Advances in hematological methods: the blood count.* CRC Press Inc., Boca Raton, Florida.
4. Dacie JV & Lewis SM (1984) *Practical Haematology,* sixth edition. Churchill Livingstone, Edinburgh.
5. England JM & Down MC (1975) Determination of the packed cell volume using ^{131}I–human serum albumin. *British Journal of Haematology,* **30**, 365–370.
6. England JM & van Assendelft OW (1986) Automated blood counters and their evaluation. In Rowan RM & England JM (Eds) *Automation and Quality Assurance in Haematology.* Blackwell Scientific, Oxford.
7. England JM, Walford DM & Waters DAW (1972) Reassessment of the reliability of the haematocrit. *British Journal of Haematology,* **23**, 247–256.

8. Furth FW (1956) Effect of spherocytosis on volume of trapped plasma in red cell column of capillary and Wintrobe hematocrits. *Journal of Laboratory and Clinical Medicine*, **48**, 421–430.

9. Garby L & Vuille J-G (1961) The amount of plasma trapping in a high speed micro-capillary hematocrit centrifuge. *Scandinavian Journal of Clinical and Laboratory Investigation*, **13**, 642–645.

10. Guthrie DL & Pearson TC (1982) PCV measurement in the management of polycythaemic patients. *Clinical and Laboratory Haematology*, **4**, 257–265.

11. International Committee for Standardization in Haematology ICSH (1978) Recommendations for reference method for haemoglobinometry in human blood and specifications for international haemiglobincyanide reference preparation. *Journal of Clinical Pathology*, **31**, 139–143.

12. International Committee for Standardization in Haematology ICSH (1980a) Recommendation for reference method for determination by centrifugation of packed cell volume of blood. *Journal of Clinical Pathology*, **33**, 1–2.

13. International Committee for Standardization in Haematology ICSH (1980b) Recommended methods for measurement of red cell and plasma volume. *Journal of Nuclear Medicine*, **21**, 793–800.

14. International Committee for Standardization in Haematology ICSH (1982) Selected methods for the determination of the packed cell volume. In van Assendelft OW & England JM (Eds) *Advances in hematological methods: the blood count*. CRC Press Inc., Boca Raton, Florida.

15. Koepke JA (1986) The College of American Pathologists Survey Programme. In Rowan RM & England JM (Eds) *Automation and Quality Assurance in Haematology*. Blackwell Scientific, Oxford.

16. Lampasso JA (1965) Error in hematocrit value produced by excessive ethylenediaminetetraacetate. *American Journal of Clinical Pathology*, **44**, 109–110.

17. Lampasso JA (1968) Changes in hematologic values induced by storage of ethylenediaminetetraacetate human blood for varying periods of time. *American Journal of Clinical Pathology*, **49**, 443–447.

18. Lewis SM (1982) Visual hemocytometry. In: van Assendelft OW & England JM (Eds) *Advances in hematological methods: the blood count*. CRC Press Inc., Boca Raton, Florida.

19. Lines RW & Grace E (1984) Choice of anticoagulant for packed cell volume and the mean cell volume determination. *Clinical and Laboratory Haematology*, **6**, 305–306.

20. Mohandas N, Kim YR, Tycko D, Orlik J. Wyatt J & Groner W (1986) Accurate and independent measurement of volume and haemoglobin concentration of individual red cells by laser light scattering. *Blood*, **68**, 506–513.

21. Pearson TC & Guthrie DL (1983) Trapped plasma in the microhematocrit. *American Journal of Clinical Pathology*, **78**, 770–772.

22. Pearson TC & Wetherley-Mein G (1978) Vascular occlusive episodes and venous haematocrit in primary proliferative polycythaemia. *Lancet*, **ii**, 1219–1222.

23. Pennock CA & Jones KW (1966) Effects of ethylene-diamine-tetra-acetic acid (dipotassium salt) and heparin on the estimation of the packed cell volume. *Journal of Clinical Pathology*, **19**, 196–199.

24. Reardon DM, Hutchinson D, Preston FE & Trowbridge EA (1985) The routine measurement of platelet volume: a comparison of aperture-impedance and flow cytometric systems. *Clinical and Laboratory Haematology*, **7**, 251–257.

25. Rowan RM (1983) *Blood cell volume analysis*. Albert Clark and Company Limited, London.

26. Solomon HM & Grindon AJ (1986) The effect of capillary tube diameter on microhematocrit value. *Transfusion*, **26**, 199–202.

27. Tycko DH, Metz MH, Epstein EA & Grinbaum A (1985) Flow-cytometric light scattering measurement of red blood cell volume and haemoglobin concentration. *Applied Optics*, **24**, 1355–1365.

28. van Kampen EJ & Zijlstra WG (1983) Spectrophotometry of hemoglobin and hemoglobin derivatives. *Advances in Clinical Chemistry*, **23**, 199–257.

29. von Feltan U, Furlan M, Frey R & Bucher U (1978) Test of a new method for hemoglobin determinations in automatic analyzers. *Medical Laboratory*, **31**, 223–231.

3. Morphology of blood cells

EXAMINING THE BLOOD FILM

Blood films should be examined in a systematic manner, as follows.

First, patient identification should be checked and confirmed and the microscope slide matched with the corresponding full blood count report. The sex and age of the patient should be noted since the blood film cannot be interpreted without this information. In a multiracial community it is helpful also to know the ethnic origin of the patient.

Second, the film should be examined macroscopically to confirm adequate spreading and to look for any unusual spreading or staining characteristics. When pronounced, agglutination of red cells may be visible macroscopically (Fig.3.1). The presence of high levels of plasma proteins (for example either a monoclonal or polyclonal increase of immunoglobulins) causes an increased uptake of basic dyes such as methylene blue; this increased blue staining is visible macroscopically, when the blood film is compared with others stained in the same batch (Fig.3.2), and also microscopically. The presence of foreign substances, such as heparin or the vehicles of certain intravenous drugs, can also cause abnormal staining (Fig.3.3).

Third, the film should be examined microscopically first under a low power (for example with the ×10 or ×25 objective) and then under a higher power (×40 or ×50 objective), with an eyepiece magnification of ×10 or ×12. It is only necessary to use oil immersion and a

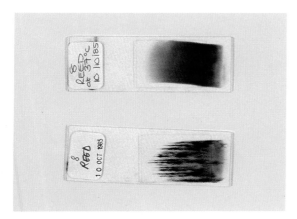

Fig.3.1 Blood films from a patient with a potent cold agglutinin. The lower film, which shows marked agglutination, was prepared from EDTA-anticoagulated blood which had been standing at room temperature. The upper film, which shows no macroscopic agglutination, was prepared from blood warmed to 37°C.

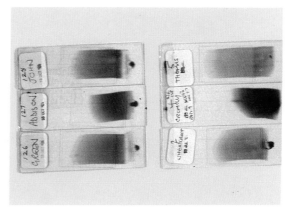

Fig.3.2 Macroscopic photograph of the blood films from two patients with multiple myeloma (centre films) compared with blood films from other patients stained in the same batch. The high levels of immunoglobulin have caused increased uptake of the basic component of the stain.

×100 objective when observation of fine detail is required. Laboratories using unmounted films may find it useful to have a ×50 oil immersion objective in addition to a ×100. The use of a relatively low power objective is important since it allows rapid scanning of a large part of the film and facilitates the detection of abnormal cells when they are present at a low frequency; it is also useful in the appreciation of rouleaux, red cell agglutination and white cell agglutination. Examination of the blood film must also include the edges and tail since large, abnormal cells are often distributed preferentially along the edges, and if clumps of platelets (Fig. 3.4) and fibrin strands (Fig. 3.5) are present they are often found in the tail.

On placing the film under the microscope the first decision to be made is whether or not it is suitable for further examination. Spreading, fixation and staining must be satisfactory and there should be no artefactual changes produced by excess EDTA or prolonged storage (see page 86). It is unwise to form an opinion on an inadequate blood film. A well spread film should have an appreciable area where cells are in a monolayer, that is, where they are touching but not overlapping. White cells should be distributed regularly throughout the film without undue concentration along the edges or in the tail, such as occurs when a film is spread too thinly.

Granulocytes are found preferentially along the edges and in the tail of a wedge-spread film and lymphocytes are preferentially in the centre, but in a carefully spread film the difference is not great (see page 8). The distribution of white cells is more even in a blood film prepared by centrifugation than in a wedge-spread film but nevertheless there is no consistent difference between differential counts on the two types of films and the increase in precision achieved by using films prepared by centrifugation is not great.

Blood films should be examined for evidence of platelet aggregation or partial clotting of the sample since these will invalidate the platelet count; partial clotting may also invalidate other parameters. Both platelet aggregates (Fig. 3.4) and fibrin strands (Fig. 3.5) may be seen; if platelets have discharged their granules following aggregation the aggregates may appear as pale blue masses not immediately identifiable as platelets.

If the blood film is judged as suitable for full examination then all cell types and also the background staining should be assessed systematically. The film appearances should be compared with the full blood count and a judgement made as to whether the results of the haemoglobin concentration, MCV, WBC and platelet count are consistent with the film, or whether

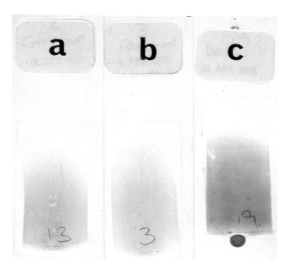

Fig. 3.3 *Macroscopic photograph of blood films showing (a,b) two films from normal blood in comparison with (c) the film from a specimen which had been inadvertently contaminated with heparin during venesection, the heparin having produced abnormal staining characteristics.*

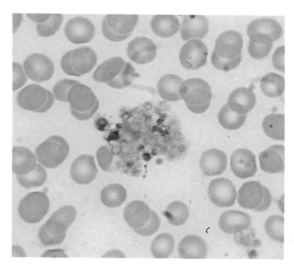

Fig. 3.4 *Platelet aggregates or agglutinates in a blood film. Some platelets in the agglutinate still have normal granularity while others have discharged their granules. × 960.*

there is some unusual feature which could invalidate them. If the full blood count and film are inconsistent with each other the blood specimen should be inspected and the full blood count — and, if necessary, the blood film — repeated as an initial step in seeking an explanation for the discrepancy. Such discrepancies may be due to: a poorly mixed or partly clotted blood sample; a sample which is too small so that the instrument aspirates an inadequate volume; the blood count and the blood film being derived from different blood samples.

Once such technical errors have been eliminated, then discrepancies may be due to an abnormality of the specimen, such as hyperlipidaemia or the presence of a cold agglutinin. Hyperlipidaemia may be suspected when there are blurred cell outlines in the stained film (Fig.3.6) and agglutinates are commonly seen in the film when a cold agglutinin is present (Fig.3.7). The validation of a blood count by comparison with the blood film and by other means is dealt with in detail in Chapter 5.

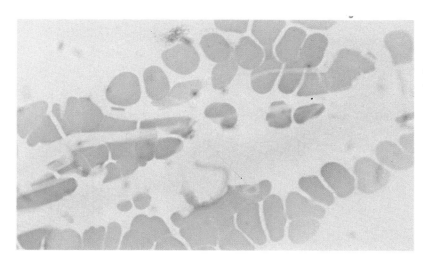

Fig.3.5 *Fibrin strands in a blood film. The fibrin strands are very faintly basophilic and cause deformation of red cells between which they pass. × 960.*

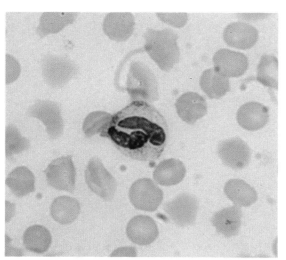

Fig.3.6 *A blood film from a patient with hyperlipidaemia showing 'fuzzy' red cell outlines consequent on the high concentration of lipids. × 960.*

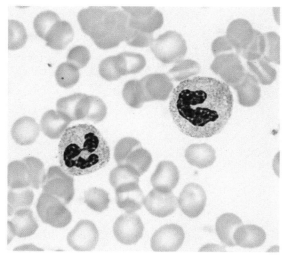

Fig.3.7 *Red cell agglutinates in the blood film of a patient with high titre cold agglutinins. × 960.*

LEUCOCYTES

Normal peripheral blood leucocytes are classified into polymorphonuclear leucocytes and mononuclear cells, the latter term indicating lymphocytes and monocytes. Polymorphonuclear leucocytes can also be referred to as polymorphonuclear granulocytes, polymorphs or granulocytes. The term granulocyte has also been used to refer more generally to both the mature polymorphonuclear granulocytes normally seen in the peripheral blood and also their granulated precursors. Polymorphs have lobulated nuclei which are very variable in shape (hence polymorphic), and have prominent cytoplasmic granules which differ in staining characteristics in the three classes: neutrophil, eosinophil and basophil. Mononuclear cells may also have granules; in the case of the monocyte they are inconspicuous, whereas in the lymphocyte they may be prominent but are small in number. In pathological states and in certain physiological states — such as pregnancy and during the neonatal period — precursors of polymorphs may appear in the peripheral blood. A variety of abnormal leucocytes may also be seen in certain disease states.

THE NEUTROPHIL

The mature neutrophil measures 12–15 μm in diameter. The cytoplasm is acidophilic with many fine granules. The nucleus has clumped chromatin and is divided into two to five distinct lobes by filaments which are narrow strands of dense heterochromatin bordered by nuclear membrane (Fig.3.8). The nucleus tends to follow an approximately circular form since in the living cell the nuclear lobes are arranged in a circle around the centrosome. In normal females a 'drumstick' may be seen protruding from the nucleus of a proportion of the cells (Fig.3.9). A normal neutrophil has granules spread evenly through the cytoplasm but there may be some agranular cytoplasm protruding at one margin of the cell — this represents the advancing edge of a cell in active locomotion.

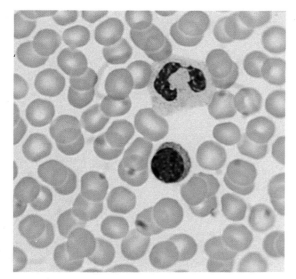

Fig.3.8 *Normal polymorphonuclear neutrophil and normal small lymphocyte. The disposition of the neutrophil lobes around the circumference of a circle is apparent. × 960.*

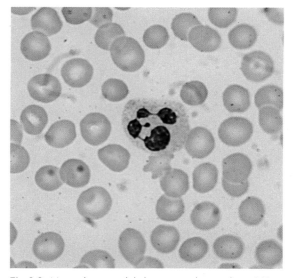

Fig.3.9 *Normal neutrophil showing a drumstick. × 960.*

Abnormalities of neutrophil morphology are summarized in Figs 3.10, 3.11 and 3.12.

ALTERATIONS AND ABNORMALITIES OF NEUTROPHIL NUCLEI	
Abnormality	**Occurrence**
Left shift	pregnancy infection, hypoxia and hypotension
Hypersegmentation	megaloblastic erythropoiesis iron deficiency uraemia infection hereditary neutrophil hypersegmentation
Hyposegmentation	Pelger–Huët anomaly bilobed neutrophils with reduction of specific 　　granules (lactoferrin deficiency)[127] non-lobed neutrophils with other congenital 　　anomalies[105] pseudo-Pelger–Huët anomaly (myelodysplastic 　　syndromes and acute myeloid leukaemia)
Increased nuclear 　　projections	trisomy D syndrome[63] associated with large platelets (single family)[46] associated with large Y chromosome 　　(drumstick-like)[91] as an isolated defect[117] in myelodysplastic syndromes
Ring nuclei	chronic granulocytic leukaemia[76] acute myeloid leukaemia[124] chronic neutrophilic leukaemia[68]
Botryoid nucleus	heat stroke[57] hyperthermia[93]
Dense chromatin clumping	myelodysplastic syndromes[50]
Nuclear fragments within 　　the cytoplasm	dysplastic granulopoiesis due to 　　immunosuppressive or 　　chemotherapeutic drugs,[7]

Fig.3.10 *Some alterations and abnormalities which may be present in neutrophil nuclei.*

ALTERATIONS AND ABNORMALITIES OF NEUTROPHIL CYTOPLASM	
Abnormality	**Occurrence**
Reduced granulation	myelodysplastic syndromes congenital lactoferrin deficiency
Increased granulation	'toxic' granulation (pregnancy, infection and inflammation) aplastic anaemia hypereosinophilic syndrome Alder–Reilly anomaly chronic neutrophilic leukaemia[68]
Abnormal granulation	Chédiak–Higashi syndrome and related anomalies[42,95] Alder–Reilly anomaly acute myeloid leukaemia[135] and myelodysplastic syndromes
Vacuolation	infection acute alcohol poisoning[26] Jordans' anomaly[67,112] carnitine deficiency[52] kwashiorkor[116]
Döhle bodies or similar inclusions	May–Hegglin anomaly isolated defect, familial[47] pregnancy infection, inflammation, burns myelodysplastic syndromes acute myeloid leukaemia kwashiorkor[116] Fechtner syndrome[104]

Phagocytosed material:
  bacteria and fungi
  cryoglobulin
  mucopolysaccharide
  nucleoprotein
  melanin
  bilirubin crystals
    or amorphous deposits
  cystine crystals
  red blood cells
	bacterial and fungal infections
	cryoglobulinaemia[136]
	various malignant tumours[96]
	systemic lupus erythematosus[18]
	melanoma[139]
	
	severe hyperbilirubinaemia[118,123]
	cystinosis[88]
	autoimmune haemolytic anaemia, paroxysmal
	  cold haemoglobinuria, incompatible transfusion,
	  potassium chlorate poisoning[58]

Fig.3.11 *Some alterations and abnormalities which may be present in neutrophil cytoplasm.*

INHERITED CONDITIONS IN WHICH LEUCOCYTES HAVE ABNORMAL GRANULES OR CYTOPLASMIC INCLUSIONS					
Abnormality	Inheritance	Associated features	Morphology of granules or inclusions	Nature of granules or inclusions	Cells affected
Chédiak–Higashi anomaly	AR*	anaemia neutropenia thrombocytopenia albinism jaundice neurological abnormalities recurrent infections	giant granules with colour ranging from grey to red	abnormal primary granules (specific granules are normal)	neutrophil eosinophil basophil monocyte lymphocyte melanocyte renal tubule many other body cells
Alder–Reilly anomaly	AR*†	Tay–Sach's disease, mucopolysaccharidoses such as Hunter's†, Hurler's, Sanfilippo, Morquio's, Scheie's, and Maroteaux–Lamy syndromes	dark purple or red inclusions which may resemble toxic granules; inclusions or vacuoles in lymphocytes	mucopolysaccharide or other abnormal carbohydrate	neutrophil eosinophil basophil monocyte (rarely) lymphocyte
May–Hegglin anomaly	AD‡	thrombocytopenia giant platelets	resemble Döhle bodies	amorphous area of cytoplasm containing structures related to ribosomes	neutrophil eosinophil basophil monocyte

*AR = autosomal recessive inheritance   ‡AD = autosomal dominant inheritance
†Hunter's syndrome is sex-linked recessive

Fig.3.12 *Inherited conditions in which leucocytes have abnormal granules or cytoplasmic inclusions.*

The neutrophil band form and left shift

A cell which otherwise resembles a mature neutrophil but which lacks nuclear lobes is referred to as a neutrophil band form (Fig.3.13), or a 'stab' form (from the German 'stabzelle' referring to a shepherd's staff or crook). The Committee for the Clarification of Nomenclature of Cells and Diseases of the Blood Forming Organs has defined a band cell as 'any cell of the granulocytic series which has a nucleus which could be described as a curved or coiled band, no matter how marked that indentation, if it does not completely segment the nucleus into lobes separated by a filament'. A filament is a thread-like connection with 'no significant nuclear material'.[86] A band cell is differentiated from a metamyelocyte (see below) by having an appreciable length of nucleus with parallel sides. Small numbers of band cells are seen in healthy subjects. An increase in number of band cells in relation to mature neutrophils is described as a left shift. When a left shift occurs neutrophil precursors more immature than band forms (metamyelocytes, myelocytes, promyelocytes and blasts) may also be released into the blood. A left shift is a physiological occurrence in pregnancy. In the nonpregnant patient it commonly indicates a response to infection or inflammation, or some other stimulus to the bone marrow.

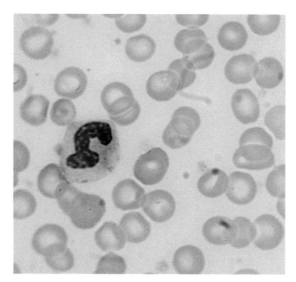

Fig.3.13 *Neutrophil band form. The nucleus is nonsegmented and also has chromatin which is less condensed than that of the majority of segmented neutrophils. Two Döhle bodies (see page 9) are present in the cytoplasm. × 960.*

The actual percentage or absolute number of band cells, or the ratio of band forms to neutrophils, which is regarded as normal is dependent on the precise definition used and on how it is applied in practice. Inconsistency between laboratories with regard to both these points is common.

Band cell counts have been employed in the detection of infection in neonates,[2,20] but again various definitions of a band form have been applied. For example, Akenzua et al.[2] defined a (segmented) neutrophil as a cell with lobes separated by a thin filament whose width is less than one-third the maximum diameter of the lobes whereas Christensen et al.[20] required the lobes to be separated by a definite nuclear filament.

The neutrophil lobe count and right shift

In normal blood, neutrophils have one to five lobes, with six-lobed neutrophils being seen very rarely. A right shift is said to be present if the average lobe count is increased (Fig.3.14). The average lobe count of normal subjects varies between observers, with values of 2.5 to 3.3 having been obtained in different studies.[17] In practice a formal lobe count is time consuming and the presence of more than 3 percent of five-lobed neutrophils is a more practical indication of right shift. This is also a more sensitive index of hypersegmentation than the average lobe count and allows the documentation of neutrophil hypersegmentation in patients whose average lobe count is normal, since they have a simultaneous increase in band forms. A further index of right shift which has been found to be more sensitive than either of the above criteria is the segmentation index, obtained by dividing the number of neutrophils with five lobes or more (× 100), by the number of neutrophils with four lobes. Values of greater than 16.9 are abnormal.[33]

A right shift or neutrophil hypersegmentation is seen in megaloblastic anaemia and in occasional patients with iron deficiency, infection or uraemia. It also occurs as a rare hereditary characteristic with an autosomal inheritance.[27]

The presence of macropolycytes (see page 47) is not an indication of right shift since the increased number of lobes is consequent on increased DNA content rather than on any abnormality of nuclear segmentation.

The neutrophil drumstick and sessile nodules

Some neutrophils in normal females have a drumstick-shaped nuclear appendage about 1.5 μm diameter which is linked to the rest of the nucleus by a filament[29]

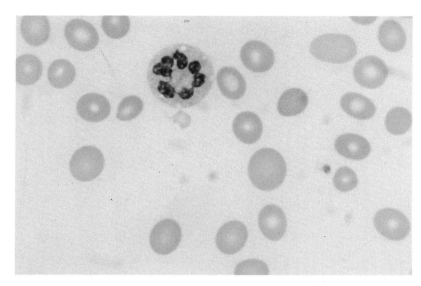

Fig.3.14 *Hypersegmented neutrophil showing seven nuclear lobes. The film also shows anisocytosis with both microcytes and macrocytes being present.* ×960.

(Fig.3.9). These drumsticks represent the inactive X chromosome of the female. Similar projections with central pallor (racquet forms) are not drumsticks and do not have the same significance. In cells without drumsticks the inactive X chromosome may be condensed beneath the nuclear membrane, where it may be detected in some neutrophil band forms,[92] or it may protrude from the nucleus as a sessile nodule (Fig.3.15). Like drumsticks, sessile nodules are usually only found in females. In one study the frequency of drumsticks was found to vary from one in 38 to one in 200 neutrophils, and to be characteristic of the individual but also proportional to the lobe count.[28,29] If a left shift occurs, the proportion of cells with drumsticks lessens, whereas in macropolycytes (see page 47), and where there is right shift due to megaloblastic anaemia or hereditary hypersegmentation of neutrophils, the frequency of drumsticks is increased.

The presence and frequency of drumsticks is related to the number of X chromosomes. They do not occur in normal males, nor in individuals with the testicular feminization syndrome who are phenotypically female but genetically male (XY), nor in Turner's syndrome (XO). In males with Klinefelter's syndrome (XXY) drumsticks are found but in lower numbers than in females. Paradoxically XXX females rarely have cells with double drumsticks and on average their lobe count and incidence of drumsticks are lower than those of normal females; they have an increased incidence of sessile nodules and it has been suggested that the presence of an extra X chromosome inhibits nuclear segmentation.[90] Females with an isochromosome of the long arms of the X chromosome have larger and more frequent drumsticks, whereas females with deletions from the X chromosome have smaller drumsticks.[27]

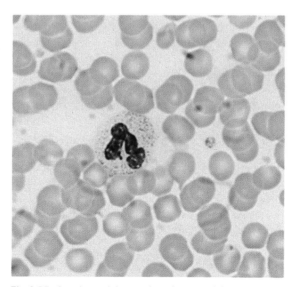

Fig.3.15 *Sessile nodule in a band neutrophil.* × 960.

Natural human chimaeras whose red cells are a mixture of cells of male and female origin also have a drumstick frequency consistent with a male/female mixture of neutrophils[28] and, similarly, an alteration of the drumstick count may be seen after bone marrow transplantation, when bone marrow from a female has been transplanted into a male or vice versa.

The proportion of neutrophils with drumsticks and with sessile nodules is reduced in women with chronic granulocytic leukaemia but returns to normal when the WBC count falls on treatment.[129]

The drumstick count (and the average lobe count) are reduced in Down's syndrome.[3]

In addition to drumsticks and sessile nodules, neutrophil nuclei may have other nuclear projections which may have the shape of clubs, hooks or tags (see Fig.3.10). These projections may also be seen in the neutrophils of males.

Other abnormalities of neutrophil nuclei (see Fig.3.10)

Reduced neutrophil segmentation which is not consequent on temporary bone marrow stimulation with release of immature cells may be seen as an inherited anomaly (the Pelger–Huët anomaly) or as an acquired anomaly (the pseudo-Pelger–Huët anomaly). The Pelger–Huët anomaly was first described by Pelger in 1928 and its familial nature was recognized by Huët in 1931.[14] It is inherited as an autosomal dominant characteristic with a prevalence of between 1 in 1000 and 1 in 10 000 in different communities.[122] It has been recognized in many ethnic groups including Caucasians, Blacks, Chinese, Japanese and Indonesians. The abnormality is distinctive: the majority of neutrophils have bilobed nuclei (Fig.3.16a), the lobes being rounder than normal and the chromatin more condensed; a characteristic spectacle or *pince-nez* shape is common. Other nuclei have a peanut shape (Fig.3.16b). A small proportion of neutrophils, usually not more than 4 percent, have non-lobed nuclei (Fig.3.16c); they are distinguishable from myelocytes by a lower nucleocytoplasmic ratio and by the maturity of the cytoplasm and the condensation of the chromatin. In the rare homozygotes for the Pelger–Huët anomaly all the neutrophils have round or oval nuclei, no lobes being found. The distinction between the Pelger–Huët anomaly and a left shift is important, since the inherited condition is of no clinical significance. If a left shift occurs in a patient with the Pelger–Huët anomaly the proportion of non-lobed neutrophils is further increased. If a subject with

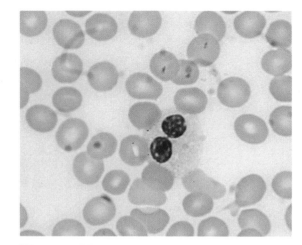

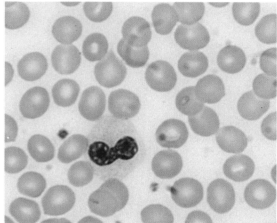

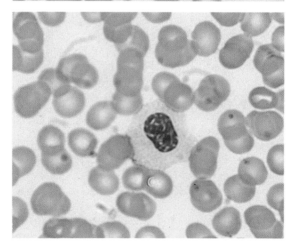

Fig.3.16 *Three neutrophils from a subject with the Pelger–Huët anomaly showing (upper) bilobed (middle) peanut shaped and (lower) non-lobed nuclei. The very round lobes of the bilobed nucleus are characteristic. × 960.*

the Pelger–Huët anomaly becomes megaloblastic then a right shift occurs and neutrophils with three, four or even five lobes are seen;[4] megaloblastosis also causes loss of the characteristic dense clumping of the nuclear chromatin and drumsticks may become identifiable. Subjects with the Pelger–Huët anomaly also show reduced lobulation of eosinophils and basophils.[72]

In another congenital anomaly, sometimes designated lactoferrin deficiency, neutrophils with bilobed nuclei also have markedly reduced numbers of the normally-occurring specific granules. This is associated with a deficiency of lactoferrin, vitamin B_{12}-binding protein and neutrophil alkaline phosphatase.[99,127]

A single patient has been described in whom non-lobed neutrophils were associated with skeletal malformations, microphthalmia and mental retardation.[105]

An acquired pseudo-Pelger–Huët anomaly is common in myelodysplastic syndromes and in acute myeloid leukaemias. Features which may help in making the distinction from the inherited Pelger–Huët anomaly are the smaller percentage of neutrophils which show the characteristic abnormal features and the commonly-associated neutropenia and reduction of neutrophil granules (Fig.3.17). Furthermore, Döhle bodies (page 9) may be a feature of cells showing the pseudo-Pelger–Huët anomaly (Fig.3.17),[1] whereas they do not occur with the inherited anomaly unless there is some complicating factor. The acquired Pelger–Huët anomaly is occasionally seen in chronic granulocytic leukaemia, in idiopathic myelofibrosis and in multiple myeloma; in the latter condition it is likely to indicate the presence of a preleukaemic myelodysplastic state.

Reduced lobulation is rarely seen in other circumstances but has been described in association with colchicine therapy, infectious mononucleosis, malaria, myxoedema, metastatic carcinoma of the bone marrow, chronic lymphocytic leukaemia and acute enteritis.[27]

Neutrophils with ring or doughnut nuclei are seen occasionally in normal subjects. Their frequency is increased in chronic granulocytic leukaemia, in chronic neutrophilic leukaemia, and probably in the myelodysplastic syndromes;[76] occasionally they are prominent in acute myeloid leukaemia.[124]

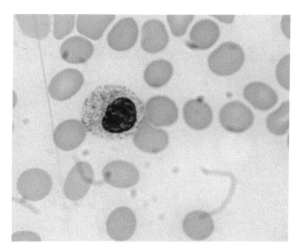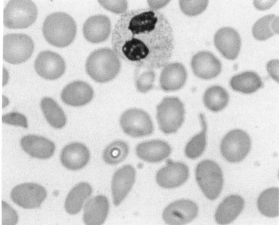

Fig.3.17 Two neutrophils from a patient with the acquired Pelger–Huët anomaly as part of a postchemotherapy myelodysplasia. The nuclei are (left) non-lobed and (right) bilobed with very rounded lobes. One cell (left) also shows Döhle bodies. × 960.

Another acquired defect of the neutrophil nucleus is radial segmentation to form a 'botryoid' nucleus (Fig.3.18), that is, a nucleus the shape of which resembles a bunch of grapes. This change is consequent on contraction of microfilaments radiating from the centriole. It has been demonstrated in heat stroke[57] and in hyperthermia arising from brainstem haemorrhage.[93]

Excessive dense clumping of the nuclear chromatin of neutrophils has been noted in myelodysplasia.[50]

Rarely, neutrophils may contain detached fragments of nuclear material equivalent to the Howell–Jolly bodies (see page 171) of erythrocytes (Fig.3.19); their nature may be confirmed by a Feulgen stain for DNA.[7] These inclusions are the result of dysplastic granulopoiesis; they are seen mainly in patients on immunosuppressive and antitumour chemotherapeutic drugs.

Abnormalities of neutrophil cytoplasm (see Fig.3.11)
Reduced granulation of neutrophils is most commonly observed in myelodysplastic conditions (Figs 3.17 and 3.20). Rarely it occurs as a congenital anomaly, for example in lactoferrin deficiency.

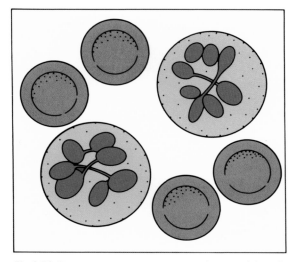

Fig.3.18 *Diagrammatic representation of neutrophils with botryoid nuclei.*

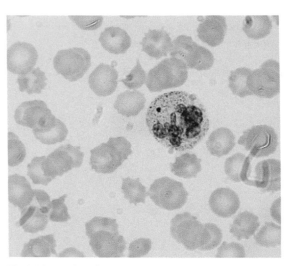

Fig.3.19 *Nuclear fragment within the cytoplasm of a neutrophil, in the blood film of a patient taking azathioprine. × 960.*

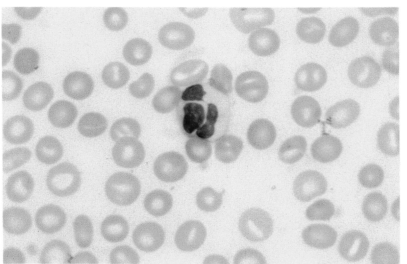

Fig.3.20 *Hypogranular neutrophil in a patient with myelodysplasia. The film also shows anisocytosis, poikilocytosis and occasional macrocytes. × 960.*

Increased granulation of neutrophils with granules appearing both larger and more basophilic than normal is designated toxic granulation (Fig.3.21). When normal maturation occurs in the neutrophil line the azurophilic, or primary, granules become less strongly azurophilic so that, rather than staining reddish-purple, they may stain violet or may fail to stain at all. In a neutrophil showing toxic granulation the primary granules remain strongly azurophilic; this may be related to a higher concentration of acid mucosubstances than in normal neutrophils.[115] Neutrophils showing toxic granulation may have reduced specific (neutrophilic) granules due to degranulation. Note that toxic granulation is not necessarily indicative of a pathological state since it is also found in normal pregnancy.

Heavy neutrophil granulation may also be seen in patients with aplastic anaemia (in the absence of overt infection) and in patients with the hypereosinophilic syndrome (Fig.3.22).

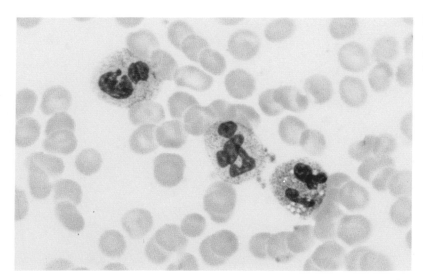

Fig.3.21 *Three neutrophils from a patient with bacterial infection showing toxic granulation and vacuolation.* ×960.

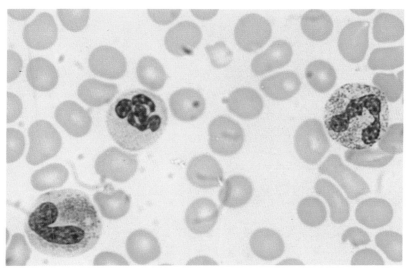

Fig.3.22 *A heavily granulated neutrophil (right) in a patient with the hypereosinophilic syndrome. A normal neutrophil (centre) has been included for comparison. The photograph also shows a hypogranular band eosinophil (left).* × 960.

Abnormal neutrophil granulation is seen in the Chédiak–Higashi anomaly and in the Alder–Reilly anomaly, the latter either occurring as an isolated anomaly or being a feature of the mucopolysaccharidoses, of Tay–Sachs disease, or of Batten–Spielmeyer–Vogt disease (see Fig.3.12). In the Chédiak–Higashi anomaly (Fig.3.23) the abnormal inclusions are quite variable in their staining characteristics and some may resemble Döhle bodies (see page 9); at the ultrastructural level, however, they are abnormal granules rather than rough endoplasmic reticulum, being formed by the fusion of primary granules with each other and with secondary granules. There have been reports of

patients with abnormal neutrophil granulation resembling that of the Chédiak–Higashi syndrome but with atypical features.[42,95] In an apparently distinct syndrome abnormal granulation of all mature myeloid cells was associated with bile duct atresia and livedo reticularis.[123] Occasional patients with the myelodysplastic syndrome or with acute myeloid leukaemia have giant granules in neutrophils, which are morphologically similar to those of the Chédiak–Higashi syndrome.[135] In the Alder–Reilly anomaly neutrophils may have heavy granulation resembling toxic granulation, or may have large, clearly abnormal granules (Fig.3.24).

Neutrophil vacuolation may occur as the result of fusion of granules with a phagocytic vacuole with subsequent exocytosis of the contents of the secondary lysosome. This is usually a feature of infection (Fig.3.21) and may be associated with partial degranulation of the neutrophil. Neutrophil vacuolation commonly occurs together with neutrophilia, left shift, toxic granulation and formation of Döhle bodies (see page 190). In one patient with *Clostridium perfringens* infection, neutrophil vacuolation was associated with intracellular spore formation.[75]

Vacuolation of neutrophils may occur as a toxic effect following ethanol ingestion[26] but this is much less commonly observed than ethanol-induced vacuolation of bone marrow myeloid precursors.

A rare cause of neutrophil vacuolation (together with vacuolation of neutrophil precursors, monocytes and some eosinophils, basophils and lymphocytes) is a familial defect designated Jordans' anomaly;[67,112] the

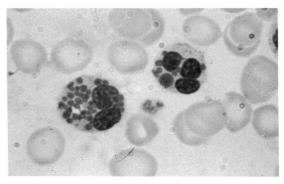

Fig.3.23 *Two granulocytes from a patient with the Chédiak–Higashi syndrome showing grossly abnormal granules, some of which are giant. × 960. Courtesy of Professor J. Stewart.*

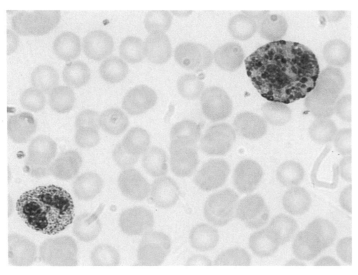

Fig.3.24 *The Alder–Reilly anomaly associated with the Maroteaux–Lamy syndrome. The neutrophil has granules which resemble toxic granules. The other granulocyte may be an eosinophil with granules having very abnormal staining characteristics. × 960.*

vacuoles are due to the dissolution of lipid.[112] Inheritance appears to be autosomal recessive.[112] Jordans' anomaly may represent carnitine deficiency.[52]

Döhle bodies are small, pale blue or blue-grey cytoplasmic inclusions, single or multiple, often found towards the periphery of the cell (see Figs 3.13 and 3.25). They usually measure only 1–2 μm in diameter, but may be up to 5 μm. At the ultrastructural level they are composed of stacks of rough endoplasmic reticulum together with some glycogen granules. Their ribosomal component is indicated by pink staining with a methyl green-pyronin stain and by destruction by ribonuc-

lease; they are seen better in films made from non-anticoagulated blood.[1] Döhle bodies are associated with pregnancy, infective and inflammatory states, and burns. They may be seen in myelodysplastic syndromes (see Fig.3.17a) and in acute myeloid leukaemia, and have also been reported in pernicious anaemia, polycythaemia vera, chronic granulocytic leukaemia, haemolytic anaemia, Wegener's granulomatosis, and following use of anti-cancer chemotherapeutic agents.[64]

Large inclusions resembling Döhle bodies, often numerous and sharply defined, are a feature of the May–Hegglin anomaly[14] (see Figs 3.11 and 3.26); they

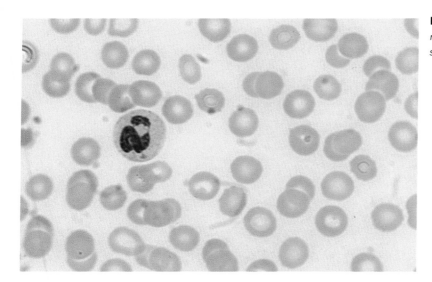

Fig.3.25 A Döhle body in a neutrophil of a patient with septicaemia. × 960.

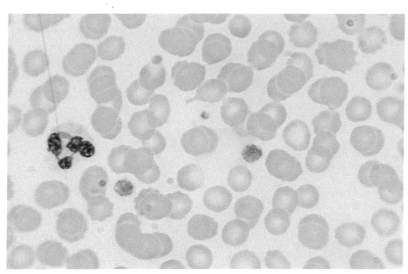

Fig.3.26 A large inclusion resembling a Döhle body in a neutrophil of a patient with the May–Hegglin anomaly. Thrombocytopenia and giant platelets are also apparent. × 960.

are often spindle- or crescent-shaped, randomly distributed in the cell rather than near the cell margin, and more intensely staining than the Döhle body of inflammatory conditions.[65,69] At the ultrastructural level these inclusions differ from the Döhle bodies of reactive states; they appear as an amorphous area largely devoid of organelles, often incompletely surrounded by a single strand of rough endoplasmic reticulum and containing a few dense rods and spherical particles which are probably ribosomes.[65]

Inclusions resembling Döhle bodies but differing from them ultrastructurally have also been reported in association with the features of Epstein's syndrome (see Fig.3.62); the name Fechtner syndrome has been proposed.[104] In normal subjects Döhle bodies are rare.

In one study they were seen in three of 20 healthy subjects with an average frequency of 0.1 per 100 cells.[64] In pregnancy the number of Döhle bodies per 100 cells increases in parallel with the increase in the leucocyte count;[1] the increased frequency persists into the postpartum period.

Rarely a variety of other inclusions may appear within the cytoplasm of neutrophils (see Fig.3.12). The finding of microorganisms within neutrophils is highly significant (Fig.3.27) (see page 191). Neutrophils may ingest cryoglobulin (Fig.3.28) to give cells with either multiple inclusions or a single, large, homogeneous pale-blue inclusion which displaces the nucleus; phagocytosis of cryoglobulin occurs not *in vivo* but *in vitro* if the blood is left standing.[136] Abnormal mucopolysac-

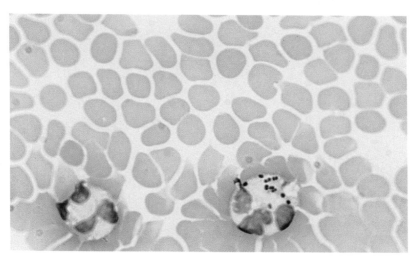

Fig.3.27 *A neutrophil containing diplococci from a patient with fatal Neisseria meningitidis septicaemia.*
× 960.

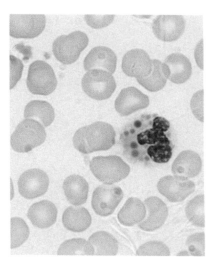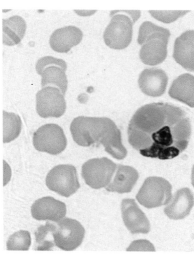

Fig.3.28 *Cryoglobulin which has been ingested by neutrophils to give (left) small round inclusions (right) large masses which fill the cytoplasm and displace the nucleus. Some extracellular cryoglobulin is also present (right).* × 960.

charide, which circulates in the blood of patients with certain malignant diseases, may be ingested by neutrophils; the blood film may also show amorphous or fibrous deposits.[96] Malarial pigment is occasionally observed in neutrophils (Fig.3.29) but is more commonly present in monocytes. The formation of LE (lupus erythematosus) cells is usually an *in vitro* phenomenon but they have been seen in the peripheral blood in patients with severe lupus erythematosus.[18] The square or rectangular crystals which may be seen in the peripheral blood leucocytes in cystinosis are more readily seen with phase-contrast microscopy.[88] Large inclusions were observed in a case of colchicine poisoning.[108]

Other abnormalities of neutrophil morphology

These abnormalities include macropolycytes, necrobiotic neutrophils and neutrophil aggregation.

A macropolycyte is about twice the size of a normal neutrophil (Fig.3.30); its diameter is 15–25 μm rather than 12–15 μm and analysis of its DNA content shows that it is tetraploid rather than diploid, the number of lobes present being increased approximately. Occasional macropolycytes are seen in the blood of healthy subjects. Increased numbers are seen as an inherited (autosomal dominant) condition in which 1–2 percent of neutrophils are giant with six- to ten-lobed nuclei, or with twin mirror-image nuclei.[69] Macropolycytes have also been reported in chronic infection, chronic

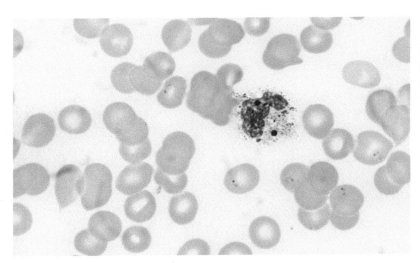

Fig.3.29 *A neutrophil containing malarial pigment. The patient had malaria due to Plasmodium falciparum and ring forms of the parasite are present in the red cells.* × 960.

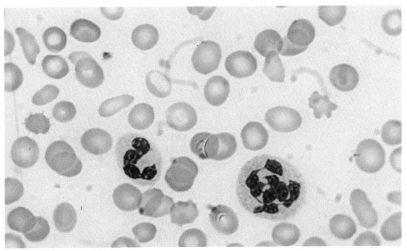

Fig.3.30 *A normal neutrophil and a macropolycyte in a blood film from a patient with myelodysplasia. The macropolycyte is about twice the size of the normal neutrophil and has increased nuclear segmentation. The film also shows anisochromasia.* × 960.

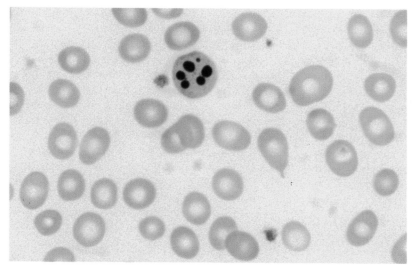

Fig.3.31 *A necrobiotic neutrophil in a blood film from a patient with megaloblastic anaemia. The neutrophil nucleus has degenerated into rounded pyknotic masses. The film also shows anisocytosis, macrocytosis and a tear drop poikilocyte. × 960.*

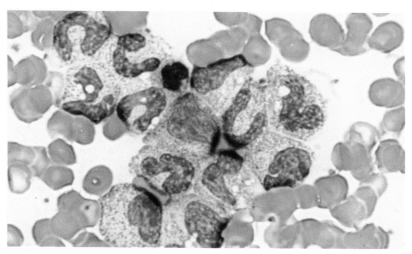

Fig.3.32 *Neutrophil aggregation* **(a)** *as a feature of overwhelming infection; the neutrophils also show toxic granulation and vacuolation and band forms are increased. ×960.*

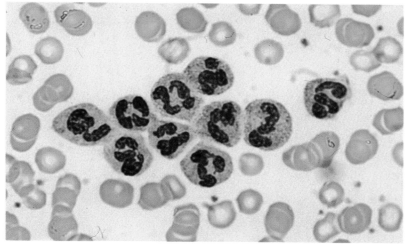

(b) *as a persistent feature in a patient with rheumatoid arthritis. × 960.*

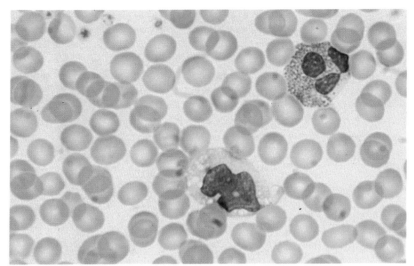

Fig.3.33 A normal eosinophil in the blood film of a healthy subject. The majority of eosinophils have bilobed rather than trilobed nuclei. The film also shows a monocyte (lower cell). × 960.

granulocytic leukaemia and other myeloproliferative conditions, megaloblastosis, and following the administration of cytotoxic drugs and antimetabolites. Most macropolycytes have staining characteristics which are the same as those of other neutrophils but in megaloblastic anaemia macropolycytes may be seen which have a more open chromatin pattern and do not have an increased number of lobes.[22]

Necrobiotic neutrophils are cells which have died in the peripheral blood. Occasional such cells are seen in the blood of healthy subjects and are recognized by their dense, homogeneous (pyknotic) nucleus which eventually becomes completely round or breaks up into multiple dense round masses; the cytoplasm shows prominent acidophilia (Fig.3.31). The frequency of necrobiotic leucocytes is increased in some patients with acute myeloid leukaemia. If blood is left at room temperature for prolonged periods of time a similar change may occur as an *in vitro* artefact (page 86). Leucocytes which have degenerated to the extent that nuclear material is no longer apparent have been designated as necrotic; this is generally an artefact consequent on prolonged storage.

Aggregation of neutrophils with or without aggregation of platelets may develop *in vitro* when EDTA-anticoagulated blood is allowed to stand. On some occasions this is an acute phenomenon which has occured in association with infectious mononucleosis[49] or with acute bacterial infection (Fig.3.32a). On other occasions it is observed in the same patient over many months, and in these patients the phenomenon may be associated with autoimmune disease (Fig.3.32b). In

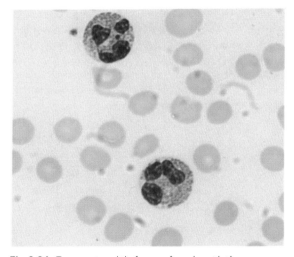

Fig.3.34 Two eosinophils from a female with the hypereosinophilic syndrome. The upper cell shows a drumstick. × 960.

some patients in whom the phenomenon is due to a cold antibody, red cell agglutinates coexist.

THE EOSINOPHIL

The eosinophil (Fig.3.33) is slightly larger than the neutrophil with a diameter of 12–17 μm. The nucleus is usually bilobed but occasional nuclei are trilobed, the average lobe count being about 2.3. In females, eosinophils may have drumsticks (see page 38) (Fig.3.34), but as the frequency of drumsticks is related to the degree of lobulation of a nucleus they are quite infrequent. Eosinophil granules are spherical and considerably larger than those of neutrophils; they pack the cytoplasm and stain reddish-orange. The cytoplasm of eosinophils is weakly basophilic, ribosomes and rough endoplasmic reticulum being more abundant than in mature neutrophils; when degranulation occurs the pale blue cytoplasm is seen. Very occasional eosinophils in healthy subjects contain some granules which are basophilic.

Alterations and abnormalities of eosinophils

Abnormal eosinophil inclusions may be seen, together with neutrophil inclusions, in a variety of inherited conditions (Fig.3.12). A further abnormality, confined to eosinophils and basophils, has been noted in one family, the inheritance being autosomal dominant;[130] inclusions were grey or blue-grey. Other morphological abnormalities which may occur in eosinophils include nuclear hypersegmentation (Fig.3.35), lack of nuclear segmentation (Fig.3.36), and, rarely, ring-shaped nuclei (Fig.3.37). Cytoplasm may be completely (Fig.3.36) or partly (Fig.3.35) degranulated, or may be vacuolated (Fig.3.35). All these changes are characteristic of the idiopathic hypereosinophilic syndrome (see page 201)

but are seen also, to a lesser extent, in reactive conditions (see Chapter 8). Hypersegmentation of eosinophil nuclei may also occur as a hereditary condition;[27] in one family hypersegmented eosinophils were also very poorly granulated[110] without any apparent clinical defect. Reduced eosinophil lobulation has been observed in congenital lactoferrin deficiency[127] and as an acquired defect in myeloproliferative disorders including idiopathic myelofibrosis, and in myelodysplasia (Fig.3.38). In the latter group the chromatin may be clumped and the nuclei entirely or largely non-lobed;[71] this may be regarded as a pseudo-Pelger–Huët anomaly restricted to eosinophils. The presence of basophilic granules in eosinophils is a sign of cytoplasmic immaturity (Fig.3.39). It is more common in leukaemia (chronic granulocytic leukaemia, eosinophilic leukaemia, and certain acute myeloid leukaemias which are associated with eosinophilia) than in healthy subjects. Recent evidence has shown that patients with chronic granulocytic leukaemia may also produce hybrid cells with a mixture of granules characteristic of the eosinophil and the basophil respectively.[138] In the Alder–Reilly anomaly eosinophils have granules with abnormal staining properties; they may be grey-green or purple on a Romanowsky stain.[14]

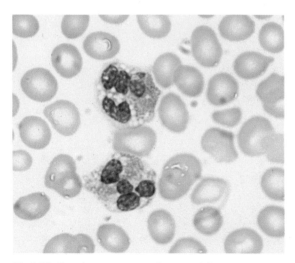

Fig.3.35 *Two hypersegmented eosinophils in a patient with the hypereosinophilic syndrome.* × 960.

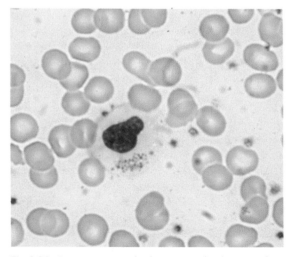

Fig.3.36 *A nonsegmented, almost completely agranular eosinophil in a patient with the hypereosinophilic syndrome.* × 960.

THE BASOPHIL

The basophil (Fig.3.40) is of similar size to the neutrophil (10–14 μm in diameter). The nucleus is usually obscured by purple-black granules which are intermediate in size between those of the neutrophil and those of the eosinophil. Basophils have abnormal granules in various inherited conditions (see Fig.3.12): granules

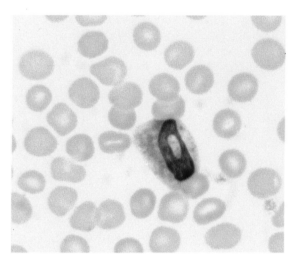

Fig.3.37 An eosinophil with a ring shaped nucleus from a patient with cyclical oedema with eosinophilia. × 960.

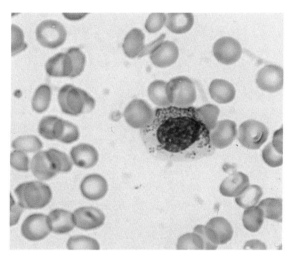

Fig.3.38 A nonsegmented hypogranular eosinophil in a blood film from a patient with myelodysplasia. × 960.

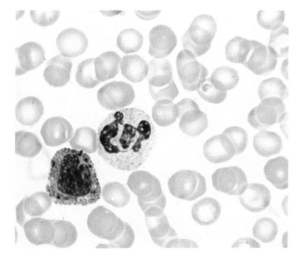

Fig.3.39 An eosinophil and a neutrophil in a patient with chronic granulocytic leukaemia; the eosinophil has some basophilic granules. × 960.

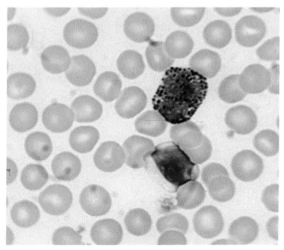

Fig.3.40 A normal basophil and a normal small lymphocyte in a blood film from a healthy subject. × 960.

can be reduced in number in myeloproliferative disorders and in myelodysplasias (Fig. 3.41), and degranulation can occur in acute allergic conditions (such as urticaria and anaphylactic shock), and during postprandial hyperlipidaemia. A reduction of granules can also be artefactual since basophil granules are highly water-soluble.

THE LYMPHOCYTE

Peripheral blood lymphocytes vary in diameter from 10–16 μm. The smaller lymphocytes (10–12 μm), which predominate, usually have scanty cytoplasm and a round nucleus with largely condensed chromatin (Fig. 3.42). The larger lymphocytes (12–16 μm), which make up about 10 percent of circulating lymphocytes, have more abundant cytoplasm and the nuclear chromatin is somewhat less condensed (Fig. 3.43). The smaller lymphocytes are usually circular in outline, whereas larger ones may be somewhat irregular. The cytoplasm, being weakly basophilic, stains pale blue. Lymphocytes may have small numbers of azurophilic granules which contain lysosomal enzymes; occasional larger cells with more abundant cytoplasm have a dozen or so quite prominent azurophilic granules; such cells have been designated 'large granular lymphocytes'

(Fig.3.44). The lymphocyte nucleus appears approximately round, but there may be a slight indentation on one side. Mature lymphocytes have a nucleolus but it is usually undetectable by light microscopy. Since the nuclear chromatin of most lymphocytes is condensed, the sex chromatin is difficult to detect; however in those lymphocytes with more dispersed chromatin it may be discernable, condensed beneath the nuclear membrane.[92] The lymphocytes of infants and children are larger than those of adults. In general the different functional subsets of lymphocytes cannot be distinguished morphologically, but natural killer (NK) lymphocytes have been found to be among the large granular lymphocytes.

Morphological abnormalities of lymphocytes in inherited conditions

Inclusions may be found in lymphocytes in the Chédiak–Higashi syndrome and in the Alder–Reilly anomaly (see Fig.3.12). In the Chédiak–Higashi syndrome the lymphocyte inclusions can be very large but in the Alder–Reilly anomaly they are only a little larger than the granules of normal large lymphocytes. Heterozygous carriers of the Chédiak–Higashi anomaly may also have inclusions, but in only a small percentage

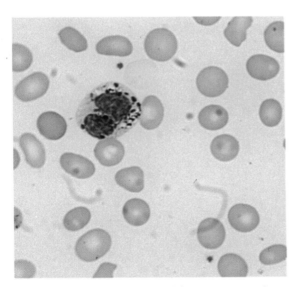

Fig.3.41 A hypogranular basophil from a patient with myelodysplasia. × 960.

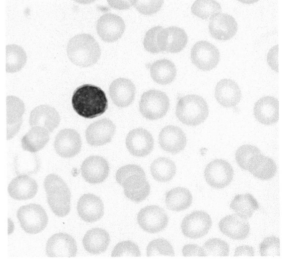

Fig.3.42 A normal small lymphocyte in the blood film of a healthy subject. × 960.

of peripheral blood lymphocytes.[31] Occasionally in the Alder–Reilly anomaly inclusions may be found in the lymphocytes in the absence of neutrophil inclusions. Lymphocyte inclusions are found when the Alder–Reilly anomaly is consequent on Tay–Sachs disease or on the mucopolysaccharidoses, although they are rare in Morquio's syndrome. The inclusions of the Alder–Reilly anomaly may be round or comma-shaped; they are sometimes surrounded by a halo, and tend to be clustered at one pole of the cell (Fig.3.45). When the Alder–Reilly anomaly is due to one of the mucopolysaccharidoses the inclusions stain metachromatically (that is, give varying colours) with toluidine blue (Fig.3.46). When the Alder–Reilly anomaly is due to Tay–Sachs disease the inclusions do not stain with toluidine blue. In Tay–Sachs disease heterozygous carriers also have lymphocyte inclusions,[14] but in a much smaller proportion of cells than in the homozygotes.

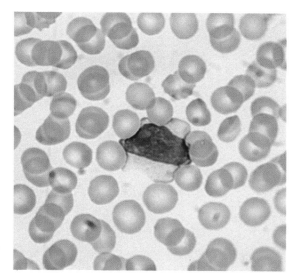

Fig.3.43 A normal large lymphocyte in the blood film of a healthy subject. × 960.

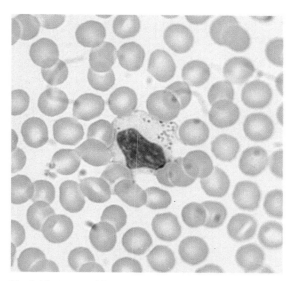

Fig.3.44 A normal large granular lymphocyte in the blood film of a healthy subject. × 960.

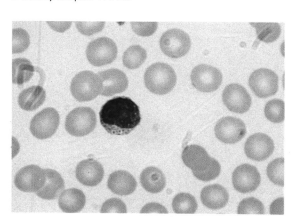

Fig.3.45 Abnormal inclusions in a small lymphocyte in the blood film of a patient with the San Filippo syndrome. The inclusions are surrounded by a halo. × 960.

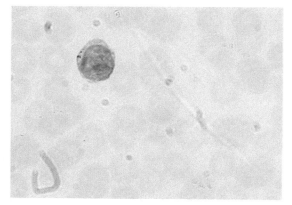

Fig.3.46 Toluidine blue stain in lymphocytes of a patient with the San Filippo syndrome showing purple staining of the cytoplasmic inclusions. × 960.

Patients with the mucopolysaccharidoses and with Tay–Sachs and Batten–Spielmeyer–Vogt diseases may have lymphocyte vacuolation possibly consequent on dissolution of abnormal granules. In the latter two conditions heterozygous carriers may also have abnormal lymphocyte vacuoles. Lymphocyte vacuolation is a feature of Jordans' anomaly (see page 44), Niemann–Pick disease, Wolman's disease, Pompe's disease and of several other rare congenital metabolic disorders.[14,48,73]

In Wolman's disease the vacuole contents are lipid and stain with Oil Red O, whereas in Pompe's disease the vacuole contents are glycogen and stain with the periodic acid-Schiff stain.[52]

Lymphocyte inclusions and vacuoles are not confined to inherited disorders of metabolism; they may also occur in reactive conditions such as infectious mononucleosis and in lymphoproliferative disorders (Fig.3.47) (see below).

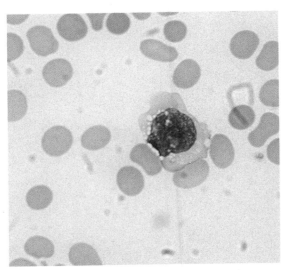

Fig.3.47 *Vacuolated lymphocyte in a patient with non-Hodgkin's lymphoma — these are circulating lymphoma cells. × 960.*

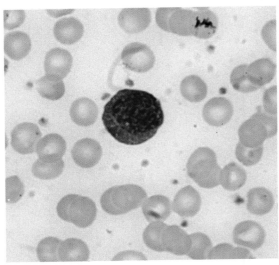

Fig.3.48 *A plasmacytoid lymphocyte in the postoperative blood film of a patient who had had a limb amputation. × 960.*

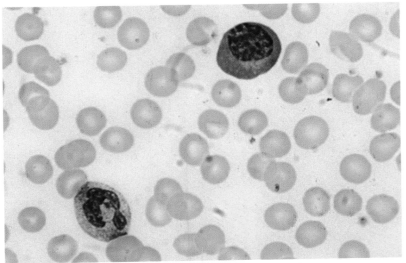

Fig.3.49 *A plasma cell in the blood film of the same patient as shown in Fig.3.48; the neutrophil shows toxic granulation and a drumstick. × 960.*

Reactive changes in lymphocytes

Lymphocytes may respond to viral infections and other immunological stimuli by alteration of morphology. Such alteration may include an increase of size, increasing cytoplasmic basophilia, acquisition of a more diffuse chromatin pattern or of a nucleolus, and vacuolation of the cytoplasm. Lymphocytes may transform into blast cells or differentiate to plasmacytoid lymphocytes or plasma cells. A plasmacytoid lymphocyte (Fig.3.48) is a cell with cytoplasmic basophilia but without the eccentric nucleus and fully developed Golgi zone of the plasma cell (Fig.3.49). The term 'Türk cell' has been applied to a lymphocyte showing differentiation in the direction of a plasma cell, and the term 'Mott cell', morular cell or grape cell to a plasmacytoid lymphocyte with abundant globular cytoplasmic inclusions (Fig.3.50). The appearance of these cells has no particular significance beyond indicating that differentiation to plasma cells is occurring.

Reactive changes of all types are much commoner in children than in adults, and in both children and adults may be accompanied by a lymphocytosis. The assessment of blood films showing abnormal lymphocyte morphology which is thought to be reactive is discussed in Chapter 8.

Lymphocyte abnormalities in lymphoproliferative disorders

Abnormal features which may be noted in lymphoproliferative disorders include increased cell size, nuclear abnormalities, cytoplasmic abnormalities, and cell smearing (see page 59) as a consequence of cell fragility. Nuclear abnormalities include clefting or lobulation, radial segmentation and deep infolding (cerebriform nucleus), a diffuse chromatin pattern with or without a nucleolus, and hyperchromaticism or dense staining of the nucleus. Cytoplasmic abnormalities include abundant cytoplasm, increased cytoplasmic basophilia, irregular cytoplasmic margins, prominent azurophilic granules, and cytoplasmic crystals, vacuolation or the presence of other inclusions. Some of the changes which occur in lymphoproliferative disorders are also seen as reactive changes. The interpretation of morphological abnormalities of lymphocytes in lymphoproliferative disorders is discussed in Chapter 8.

THE MONOCYTE

The monocyte (Fig.3.51a,b) is the largest normal peripheral blood cell with a diameter of about 12–20 μm; it has an irregular, often lobulated nucleus and opaque greyish-blue cytoplasm with fine azurophilic

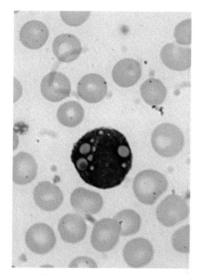

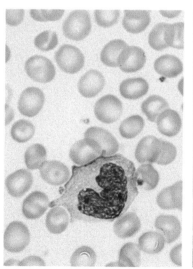

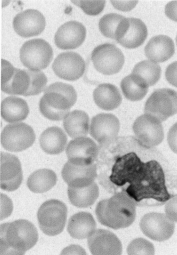

Fig.3.50 A Mott cell in the blood film of the same patient as shown in Fig.3.48. × 960.

Fig.3.51 Monocytes from the blood films of healthy subjects; both cells have lobulated nuclei and one (right) has cytoplasmic vacuolation. × 960.

granules. The cell outline is often irregular and the cytoplasm may be vacuolated. Sex chromatin may be detected condensed beneath the nuclear membrane of some monocytes.[92]

Monocytes may have abnormal inclusions in various inherited conditions (see Figs 3.12 and 3.52). Since they are phagocytic they may be found, uncommonly, to contain red cells (for example in autoimmune haemolytic anaemia, sickle cell anaemia and acute haemolytic anaemias of various aetiologies),[35] bacteria, fungi such as *Histoplasma capsulatum*,[66] parasites such as *Leishmania donovani* (Fig. 3.53a,b), cryoglobulin (Fig. 3.53c) and, rarely, melanin[139] or bilirubin.[123] Following the ingestion and breakdown of malarial parasites, residual pigment may be seen in the cytoplasm.

Monocytes usually develop into macrophages (also designated histiocytes) in tissues rather than in the peripheral blood. However, phagocytic cells which more closely resemble tissue histiocytes than they do monocytes may appear in the blood in a variety of conditions including infective and inflammatory states (such as subacute bacterial endocarditis and tuberculosis), malignant disease and parasitic disease. They may be little larger than a monocyte or they may be very large and multinucleated;[88] contents include amorphous debris, haemopoietic cells and recognizable cellular debris. In certain inherited metabolic disorders foamy macrophages containing lipid circulate in the peripheral blood.[73]

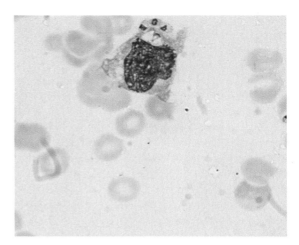

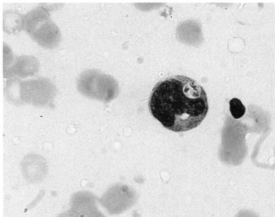

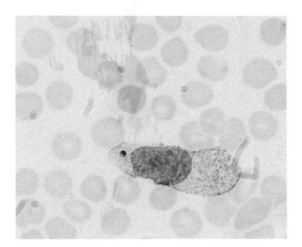

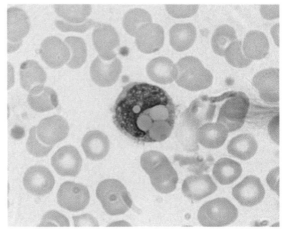

Fig.3.52 *A monocyte in the blood film of a patient with Maroteaux–Lamy syndrome showing an abnormal cytoplasmic inclusion.* × 960.

Fig.3.53 *Monocytes containing phagocytosed material; (upper and middle) parasites of* Leishmania donovani *(lower) cryoglobulin; (upper) and (lower) are bone marrow monocytes, but similar cells can sometimes be found in the peripheral blood.* × 960.

Circulating phagocytic cells may also be seen in malignant histiocytosis and familial histiocytic reticulosis.

GRANULOCYTE PRECURSORS

Granulocytes are normally produced in the bone marrow from myeloblasts, with the intervening stages being promyelocytes, myelocytes and metamyelocytes. On occasion these normal bone marrow cells may be seen in the peripheral blood. The appearance of appreciable numbers of such immature cells may be designated a left shift and if nucleated red blood cells are also present then the blood film is described as leucoerythroblastic.

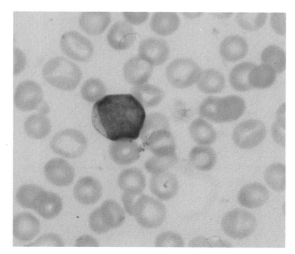

Fig.3.54 A myeloblast from the blood of a patient with myelodysplasia. × 960.

The myeloblast measures 12–20 μm and has a high nucleocytoplasmic ratio and a round or, more usually, slightly oval nucleus (Fig.3.54). The cell is usually somewhat oval and the outline may be slightly irregular. The nucleus has one to five (most often two or three) not very prominent nucleoli. The cytoplasm is pale blue. A myeloblast is usually defined as a cell which has a diffuse chromatin pattern and appears agranular on light microscopy, whereas a promyelocyte has some condensation of the chromatin and has azurophilic granules. Occasional cells are seen which have no chromatin condensation and yet have a few azurophilic granules; it appears more satisfactory to classify these cells as myeloblasts rather than promyelocytes. Electron microscopy and staining for peroxidase activity have shown that myeloblasts do have some granules even though none is usually visible by light microscopy. The distinction betwen a myeloblast and a promyelocyte is further discussed on page 206. Although a myeloblast does have characteristic morphology it is not always possible to make the distinction between a myeloblast and a lymphoblast by light microscopy alone (see Chapter 8).

The promyelocyte is larger than the myeloblast and has a diameter of 15–25 μm (Fig.3.55). In comparison with the myeloblast the nucleocytoplasmic ratio is lower and the cytoplasm is more basophilic. The nuclear chromatin pattern shows only slight condensation and one to five (most often two or three) nucleoli may be present. The nucleus is oval with an indentation on one side. The Golgi zone is apparent as a much less basophilic area adjacent to the nuclear indentation. The promyelocyte contains primary or azurophilic granules

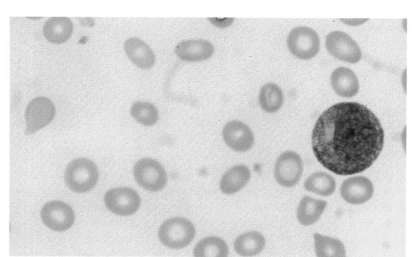

Fig.3.55 A promyelocyte from the blood of a patient with megaloblastic anaemia. The nucleolus and the Golgi zone are readily detectable. The blood film also shows anisocytosis and tear drop poikilocytes. × 960.

which surround the Golgi zone and are scattered throughout the remainder of the cytoplasm.

The myelocyte is smaller than the promyelocyte, measuring 10–20 μm in diameter (Fig.3.56). It can be identified as belonging to the neutrophil, eosinophil or basophil series by the presence of specific or secondary granules with the staining characteristics of these cell lines. The nucleus is oval with sometimes a slight indentation in one side and the chromatin shows a moderate degree of coarse clumping. (The clumped chromatin, or heterochromatin, is genetically inactive chromatin, whereas diffuse euchromatin is genetically

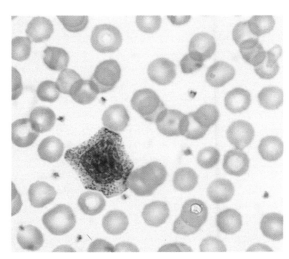

Fig.3.56 A myelocyte from the blood of a healthy pregnant woman. × 960.

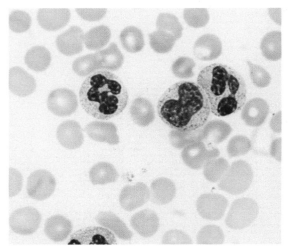

Fig.3.57 A metamyelocyte and two neutrophils in the blood film of a patient with chronic granulocytic leukaemia. × 960.

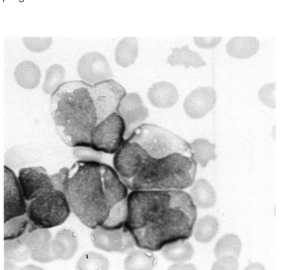

Fig.3.58 A group of leukaemic blast cells, one of which contains two Auer rods; from the blood of a patient with acute myelomonocytic leukaemia. × 960.

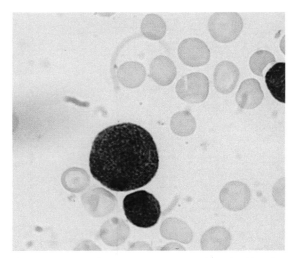

Fig.3.59 A hypergranular promyelocyte from the blood of a patient with hypergranular promyelocytic leukaemia; the cytoplasm as well as being packed with granules contains one giant granule. The smaller cell is also a hypergranular leukaemic cell. × 960.

active). The cytoplasm is more acidophilic than that of a promyelocyte and the Golgi zone is less apparent.

The metamyelocyte measures 10–12 μm in diameter. Its chromatin is clumped and the nucleus is definitely indented or 'U' shaped (Fig.3.57). Protein synthesis has stopped, and in the case of a neutrophil metamyelocyte the cytoplasm is acidophilic.

Abnormalities of granulocyte precursors

The appearance in the peripheral blood film of leucocytes of an earlier stage of development than the metamyelocytes can generally be regarded as an abnormal finding, exceptions being when the blood is from a pregnant woman (page 84) or a neonate (see page 85). If buffy-coat preparations are made, however, metamyelocytes and/or myelocytes are found in about 80 percent of healthy subjects with a frequency of about one per 1000 granulocytes.[34] Granulocyte precursors in the peripheral blood may show morphological abnormalities. In acute myeloid leukaemia and related conditions myeloblasts may contain Auer rods, which are formed by the fusion of primary granules and have the same staining characteristics (Fig.3.58). The finding of a single myeloblast containing an Auer rod is of considerable significance since these inclusions are seen only in acute myeloid leukaemia and related conditions. A similar importance attaches to the finding of hypergranular promyelocytes (Fig.3.59) since these are associated only with acute promyelocytic leukaemia.

DISINTEGRATED CELLS

The finding of more than a small percentage of disintegrated cells in a blood film is of significance. It may indicate that several days have elapsed since the blood was taken from the patient and the specimen is unfit for testing. When disintegration of cells is due to prolonged storage the granulocytes are smeared preferentially and, if an attempt is made to perform a differential count, there will appear to be a neutropenia. If disintegration of cells occurs on making a blood film from fresh blood, it indicates that the cells are abnormally fragile. Disintegrated lymphocytes, usually designated 'smear cells' or 'smudge cells', are common in chronic lymphocytic leukaemia (Fig.3.60); their presence is of diagnostic use since they are not common in non-Hodgkin's lymphoma, from which it may be necessary to make a distinction. The fact that these cells are intact *in vivo* but are smeared during the preparation of the standard blood film is demonstrated by the fact that they are not present in a film of the same blood made by centrifugation. Although smeared lymphocytes are characteristic of chronic lymphocytic leukaemia they may also be seen in reactive conditions, for example in whooping cough. Cells other than lymphocytes, for example the cells of acute myeloid leukaemia, may also disintegrate on spreading the blood film. 'Basket cell' is another term which has been applied to a very spread out disintegrated cell.

If the nature of disintegrated cells is obvious, they should be included in the differential count with the class of cell to which they belong. Otherwise, if they are numerous, they should be included in the differential count as a separate category; their omission will cause the differential count and the absolute counts of all cell classes to be inaccurate.

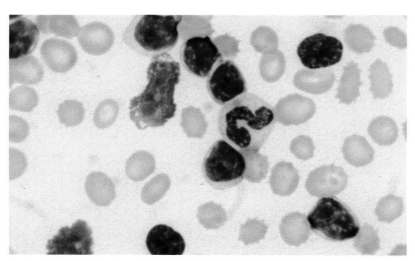

Fig.3.60 *Disintegrated cells (and intact lymphocytes) in the blood of a patient with chronic lymphocytic leukaemia.* × 960.

PLATELETS AND CIRCULATING MEGAKARYOCYTES

When platelets are examined in a blood film an assessment should be made of their number (by relating them to the number of red cells), their size, and their morphology, and the film should be examined for the presence of platelet aggregates or platelet satellitism. Megakaryocytes are seen, though rarely, in the peripheral blood of healthy subjects. Their numbers are increased in certain disease states.

NORMAL PLATELET SIZE AND MORPHOLOGY

The normal platelet measures 1–3 μm in diameter. Platelets contain fine azurophilic granules which may be dispersed through the cytoplasm or may be concentrated in the centre; in the latter case the central granule-containing cytoplasm is known as the granulomere and the peripheral, weakly basophilic cytoplasm as the hyalomere (Fig.3.61). Platelets contain several different types of granule of which the alpha granules are equivalent to the azurophilic granules detectable by light microscopy.

In EDTA-anticoagulated blood, platelets generally remain separate from one another whereas in native blood they show a tendency to aggregate (see Figs 1.3–1.5). In Glanzmann's thrombasthenia, a severe inherited defect of platelet function, the normal tendency of platelets to aggregate when films are made from native blood is completely absent.

ABNORMALITIES OF PLATELET SIZE

Platelet size can be assessed by comparing the diameter of the platelets with the diameter of erythrocytes, or platelet diameter can be measured by means of an ocular micrometer. Platelets with a diameter of more than 4 μm can be regarded as increased in size.

Platelet size in healthy subjects varies inversely with the platelet count (see page 134) but this variation is not sufficiently great to be detected in a blood film using light microscopy. A size increase sufficient to be detected when examining the blood film occurs in certain congenital megakaryocytic abnormalities and in various disease states (Fig.3.62). Large platelets (with diameter greater than 4 μm) are designated macrothrombocytes and if particularly large, with diameters similar to those of red cells or lymphocytes, the descriptive term giant platelet may be used (Fig.3.63). The differential diagnosis of increased platelet size is discussed on page 37. The absence of large platelets despite thrombocytopenia is of diagnostic significance and should therefore be noted. Decreased platelet size is less commonly detected than increased platelet size but may be apparent in the Wiskott–Aldrich syndrome (Fig.3.64).

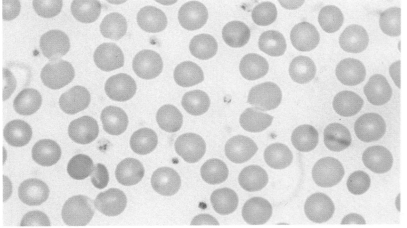

Fig.3.61 *A blood film from a healthy subject showing normal red cells and platelets. Some of the platelets show granules dispersed through the cytoplasm while others have a granulomere and a hyalomere. × 960.*

MORPHOLOGY OF BLOOD CELLS

Fig.3.62 *Some of the causes of large platelets.*

SOME CAUSES OF LARGE PLATELETS	
congenital	**inheritance**
Bernard–Soulier syndrome* (giant platelets with defective ristocetin induced aggregation)	AR
heterozygous carriers of Bernard–Soulier syndrome[59]	
Epstein's syndrome*[37] (associated with hereditary deafness and nephritis)	AD
Mediterranean macrothrombocytosis*[137]	uncertain
Chédiak–Higashi anomaly* (see Fig. 3.12)	AR
May–Hegglin anomaly* (see Fig. 3.12)	AD
associated with increased nuclear projections in neutrophils[46]	AD
in occasional families with Marfan's syndrome and other inherited connective tissue defects[38]	varied
grey platelet syndrome*[111]	AR
hereditary thrombocytopenia with giant platelets but without other morphological abnormality or associated disease*	AR or AD
acquired	
immune thrombocytopenic purpura* (primary and secondary)	
myeloproliferative disorders: polycythaemia vera chronic granulocytic leukaemia* chronic granulocytic leukaemia in transformation* myelofibrosis* essential thrombocythaemia	
myelodysplasia*	
megakaryoblastic leukaemia*	
postsplenectomy and hyposplenic states (including sickle cell anaemia)	
disseminated intravascular coagulation*	
thrombotic thrombocytopenic purpura*	

*may also have thrombocytopenia
AR=autosomal recessive inheritance
AD=autosomal dominant inheritance

ABNORMALITIES OF PLATELET MORPHOLOGY

Platelets which are lacking in alpha granules appear grey or pale blue. This occurs as a rare congenital defect which has been designated the grey platelet syndrome[111] (Fig.3.65) but more commonly it is consequent on discharge of platelet granules *in vivo* or *in vitro* or on formation of defective platelets by dysplastic megakaryocytes. Some agranular platelets are commonly present in myelodysplasia and in myeloproliferative disorders. Cardiopulmonary bypass may cause discharge of alpha granules with the agranular platelets continuing to circulate. In hairy cell leukaemia agranular platelets are probably formed by degranulation *in vivo* within the abnormal vascular channels, the splenic pseudosinuses lined by hairy cells, which are a feature of the disease. If venepuncture is difficult, stimulation of platelets may cause discharge of platelet granules and platelet aggregation so that masses of agranular platelets are seen. Rarely, a similar phenomenon is caused by a plasma factor causing platelet degranulation and aggregation *in vitro*;[85] in one patient the factor originated from a leiomyosarcoma.[125] In the May–Hegglin anomaly platelets are not only large but may

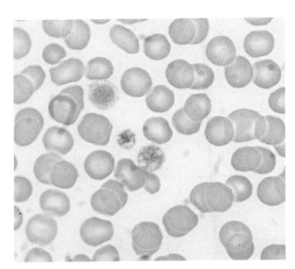

Fig.3.63 *Giant platelets in a patient with the Bernard–Soulier syndrome.* × 960.

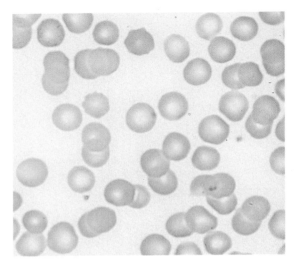

Fig.3.64 *Small platelets in a patient with the Wiskott–Aldrich syndrome.* × 960.

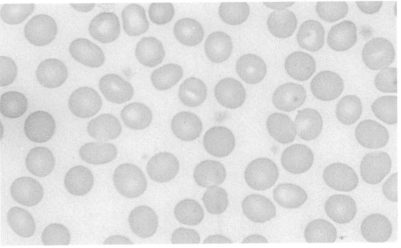

Fig.3.65 *Agranular platelets in a patient with the grey platelet syndrome.* × 960.

also be of abnormal shape, for example cigar-shaped.[51] In myelodysplastic syndromes and in idiopathic myelofibrosis, dysplastic megakaryocytes may produce not only agranular platelets but also giant platelets and platelets of abnormal shape.

Various particles, for example the parasites of *Plasmodium vivax*,[41] may be found within platelets. This phenomenon is unlikely to represent phagocytosis; it is probably equivalent to emperipolesis, a phenomenon observed in megakaryocytes in which cells and other particles enter the surface connected system – the system of platelet demarcation membranes which connect with the surface of the platelet.

Platelet aggregation (see Fig.3.4) may represent incipient blood clotting following platelet stimulation during skin prick or venepuncture but it can also be a consequence of a platelet cold agglutinin or of a plasma factor which causes aggregation *in vitro* in EDTA-anticoagulated blood. Aggregated platelets may or may not be agranular. The presence of platelet aggregates in EDTA-anticoagulated blood is often associated with a factitiously low platelet count (page 136).

Platelet satellitism (Fig.3.66) is seen as an *in vitro* phenomenon occurring particularly in EDTA-anticoagulated blood; it is induced by a plasma factor, usually IgG or IgM. Platelets adhere to and encircle neutrophils and some platelets may be phagocytosed.[143] Neutrophils may be joined together by a layer of platelets. Platelet satellitism does not appear to be of any clinical significance, although it can lead to an inaccurate platelet count (page 136).

MEGAKARYOCYTES

Megakaryocytes are seen rarely in the peripheral blood of healthy adults. They are released by the bone marrow and most are trapped in the pulmonary capillaries. However, the fact that they are detectable, albeit in small numbers, in venous blood draining parts of the body lacking haemopoietic marrow indicates that some can pass through the pulmonary capillaries. Since their concentration is, on average, only 5–7 per ml they are more likely to be seen in buffy-coat preparations or when special concentration procedures are carried out. In healthy subjects, 99 percent of the megakaryocytes in peripheral venous blood are almost bereft of cytoplasm (Fig.3.67) but rare cells with copious cytoplasm are seen.[53] Peripheral blood megakaryocytes are increased in neonates and in young infants and also postpartum, postoperatively and in patients with infection, inflammation, malignancy, disseminated intravascular coagulation or myeloproliferative disorders such as chronic granulocytic leukaemia, idiopathic myelofibrosis and polycythaemia vera.[54,100–102] The proportion of peripheral blood megakaryocytes which are intact and have copious cytoplasm may be increased in infants[101] and in patients with idiopathic myelofibrosis and chronic granulocytic leukaemia.[102]

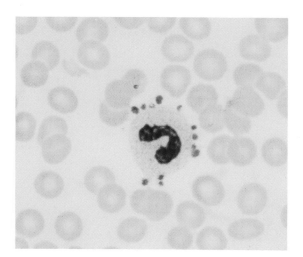

Fig.3.66 *Platelet satellitism. × 960.*

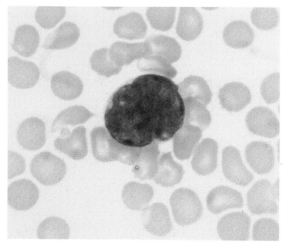

Fig.3.67 *Bare megakaryocyte nucleus in a blood film of a healthy subject; the size and lobulation of the nucleus indicates its origin from a polyploid megakaryocyte. × 960.*

Abnormal megakaryocytes and megakaryoblasts may circulate in the peripheral blood in pathological states. Micromegakaryocytes (Fig.3.68) may be detected in myelodysplastic syndromes and in certain myeloid leukaemias — particularly megakaryoblastic leukaemia and chronic granulocytic leukaemia in megakaryoblastic transformation. They are small, mononuclear cells with a diameter of 7–10 μm, which are not always immediately identifiable as belonging to the megakaryocyte lineage. Studies of DNA content show them to be diploid whereas megakaryocytes are generally polyploid. The nucleus is round or slightly irregular with dense chromatin. Cytoplasm varies from scanty to moderate in amount; when scanty the nucleus may appear 'bare' but electron microscopy shows that such cells usually have a thin rim of cytoplasm. Cytoplasm is faintly basophilic; there may be cytoplasmic vacuolation or a few or numerous azurophilic granules.

Megakaryoblasts (Fig.3.69) vary from about 10 μm in diameter up to 15–20 μm or larger. Smaller ones often resemble lymphoblasts and have no distinguishing features. Larger cells have a diffuse chromatin pattern and cytoplasm which varies from weakly to moderately strongly basophilic; cytoplasm varies from scanty to moderate in amount and may form buds or pseudopodia.

ERYTHROCYTES

The majority of normal erythrocytes, or red cells, are disciform in shape (Fig.3.70); a minority are bowl-shaped. On a stained peripheral blood film they are approximately circular in outline and show only minor variations in shape and moderate variations in size (see Fig.3.61). The average diameter is about 7.5 μm. In the area of a blood film where cells form a monolayer a paler

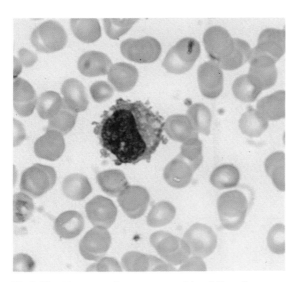

Fig.3.68 *Micromegakaryocyte in a blood film of a patient with idiopathic myelofibrosis.* × 960.

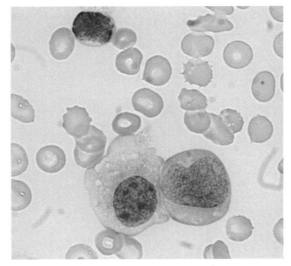

Fig.3.69 *A megakaryoblast from the blood of a patient with megakaryocytic transformation of chronic granulocytic leukaemia. This megakaryoblast has no distinguishing features on light microscopy but the adjacent cell which is showing some maturation has cytoplasm which resembles a platelet; the small cell resembling a lymphocyte also belongs to the megakaryocyte series. The nature of the cells was demonstrated by ultrastructural cytochemistry.[7]* × 960.

central area occupies approximately the middle third of the cell.

Certain terms used to describe red cell morphology require definition. Two terms are used to describe cells of normal morphology. They are: normocytic, which means that the cells are of normal size; and normochromic, which means that the cells contain the normal amount of haemoglobin so that they stain normally. The other terms used to describe red cell morphology imply that the morphology is abnormal and such terms should therefore not be used, when reporting blood films, to describe normal physiological variation. For example, the cells of a neonate should not be reported as 'macrocytic' since it is normal for the cells of a neonate to be larger than those of an adult. Similarly, the red cells of a healthy pregnant woman show more variation in size and shape than the red cells of a non-pregnant woman; this should not be reported as 'anisocytosis' and 'poikilocytosis', since no abnormality is present.

Policy in laboratories varies as to whether every normal film is reported as being normocytic and normochromic, or whether a comment on the red cell morphology is made only when it is particularly significant that it is normal. Either policy is acceptable as long as it is applied consistently and the clinical staff can therefore become aware of it. If a patient is anaemic but the blood film shows no morphological abnormality of red cells then it is useful to describe the cells as normocytic and normochromic since the absence of specific abnormalities narrows the diagnostic possibilities.

ANISOCYTOSIS

Anisocytosis is an increase in the variability of erythrocyte size beyond what is observed in a blood film from a haematologically normal, healthy subject (see Fig.3.14). Anisocytosis is a common, non-specific abnormality. In automated instruments which can measure the degree of variation of red cell size anisocytosis may be expressed by various mathematical formulae (see page 29).

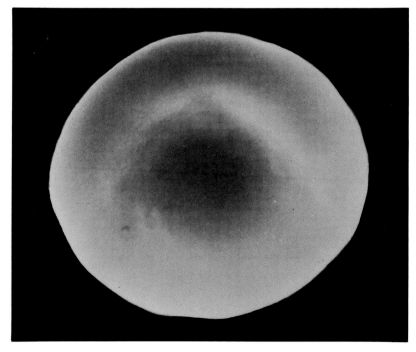

Fig. 3.70 *Scanning electron micrograph of a normal red cell (discocyte). By courtesy of Professor A. Polliack.*

MICROCYTOSIS

Microcytosis is a decrease in the size of erythrocytes. Microcytes are detected in a blood film by a reduction of red cell diameter to less than 7–7.2 μm (Fig.3.71). The nucleus of a small lymphocyte which has a diameter of approximately 8.5 μm is a useful guide to the size of a red cell. Microcytosis may be general or there maybe a population of small red cells. If all or most of the cells are microcytic then the mean corpuscular volume (MCV) will be low, but a small population of microcytes may be present without the MCV falling below the normal range. Some of the causes of a microcytic blood film are listed in Fig.3.73 and the differential diagnosis of microcytosis is discussed in Chapter 9. The red cells of healthy children are smaller than those of adults, so that the size of the cells must be interpreted in the light of the age of the subject. As a group healthy Blacks have smaller red cells than healthy Caucasians; this is likely to be consequent mainly on the high prevalence of α-thalassaemia trait in Blacks, together with a lower prevalence of haemoglobin C trait and other haemoglobinopathies often associated with microcytosis (see Chapter 9).

MACROCYTOSIS

Macrocytosis is an increase in the size of erythrocytes. It is recognized in the blood film by increased cell diameter (see Figs 3.14 and 3.72). It may be a general change, in which case the MCV will be raised, or it may affect only a proportion of the red cells. Even quite a small proportion of macrocytes may be of diagnostic importance. Macrocytes may be round or oval in outline, the diagnostic significance being somewhat different. Some of the causes of macrocytosis are listed in Fig.3.74, and the differential diagnosis of macrocytosis is discussed in Chapter 9. The cells of neonates show a considerable degree of macrocytosis if they are assessed in relation to those of adults (see page 85). A slight degree of macrocytosis is also seen as a physiological feature during pregnancy[16] and in older adults.[56]

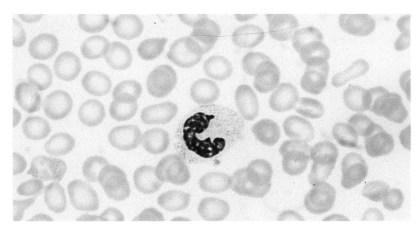

Fig.3.71 *Microcytosis in a patient with β-thalassaemia trait; the MCV was 62 fl. The blood film also shows mild hypochromia, anisocytosis and poikilocytosis.* × 960.

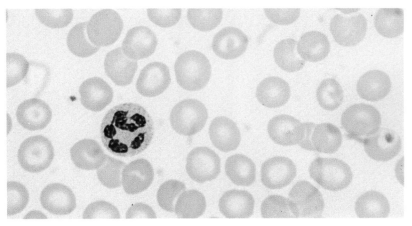

Fig.3.72 *Macrocytosis associated with liver disease. The MCV was 105 fl. Several target cells are also present.* × 960.

SOME CAUSES OF MICROCYTOSIS

iron deficiency

anaemia of chronic disease

sideroblastic anaemia

β-thalassaemia minor (heterozygosity for β thalassaemia)

β-thalassaemia major (homozygosity for β thalassaemia)

δβ- and γδβ-thalassaemia heterozygotes and homozygotes

heterozygotes and homozygotes for haemoglobin Lepore

homozygotes and some heterozygotes for hereditary persistence of fetal haemoglobin

α-thalassaemia trait (particularly α_1-thalassaemia trait) and haemoglobin Constant Spring

haemoglobin H disease

sickle cell trait [82, 120]

haemoglobin C heterozygotes [82,120] and homozygotes

haemoglobin SC disease [70]

haemoglobin E heterozygotes [40] and homozygotes [11]

haemoglobin D $^{Los Angeles}$ trait

other rare abnormal haemoglobins producing thalassaemia-like condition (Hb Tak, Hb Indianapolis)

acquired haemoglobin H disease

myelodysplasia (preleukaemia) [132]

hyperthroidism [62]

lead poisoning

cadmium poisoning [60]

aluminium poisoning

atransferrinaemia

antibody to erythroblast transferrin receptor [77]

ferrochelatase deficiency [126]

Fig.3.73 *Some causes of microcytosis.*

SOME CAUSES OF MACROCYTOSIS

Associated with reticulocytosis

haemolytic anaemia

haemorrhage

Associated with megaloblastic erythropoiesis

vitamin B_{12} deficiency

folic acid deficiency and antifolate drugs (including methotrexate, pentamidine, pyrimethamine, and trimethroprim)

drugs interfering with DNA synthesis (including adriamycin, azathioprine, cyclophosphamide, cytosine arabinoside, daunorubucin, fluorouracil, hydroxyurea, mercaptopurine, procarbazine and thioguanine)

rare inherited defects of DNA synthesis (including hereditary orotic aciduria, thiamine-responsive anaemia, Lesch–Nyhan syndrome)

Associated with megaloblastic or macronormoblastic erythropoiesis

myelodysplastic syndromes including primary acquired sideroblastic anaemia

di Guglielmo's syndrome

some acute myeloid leukaemias

multiple myeloma

ethanol intake

liver disease

phenytoin therapy

copper deficiency [107]

Associated with macronormoblastic erythropoiesis

aplastic anaemia

pure red cell aplasia of infancy (Blackfan–Diamond syndrome)

type I congenital dyserythropoietic anaemia

Uncertain mechanism

cigarette smoking [56]

Down's syndrome [32]

chronic obstructive airways disease

Fig.3.74 *Some causes of macrocytosis.*

HYPOCHROMIA

Hypochromia is a reduction of the staining of the red cell; there is an increase in central pallor to more than the normal approximate third of the cell (Fig.3.75). Hypochromia may be general or there may be a population of hypochromic cells. Severe hypochromia may be reflected in a reduction of the mean corpuscular haemoglobin concentration (MCHC) but the sensitivity of this measurement to hypochromia depends on which method is used for its measurement (see pages 23 and 25). Any of the conditions leading to microcytosis may also cause hypochromia, though in some subjects with α- or β-thalassaemia trait the blood film may show microcytosis without appreciable hypochromia, and in some of the rare patients with copper deficiency, hypochromia may be associated with macrocytosis.[107] The red cells of healthy children are often hypochromic if assessed in relation to the normal appearances of red cells from adults. Since the intensity of staining of the red cell is determined by the thickness of the cell as well as its haemoglobin concentration, hypochromia may also be noted in cells which are thinner than normal but have a normal volume and haemoglobin concentration; these cells are designated leptocytes.

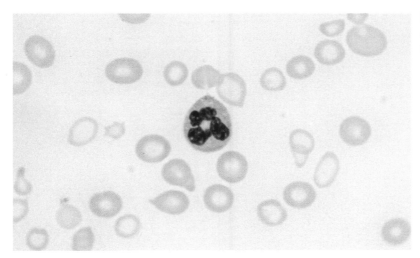

Fig.3.75 *Hypochromic red cells in a patient with iron deficiency anaemia.* × *960.*

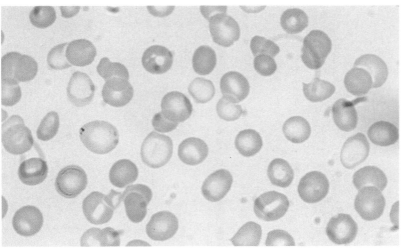

Fig.3.76 *A dimorphic blood film from a patient with sideroblastic anaemia as a consequence of myelodysplasia. One population of cells is normocytic and normochromic while the other is microcytic and hypochromic. One of the poorly haemoglobinized red cells contains some Pappenheimer bodies.* × *960.*

HYPERCHROMIA

The term hyperchromia is rarely used in describing blood films. It can be applied when cells are more intensely stained than normal but it is more useful to indicate why a cell is hyperchromic. Spherocytes (see page 276) stain more intensely than normal cells, central pallor being virtually totally lacking; an increase in the MCHC may be present indicating that the hyperchromia is related not only to the change in shape of the cell but also to a true increase in the concentration of haemoglobin. Irregularly contracted cells are also hyperchromic (see page 79). Some macrocytes are thicker than normal and this causes them to be hyperchromic without there being any increase in the concentration of haemoglobin within the red cell; central pallor may be totally lacking (see Fig.3.14).

ANISOCHROMASIA

Anisochromasia describes an increased variability in the degree of staining or the haemoglobinization of the red cells (see Fig.3.30). In practice it usually means that there is a spectrum of staining from hypochromic to normochromic. Anisochromasia commonly indicates a changing condition, such as iron deficiency responding to treatment or inflammatory disease developing or regressing.

DIMORPHISM

Dimorphism indicates the presence of two distinct populations of cells (Fig.3.76). It is most commonly applied when there is one population of hypochromic, microcytic cells and another population of normochromic cells which are either normocytic or macrocytic but the term may be applied correctly whenever there are two distinct populations. It is necessary to describe the two populations of cells since this is relevant to the diagnosis: they may differ in their size and/or their haemoglobin content. Automated counters may confirm the visual impression of dimorphism, although earlier instruments may not be able to distinguish between a difference in size and a difference in haemoglobin concentration (see page 29). Causes of a dimorphic blood film include: iron deficiency on treatment, sideroblastic anaemia, the heterozygous carrier state for sideroblastic anaemia (some subjects), transfusion of a patient with microcytosis or macrocytosis, double deficiency of iron and either vitamin B_{12} or folic acid, delayed transfusion reaction, and the treatment of megaloblastic anaemia with the unmasking of iron deficiency.

POLYCHROMASIA AND RETICULOCYTOSIS

Erythrocytes which have been newly released from the bone marrow are detected by two methods. First, on vital staining (staining of living cells) dyes such as brilliant cresyl blue or new methylene blue are taken up by ribosomal RNA to produce a reticular pattern; the cells are therefore designated reticulocytes (see Chapter 7). Secondly, the residual RNA in young erythrocytes may produce cytoplasmic basophilia with a Romanowsky stain; this basophilia, together with the eosinophilic character of haemoglobin, produces a polychromatic or polychromatophilic cell (Fig.3.77). In healthy subjects a reticulocyte stain using new methylene blue shows that up to approximately 2.5 percent of erythrocytes in men and up to approximately 4 percent of erythrocytes in women are reticulocytes.[30] The number of polychromatic cells, however, is low: usually they constitute less than 0.1 percent of erythrocytes.[103] Perotta and Finch have shown that if reticulocytes are graded as I to IV, depending on the amount of reticulin they contain, then only the cells with most reticulin are polychromatic on a Wright's stain.[103] The diameter of these early reticulocytes is, on average, 28 percent greater than that of mature erythrocytes. Similarly, polychromatic cells observed on a Wright's stain have a diameter, on average, about 27 percent larger than that of other cells. Since polychromatic cells are usually detectably macrocytic they may be described as polychromatic macrocytes. Later reticulocytes cannot

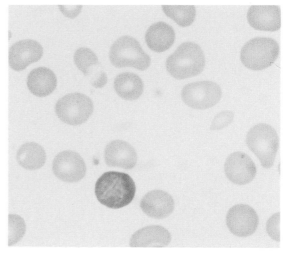

Fig.3.77 *A polychromatic cell which is also larger than normal; it may be designated a polychromatic macrocyte. The film also shows anisocytosis and poikilocytosis.* × 960.

be distinguished from mature erythrocytes on a Romanowsky-stained film since they are not polychromatic and they are only slightly larger than mature erythrocytes.

Polychromatic macrocytes or grade I reticulocytes are very infrequent in the blood of healthy subjects. They have been designated 'shift erythrocytes'[103] or 'stress reticulocytes' being either cells released prematurely from the marrow under the influence of high levels of erythropoietin, or cells which are large because of the premature termination of cell division under the influence of erythropoietin. Their numbers rise, in absolute terms, as a percentage of erythrocytes and as a percentage of reticulocytes, as a physiological response to altitude: they may increase to form 10 percent of reticulocytes at the time of peak marrow response.[103] In haemolytic anaemias they rise similarly, under the influence of erythropoietin, reaching levels of up to 38 percent of reticulocytes or 25 percent of erythrocytes. In renal failure, where there is often a failure of erythropoietin to rise in response to anaemia, polychromasia is less likely to be seen.

Polychromatic erythrocytes are also increased in myelofibrosis and in metastatic carcinoma of the bone marrow. In these conditions the number of polychromatic cells is higher than would be expected

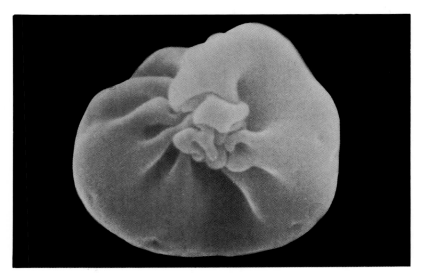

Fig. 3.78 *Scanning electron micrograph of a reticulocyte. By courtesy of Professor A. Polliack.*

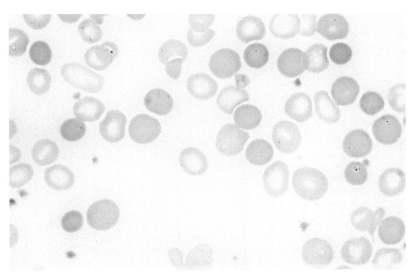

Fig.3.79 *Spherocytes in the blood film of an iron-deficient patient who has suffered a delayed transfusion reaction due to an anti-D antibody; the film is dimorphic showing a mixture of the recipient's hypochromic microcytic cells and the donor cells which have become spherocytic. × 960.*

from the degree of anaemia; the polychromatic cells may be abnormal — more deeply basophilic than is usual and not always increased in size.[103] Polychromatic erythrocytes are more adherent than mature erythrocytes and may appear as clumps in a blood film.

The more mature reticulocytes which are found in normal subjects are found on scanning electron microscopy to be cup-shaped rather than disc-shaped. The younger reticulocytes which are produced under conditions of transient or persistent erythropoietic stress have an irregular, multilobulated surface (Fig. 3.78); for this reason polychromatic cells on a Romanowsky stain lack central pallor.

POIKILOCYTOSIS

A cell of abnormal shape is a poikilocyte. Poikilocytosis is therefore a state in which there is an increased proportion of cells of abnormal shape. Poikilocytosis is a common, non-specific finding in many haematological abnormalities, it may result from production of an abnormal cell by the bone marrow or from damage to the cell after release into the bloodstream. If poikilocytosis is very marked, the possibility of myelofibrosis or a congenital or acquired dyserythropoietic anaemia should be considered. High altitude produces some degree of poikilocytosis in previously haematologically normal people.[113] The presence of poikilocytes of certain specific shapes (for example, spherocytes or elliptocytes) may have a particular significance (see below).

Spherocytosis

Spherocytes (Figs 3.79 and 3.80) are cells which, rather than being disciform, are spherical or near spherical in shape. Scanning electron microscopy shows that both in hereditary spherocytosis and in warm autoimmune haemolytic anaemia many cells are not strictly spherical but have a slight indentation on one side (Fig. 3.80). In a stained blood film spherocytes lack the normal central pallor. The diameter of a sphere is less than that of a disc-shaped object of the same volume, and thus a spherocyte may appear smaller than a discocyte. It appears preferable, however, to restrict the term microspherocyte to cells of reduced volume rather than merely reduced diameter. Spherocytes do not stack well into rouleaux. In examining a blood film for the presence of spherocytes it is important to examine that part of the film where the red cells are just touching, since normal cells may lack central pallor near the tail of the film.

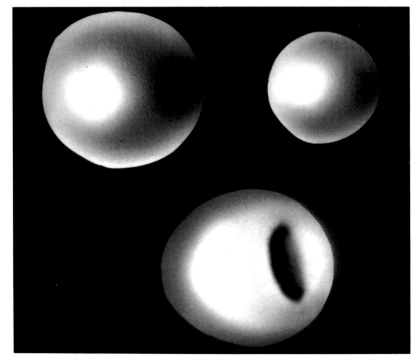

Fig. 3.80 *Artist's impression of SEM of a spherocyte, a microspherocyte and a spherostomatocyte.*

The distinction between spherocytes and irregularly-contracted cells (see below) is important since the diagnostic significance is different. However, in haemolytic anaemias associated with Heinz body formation there are usually some spherocytes in addition to the irregularly contracted cells.

Some of the causes of spherocytosis are shown in Fig.3.81 and the differential diagnosis when the blood film shows spherocytes is discussed on page 276. Spherocytosis may be consequent upon: an inherited defect of the cell membrane, hereditary spherocytosis; an acquired defect of the membrane, as when the membrane is damaged by clostridial toxin or by excessive heat; removal of part of the cell membrane when a phagocyte ingests part of the cell; the tearing of a cell in two as in microangiopathic haemolytic anaemia; or a metabolic defect when phosphate depletion leads to a fall in concentration of red cell ATP. Erythrocytes stored for transfusion become spheroechinocytes as the blood ages (see below).

Elliptocytosis and ovalocytosis

Elliptocytosis and ovalocytosis indicate respectively that the red cells are elliptical or oval in outline (Fig.3.82a,b). These terms have not been used in any consistent manner; some haematologists have used them interchangeably while others have used ovalocyte to mean a cell which is moderately elongated and elliptocyte a cell which is markedly elongated — I have adopted the latter usage. Attempts have been made to define precisely the degree of ovalocytosis in terms of the ratio of the longest to the shortest diameter of the cell[94] but this has not been generally adopted. When the abnormality of cell shape is generalized, it is likely that the subject has hereditary elliptocytosis or hereditary ovalocytosis. Smaller numbers of elliptocytes or ovalocytes may be seen in iron deficiency (the term 'pencil cell' having been used to describe a particularly long thin elliptocyte which is common in iron deficiency), in some patients with thalassaemia, in megaloblastic anaemia, in myelofibrosis, and in some patients with pyruvate kinase deficiency.[25] Oval macrocytes or macrocytic ovalocytes may be seen not only in megaloblastic anaemia but also in South-east Asian ovalocytosis (Fig.3.82b) and in dyserythropoietic states such as myelofibrosis. Elliptocytes are biconcave and thus are capable of forming rouleaux.

SOME CAUSES OF SPHEROCYTOSIS

Conditions usually associated with a large number of spherocytes

hereditary spherocytosis

warm autoimmune haemolytic anaemia

delayed transfusion reaction

ABO haemolytic disease of the newborn

burns

Clostridium welchi sepsis

drug-induced immune haemolytic anaemia (innocent bystander mechanism)

Zieve's syndrome

low red cell ATP due to phosphate deficiency[141]

haemolysis due to snake bite

bartonellosis (Oroya fever)

water dilutional haemolysis (fresh water drowning or intravenous infusion of water)

Conditions usually associated with a smaller number of spherocytes

normal neonate

splenectomy or hyposplenism

microangiopathic haemolytic anaemia

immediate transfusion reaction

acute cold autoimmune haemolytic anaemia

chronic cold haemagglutinin disease

acute attacks of paroxysmal cold haemoglobinuria

Rhesus haemolytic disease of the newborn

haemolytic anaemias associated with Heinz body formation

penicillin-induced haemolytic anaemia

homozygous hereditary elliptocytosis[109]

hereditary elliptocytosis with transient severe manifestations in infancy[5]

hereditary pyropoikilocytosis[144]

infusion of large amounts of intravenous lipid[80]

Fig.3.81 *Some causes of spherocytosis.*

Tear drop cells (dacrocytes)

Tear drop or pear-shaped cells (dacrocytes) (see Figs 3.31, 3.55 and 3.83) occur in primary idiopathic myelofibrosis, in secondary myelofibrosis consequent on bone marrow metastases or other infiltration, in megaloblastic anaemia, in thalassaemia major and other severe dyserythropoietic states, and in some haemolytic anaemias, including haemolytic anaemia associated with Heinz body formation. In both thalassaemia major and myelofibrosis the proportion of tear drop cells decreases if splenectomy is carried out, suggesting that the spleen may have a role in their formation.

Spiculated cells

The terminology applied to spiculated cells is confused. In particular, the term 'burr cell' has been used by different authors to describe different cells and therefore is better abandoned. The terminology of Bessis[9] is to be recommended since it is based on careful study of abnormal cells by scanning electron microscopy and is clear and relatively easy to apply. Bessis has divided spiculated cells into echinocytes, acanthocytes, keratocytes and schistocytes.

Echinocytes are erythrocytes which have lost their disc shape and are covered with 10–30 short, blunt spicules of fairly regular form (Fig.3.84a,b). Echinocytes may be produced *in vitro* by exposure to fatty acids or certain drugs, or simply by incubation. The change is reversed by suspending the cells in fresh plasma. The echinocytic change may be related to ATP depletion, high pH, lysolecithin formation, and the entry of calcium ions into the cell, with polymerization of spectrin. In laboratories which make films from EDTA-anticoagulated rather than native blood, by far the most common cause of echinocytosis is delay in making the blood film. This storage artefact (commonly referred to as 'crenation') is likely to be consequent on a fall of ATP or on lysolecithin formation. Echinocytes which have been observed following the development of hypophosphataemia in patients on parenteral feeding are attributable to a fall in ATP concentration and this may also be the mechanism operating when echinocytes develop

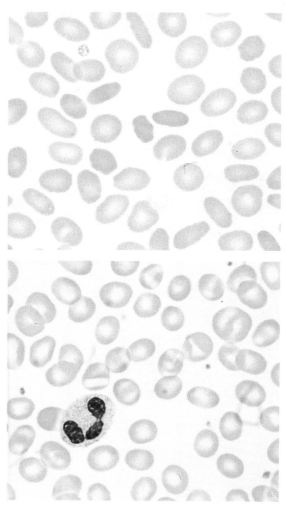

Fig.3.82 (upper) Elliptocytes in a patient with hereditary elliptocytosis. (lower) Ovalocytes in a patient with South-east Asian ovalocytosis. × 960.

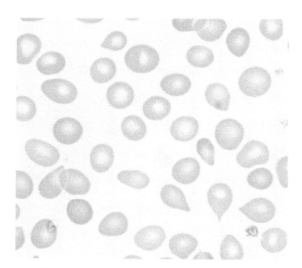

Fig.3.83 Tear drop poikilocytes in a patient with idiopathic myelofibrosis. × 960.

in hereditary pyruvate kinase deficiency and in phosphoglycerate kinase deficiency. Echinocytes developing in hypothermic, heparinized patients on cardiopulmonary bypass have been attributed to a rise of free fatty acid concentration.[13] The echinocytosis which has been noted as a delayed response in severely burned patients may be consequent on lipid abnormalities. When donor blood is stored for transfusion, cells become spheroechinocytes (Fig.3.84a) as ATP levels decrease; membrane lipid (both cholesterol and phospholipid) is then lost as microvesicles, containing small amounts of haemoglobin, which are shed from the tips of the spicules. When blood is transfused, many of the cells are capable of reverting not to discocytes but to cup-shaped

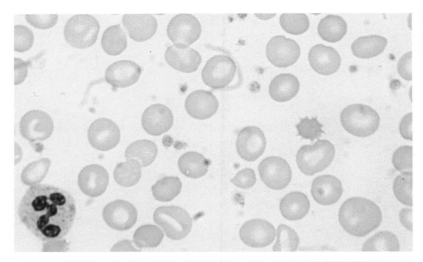

Fig.3.84 (a) *Echinocyte in a blood film taken shortly after a blood transfusion. × 960.*

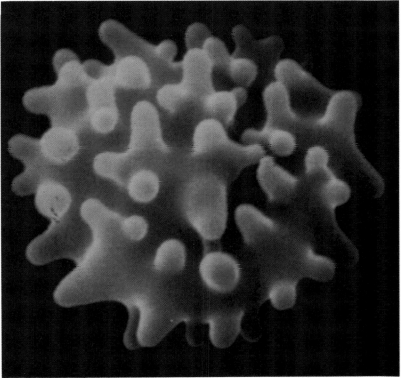

(b) *Scanning electron micrograph of an echinocyte. By courtesy of Professor A. Polliack.*

cells; those cells which have lost membrane remain as spherocytes.

The end stage of a discocyte:echinocyte transformation is a spheroechinocyte. A spheroechinocyte is also formed if a spherocyte undergoes an echinocytic change, and similarly other cells of abnormal shape, including acanthocytes may undergo an echinocytic change.

Acanthocytes (Fig.3.85a,b) are cells of approximately spherical shape bearing 2–20 spicules which are of unequal length and are distributed irregularly over the cell surface. The tips of the spicules tend to be club-shaped rather than pointed. Acanthocytes cannot form rouleaux. Unlike echinocytosis, acanthocytosis is not reversible on suspending cells in fresh plasma. This

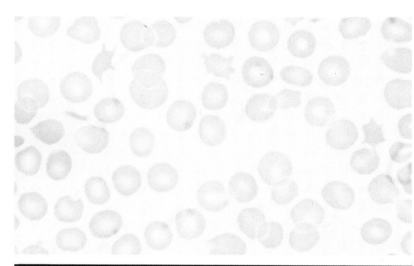

Fig.3.85 (a) *Acanthocytes in a blood film from a patient with anorexia nervosa.* × 960.

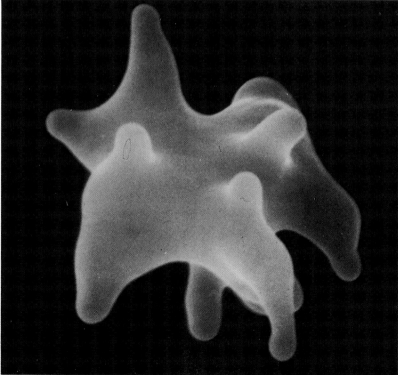

(b) *Scanning electron micrograph of an acanthocyte. By courtesy of Professor A. Polliack.*

morphological abnormality was first described in association with a hereditary condition in which there is retinitis pigmentosa, degenerative neurological disease, fat malabsorption and abetalipoproteinaemia.[8] Subsequently it was found to occur also with inherited and

acquiried hypobetalipoproteinaemia[79] and in association with various rare degenerative neurological diseases with normal betalipoproteins.[39,114] Some of the other causes of acanthocytosis are shown in Fig.3.86. In acanthocytosis due to either abetalipoproteinaemia or liver disease the cholesterol:phospholipid ratio in the red cell membrane is increased. This is in contrast to liver disease associated with target cell formation in which the cholesterol and phospholipid concentration rise in parallel.

Keratocytes (or horned cells) (Fig.3.87) are cells with pairs of spicules, usually two, but sometimes four or six, which have been formed by the fusion of opposing membranes to form a pseudovacuole with subsequent rupture of the membrane at the cell surface. Keratocytes are formed when there is mechanical damage to red cells, for example by fibrin strands or by a malfunctioning cardiac prosthesis. They have been observed in uraemia, glomerulonephritis, disseminated intravascular coagulation, microangiopathic haemolytic anaemia, and also following renal transplantation.

Schistocytes (Fig.3.88) are fragments of red cells formed following mechanical erythrocyte damage; they occur in the same conditions as keratocytes. Many schistocytes are spiculated. Others have been left with too little membrane for their cytoplasmic volume and therefore have formed microspherocytes. Bessis has designated these spheroschizocytes;[9] they may also be

SOME CAUSES OF ACANTHOCYTES
Conditions associated with large numbers of acanthocytes
hereditary abetalipoproteinaemia[8]
hypobetalipoproteinaemia (hereditary, or due to malnutrition or lipid deprivation)[79]
haemolytic anaemia associated with liver disease — 'spur cell anaemia' (usually associated with alcoholic cirrhosis but occasionally with severe viral hepatitis, cardiac cirrhosis, metastatic liver disease or neonatal hepatitis)
associated with degenerative neurological disease but with normal lipoproteins [39,114]
associated with McLeod red cell phenotype (defective formation of Kell antigens)[128]
associated with In(Lu) red cell phenotype [133]
infantile pyknocytosis[131]
vitamin E deficiency in premature neonates[98]
Conditions associated with smaller numbers of acanthocytes
anorexia nervosa and starvation
postsplenectomy and hyposplenism
myxoedema and panhypopituitarism
pyruvate kinase deficiency
heterozygotes for the McLeod phenotype
Woronets trait[10]

Fig.3.86 *Some causes of acanthocytosis.*

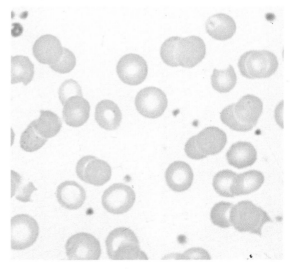

Fig.3.87 *Keratocytes in a patient with microangiopathic haemolytic anaemia.* × 960.

designated microspherocytes since they are both spherical and smaller than normal cells, being fragments of them. Schistocytes are the characteristic cells of microangiopathic haemolytic anaemia and of mechanical haemolytic anaemia (see page 286).

Target cells

Target cells are cells in which an area of increased staining appears in the middle of the area of central pallor (see Figs 3.72 and 3.89a, b). Target cells are formed as a

consequence of there being redundant membrane in relation to the volume of the cytoplasm. They may also be thinner than normal cells. *In vivo* they are bell-shaped and this shape may be demonstrated by scanning electron microscopy (Fig. 3.89b). They flatten on spreading to form the characteristic cell seen by light microscopy. Target cells may be normocytic, microcytic or macrocytic, depending on the associated condition and the mechanism of formation.

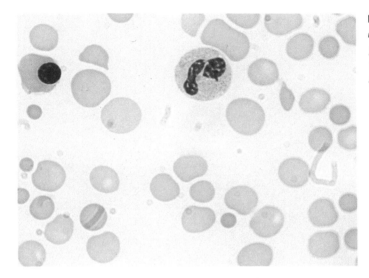

Fig. 3.88 *Fragments, including microspherocytes, in the blood film of a patient with the haemolytic uraemic syndrome; the film also shows polychromasia and a nucleated red blood cell.* × 960.

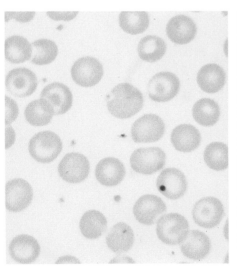
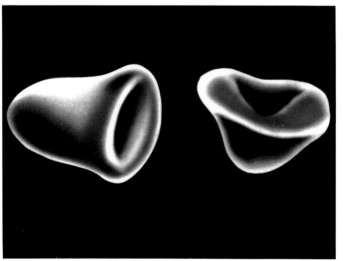

Fig. 3.89 *(left) Postsplenectomy target cells; a cell containing a Howell-Jolly body is also present. × 960. (right) Artist's impression of SEM of target cells.*

Some of the causes of target cell formation are shown in Fig.3.90 and the differential diagnosis when the blood film shows target cells is discussed in Chapter 9.

Target cells may be formed because of an excess of red cell membrane or a lack of red cell cytoplasmic contents. One mechanism of formation is that operative in obstructive jaundice, severe parenchymal liver disease, and hereditary deficiency of lecithin-cholesterol acyl transferase (LCAT). In these conditions an increase in membrane lipid causes an increase in the surface area of the cell. The ratio of membrane cholesterol to cholesterol ester is increased. Red cells lack enzymes for biosynthesis of cholesterol and phospholipid and for esterification of cholesterol, so that the changes in the red cell membrane lipids are passive, reflecting changes in plasma lipids. When LCAT activity is reduced, the ratio of cholesterol to cholesterol ester in the red cell membrane rises in consequence. There may also be an increase in total membrane cholesterol, with a proportionate increase in lecithin, and with a reduction of membrane ethanolamine. LCAT is synthesized by parenchymal cells of the liver and so it may be reduced in liver disease. In obstructive jaundice very high levels of bile salts inhibit LCAT. This does not, however, appear to be the sole mechanism of target cell formation in obstructive jaundice since patients may have target cell formation without their plasma having the ability to inhibit the LCAT activity of normal plasma. When target cells are formed as a consequence of plasma lipid abnormalities, they revert to a normal shape on being transfused into a subject with normal plasma lipids. If membrane lipid changes which would usually cause target cell formation occur in patients with spherocytosis the cells become more disciform; this phenomenon may be observed when a patient with hereditary spherocytosis develops obstructive jaundice.

A different mechanism of formation operates in another group of conditions in which formation of target cells is associated with the presence of hypochromia or microcytosis and with a reduction of cytoplasmic contents. In iron deficiency, in which small numbers of target cells may be seen, there is a reduction in the haemoglobin content of the red cell. In certain haemoglobinopathies in which target cells are common a positively charged abnormal globin chain damages the inside of the red cell membrane.[15] This leads to leakage of red cell potassium and water and thus the cytoplasmic contents are reduced relative to the amount of red cell membrane.

SOME CAUSES OF TARGET CELLS
Conditions which are often associated with large numbers of target cells
obstructive jaundice
hereditary LCAT deficiency
haemoglobin C disease
haemoglobin E disease
sickle cell anaemia
haemoglobin SC disease
haemoglobin D disease
homozygotes for haemoglobin O-Arab
Conditions which may be associated with moderate or small numbers of target cells
hepatocellular liver disease
haemoglobin C trait
haemoglobin S trait
haemoglobin E trait
splenectomy and hyposplenic states
β-thalassaemia major
β-thalassaemia trait
haemoglobin H disease
sideroblastic anaemia
iron deficiency anaemia
hereditary persistence of fetal haemoglobin
hereditary stomatocytosis (dehydrated cell variant)[81]

Fig.3.90 *Some causes of target cell formation.*

Stomatocytes

Stomatocytes are red cells which are cup-shaped rather than disc-shaped. Following the spreading of a blood film they appear to have a slit-like mouth or stoma (Fig. 3.91a,b). They can be formed *in vitro*, for example in response to low pH or exposure to cationic lipid-soluble drugs such as chlorpromazine; their formation is reversible. The end stage of a disocyte:stomatocyte transformation is a spherostomatocyte. Stomatocytes are seen: as an uncommon inherited defect of the red cell membrane, hereditary stomatocytosis;[78,89] in the Rh_{null} and Rh_{mod} syndromes;[83] in healthy Mediterranean subjects;[137] in liver disease; and as a toxic effect of alcohol. Spherostomatocytes are seen in hereditary spherocytosis and warm autoimmune haemolytic anaemia. Stomatocyte formation in hereditary stomatocytosis is related to a defect in the sodium/potassium pump. Stomatocytosis in relation to liver disease and alcohol has been related to an abnormality of membrane lipids, specifically to an increase of lysolecithin in the inner lipid layer of the cell membrane.

Irregularly contracted cells

Irregularly contracted cells (Fig. 3.92) lack central pallor and appear smaller and denser than normal red cells without being as regular in shape as spherocytes. Blood films showing irregularly contracted cells will often also have some spherocytes; such spherocytes are formed

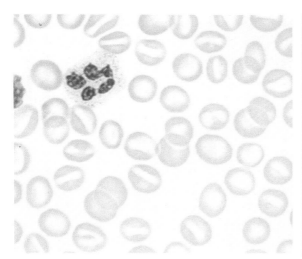

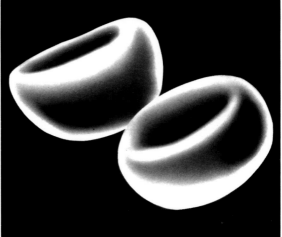

Fig.3.91 (a) *Stomatocytes.* × *960.*

(b) *Artist's impression of SEM of stomatocytes.*

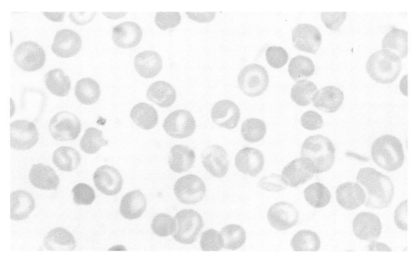

Fig.3.92 *Irregularly contracted cells in a patient with haemoglobin C disease; the blood film also shows several target cells.* × *960.*

when a red cell inclusion such as a Heinz body (precipitated haemoglobin) is removed by phagocytosis with associated loss of red cell membrane. Irregularly contracted cells are formed when cells are exposed to oxidant stress. Such damage may be due to minor degrees of oxidant stress in subjects who are deficient either in the enzyme glucose-6-phosphate dehydrogenase (G6PD), or in other enzymes involved in maintaining the reduction potential of the red cells, and may also be due to major degrees of oxidant stress in haematologically normal subjects. In practice, drugs constitute the major cause of oxidant damage to red cells of normal subjects; phenacetin and acetanilide were formerly major causes of this phenomenon but dapsone and salazopyrine are now the drugs most often incriminated.

Irregularly contracted cells are also characteristic of haemoglobin C disease and, to a lesser extent, haemoglobin E disease and the dehydrated variant of hereditary stomatocytosis;[81] smaller numbers are seen in some patients with β-thalassaemia trait and haemoglobin H disease.

CIRCULATING NUCLEATED RED BLOOD CELLS

Except in the neonatal period and occasionally in pregnancy the presence of nucleated red blood cells (NRBC) (see Fig.3.88) in the peripheral blood is abnormal, generally indicating bone marrow hyperplasia or infiltration. If granulocyte precursors are also present the blood film is designated leucoerythroblastic (see page 218). NRBC in the peripheral blood may also show specific abnormalities; for example they may be megaloblastic or show the features of iron deficiency or of sideroblastic erythropoiesis. An increased frequency of karyorrhexis in circulating NRBC may be seen in arsenic poisoning and in lead poisoning[36] and in certain dyserythropoietic states such as erythroleukaemia and severe iron deficiency anaemia. Examination of a buffy coat preparation is helpful if assessment of morphological abnormalities in circulating NRBC is required.

INCLUSIONS IN ERYTHROCYTES
Howell–Jolly bodies

Howell–Jolly bodies (Fig.3.89a) are medium sized, round, cytoplasmic red cell inclusions which have the same staining characteristics as the nucleus and can be demonstrated to be composed of DNA. A Howell–Jolly body is a fragment of nuclear material. It may arise by karyorrhexis (the breaking up of a nucleus) or by incomplete nuclear expulsion, or may represent chromosomes which have separated from the mitotic spindle

during abnormal mitosis. Some Howell–Jolly bodies are found in erythrocytes within the bone marrow in haematologically normal subjects, but as they are removed by the spleen they are not seen in the peripheral blood. They appear in the blood following splenectomy and are also present in hyposplenic states, and in normal neonates (in whom the spleen is functionally immature). The rate of formation of Howell–Jolly bodies is increased in megaloblastic and dyserythropoietic anaemias, and if the patient is also hyposplenic large numbers of Howell–Jolly bodies will be seen in the peripheral blood.

Basophilic stippling

Basophilic stippling (Fig.3.93) or punctate basophilia describes the presence in erythrocytes of considerable numbers of small basophilic inclusions which are spread through the cytoplasm of the red cell and can be demonstrated to be RNA. They are composed of aggregates of ribosomes; degenerating mitochrondria and siderosomes may be included in the aggregates but most such inclusions do not stain with Perls' acid ferrocyanide method for iron. Very occasional cells with basophilic stippling are seen in normal subjects. Increased numbers are seen in the presence of thalassaemia trait (particularly β-thalassaemia trait), thalassaemia major, megaloblastic anaemia, unstable haemoglobins, haemolytic anaemia, dyserythropoietic states in general (including sideroblastic anaemia, erythroleukaemia and myelofibrosis), liver disease, and poisoning by heavy metals such as lead, arsenic, bismuth, zinc, silver and mercury. Basophilic stippling is a prominent feature in hereditary deficiency of pyrimidine 5' nucleotidase,[134] this enzyme being required for RNA degradation. Inhibition of this enzyme may also be responsible for prominent basophilic stippling in some patients with lead poisoning.[134]

Pappenheimer bodies

Pappenheimer bodies (see Fig.3.76) are basophilic inclusions which may be present in small numbers in erythrocytes; they are often in small clusters towards the periphery of the cell and can be demonstrated to contain iron. They are composed of ferritin aggregates, or of mitochrondria or phagosomes containing aggregated ferritin. They stain on a Romanowsky stain because clumps of ribosomes are co-precipitated with the iron-containing organelles. A cell containing Pappenheimer bodies is a siderocyte; reticulocytes often contain Pappenheimer bodies. Following splenectomy in a haematologically normal subject, small numbers of Pappenheimer bodies appear, these being ferritin aggregates. In pathological conditions such as lead poisoning or sideroblastic anaemia, Pappenheimer bodies can also represent iron-laden mitochrondria or phagosomes. If the patient has also had a splenectomy the inclusions will be present in much larger numbers.

Microorganisms in red blood cells
In malaria and in other less common protozoan parasitic infections the organism is seen as an inclusion in the red cell (see page 86).

In bartonellosis or Oroya fever, a disease confined to South America, inclusions in red blood cells are the causative organism, a flagellated bacillus; associated marked spherocytosis and haemolysis are found.[69]

RED CELL AGGLUTINATION AND ROULEAUX FORMATION
Red cell agglutinates (see Fig.3.7) are irregular clumps of cells, whereas rouleaux (Fig.3.94) are stacks of cells resembling a pile of coins.

Reticulocytes may form agglutinates when their numbers are increased; this is a normal phenomenon. Mature red cells agglutinate when they are antibody coated. Small agglutinates may be seen in warm autoimmune haemolytic anaemia whereas the presence of cold agglutinins may cause massive agglutination.

Rouleaux formation is increased when there is an increased concentration of proteins of large molecular weight in the plasma. The most common causes are pregnancy (in which fibrinogen concentration is increased), inflammatory conditions (in which polyclonal immunoglobulin, α_2-macroglobulin and fibrinogen are increased) and plasma cell dyscrasia (in which monoclonal immunoglobulin is increased). Rouleaux formation may be artefactually increased if a drop of blood is left standing for too long on a microscope slide before the blood film is spread.

Abnormal clumping of red blood cells may also occur in patients receiving certain intravenous drugs which use polyethoxylated castor oils as a carrier (for example, miconazole, phytomenadione and cyclosporin).

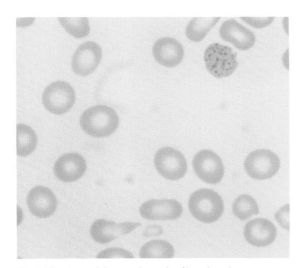

Fig.3.93 *Basophilic stippling; the film also shows anisocytosis, poikilocytosis and macrocytosis.* × 960.

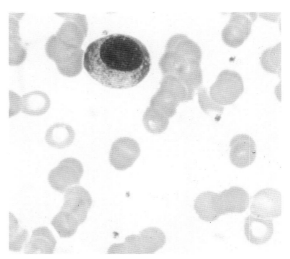

Fig.3.94 *Increased rouleaux formation consequent on multiple myeloma; the film also shows increased background staining and a circulating myeloma cell.* × 960.

OTHER CIRCULATING NUCLEATED CELLS

PLASMA CELLS

Plasma cells are usually tissue cells, but on occasions they may be present in the peripheral blood (see Figs 3.49 and 3.94). They range in size from somewhat larger than a small lymphocyte (8–10 μm) up to a diameter of about 20 μm and are oval in shape with eccentric nuclei, coarsely clumped chromatin, a moderate amount of strongly basophilic cytoplasm and a less basophilic Golgi zone adjacent to the nucleus. The clock-face chromatin pattern which is seen in tissue sections stained with haematoxylin and eosin is less apparent in circulating plasma cells stained with a Romanowsky stain.

The differential diagnosis when a blood film shows plasma cells is discussed on page 244.

ENDOTHELIAL CELLS

Endothelial cells (Fig.3.95) are most likely to be detected if a blood film is made from the first drop of blood in a needle; this was particularly noted when needles were reused and were sometimes barbed.[119] Endothelial cells may occur singly or in clusters. They are large cells, often elongated, with a diameter of 20–30 μm and a large amount of pale blue or blue-grey cytoplasm; the nucleus is round to oval with a diameter of 10–15 μm and one to three light blue nucleoli.

EPITHELIAL CELLS

When blood is obtained by skin puncture epithelial cells from the skin may occasionally be present in the blood film (Fig.3.96). They are large cells with a small nucleus and large amount of sky-blue featureless cytoplasm (Fig.3.96a); some are anucleate (Fig.3.96b).

MAST CELLS

Mast cells are tissue cells which are found extremely rarely in the peripheral blood of normal subjects.[34]

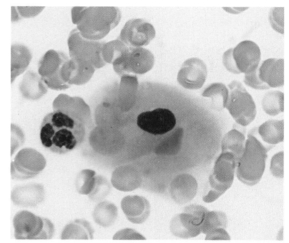

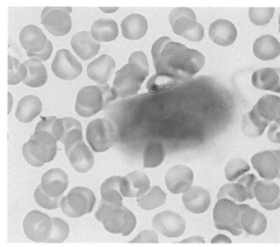

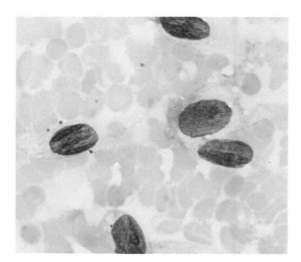

Fig.3.95 *Endothelial cells obtained by scraping the vena cava during a post-mortem examination.* × 960.

Fig.3.96 *Epithelial cells in a blood film prepared from a drop of blood obtained by a finger prick; both (upper) nucleated and (lower) anucleate epithelial cells are present.* × 960.

They may circulate in the blood in systemic mastocytosis, though even in this condition mast cell leukaemia is uncommon. Mast cells have granules which pack the cytoplasm and which, on Romanowsky stains, have similar staining properties to the granules of basophils (Fig.3.97). The cell outline is somewhat irregular. The nucleus of a normal mast cell is not obscured by the granules and is oval with a dispersed chromatin pattern; in mast cell leukaemia there may also be cells with a lobulated nucleus and a more dense chromatin pattern[23] and cells with scanty granules.

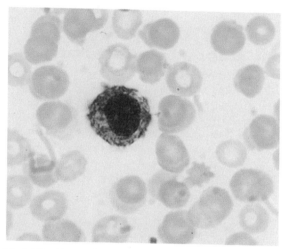

Fig.3.97 *Mast cell in the blood film of a patient with systemic mastocytosis and mast cell leukaemia. × 960.*

NON-HAEMOPOIETIC MALIGNANT CELLS

In various small-cell neoplasms of children tumour cells may circulate in the peripheral blood in appreciable numbers and may be mistaken for the lymphoblasts of acute lymphoblastic leukaemia. Such circulating cells have been described in neuroblastoma, medulloblastoma and rhabdomyosarcoma.[21, 97, 106] In rhabdomyosarcoma syncytial masses of tumour cells have been seen.[74] Carcinoma cells may circulate in the blood, but in such very small numbers that they are unlikely to be noted unless special concentration procedures are employed.[87] Rarely they may be seen on routine peripheral blood films (Fig.3.98). Even more rarely a 'leukaemia' of carcinoma cells occurs.[43] Malignant cells in the blood may be in clusters.

In patients with advanced Hodgkin's disease small numbers of Reed–Sternberg cells and mononuclear Hodgkin's cells may rarely be noted in the peripheral blood.[12] Even more rarely abnormal cells may be present in such numbers as to constitute a Reed–Sternberg cell leukaemia. In one such patient the total WBC was $140 \times 10^9/1$ with 92 percent of the cells being malignant;[121] these included typical Reed–Sternberg cells (giant cells of 12–40 μm diameter with mirror-image nuclei and giant nucleoli), and multinucleated and mononuclear Hodgkin's cells, also with giant nucleoli.

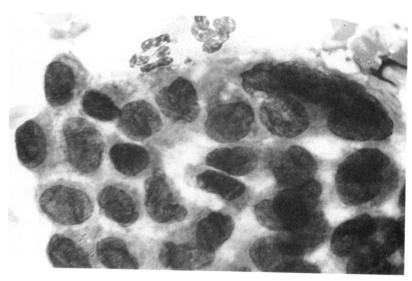

Fig.3.98 *Malignant cells in a routine peripheral blood film of a patient subsequently found to have widespread metastatic malignancy. × 960.*

THE NORMAL BLOOD FILM

The blood film of a normal adult shows only slight variation in size and shape of red cells (see Figs 3.8, 3.9 and 3.61). White cells which are normally present are neutrophils, neutrophil band forms, eosinophils, basophils, lymphocytes and monocytes. Metamyelocytes and myelocytes are rare (page 58). Megakaryocytes, usually in the form of almost bare nuclei, are very rare (page 63). Platelets are present in such numbers that the ratio of red cells to platelets is of the order of 10–40:1. The normal numbers of platelets and of the various types of white cells are discussed in Chapter 6.

THE BLOOD FILM DURING PREGNANCY

During pregnancy (see Fig.3.56) the red cells show more variation in size and shape than is seen in non-pregnant women. The average red cell size (MCV) also increases, being greatest around 35 weeks of gestation. This change occurs independently of any deficiency of vitamin B_{12} or folic acid, although there is also an increased incidence of folic acid deficiency during pregnancy. The haemoglobin level falls, the lowest level being at 30–33 weeks gestation. Although iron deficiency and folic acid deficiency have an increased incidence during pregnancy this commonly observed fall is not due to a deficiency state, and in fact occurs despite an increase in the total red cell mass. It is consequent on an even greater rise in the total plasma volume. The erythrocyte sedimentation rate (ESR) and rouleaux formation are increased. The reticulocyte count is increased, with peak levels of about 6 percent at 25–30 weeks. Polychromatic cells are more numerous.

The total WBC, neutrophil count and monocyte count rise, with neutrophils commonly showing toxic granulation and Döhle bodies. A left shift occurs: band forms, metamyelocytes and myelocytes are common, and occasional promyelocytes and even myeloblasts may be seen. The absolute lymphocyte count and the eosinophil count fall.

The platelet count and platelet size do not change during normal pregnancy, but the platelet count may fall and the mean platelet volume may rise if pregnancy is complicated by toxaemia.

Reference ranges for many haematological variables differ during pregnancy (page 144).

THE BLOOD FILM DURING INFANCY AND CHILDHOOD

In normal infants and children red blood cells are hypochromic and microcytic in comparison with those of adults and the MCV and MCH are reduced (see page 160). Iron deficiency is common in infancy and childhood but the difference from adult norms is present even when iron deficiency is not present. The male/female difference in haemoglobin concentration, PCV and RBC is not present prior to puberty.

The lymphocyte count is higher than in adults and the lymphocyte percentage commonly exceeds the neutrophil percentage ('reversed differential'). A greater proportion of large lymphocytes is commonly observed and some of these may have nucleoli visible by light microscopy. Reactive changes in lymphocytes in response to infections or other immunological stimuli are far commoner than in adults.

Reference ranges for haematological parameters in children are shown on page 158.

THE BLOOD FILM IN HYPOSPLENISM

In normal adults splenectomy produces characteristic abnormalities in the blood count and film. The same abnormalities are seen if the spleen is congenitally absent or if it suffers atrophy or extensive infarction or becomes non-functional for any reason. Occasionally features of hyposplenism may be seen in the presence of splenomegaly, if the spleen is heavily infiltrated by abnormal cells. Some of the causes of hyposplenism are shown in Fig. 9.35 and its differential diagnosis is discussed on page 294.

Immediately after splenectomy there is a thrombocytosis and a marked neutrophil leucocytosis. If infection occurs postsplenectomy the neutrophilia and left shift are very marked. After recovery from surgery the neutrophil count falls to near normal levels and the platelet count falls to high normal or somewhat elevated levels — platelet counts of around $500–600 \times 10^9/l$ may persist. A lymphocytosis and a monocytosis persist indefinitely — the lymphocytosis is usually moderate but levels up to $10 \times 10^9/l$ are occasionally seen.[140] In normal subjects the haemoglobin concentration does not change postsplenectomy but the red cell morphology is altered (see Figs 3.89a and 3.99). Abnormal features include target cells, acanthocytes, Howell–Jolly bodies, small numbers of Pappenheimer bodies (the presence of siderotic granules being confirmed on a stain for iron), occasional nucleated red cells and small numbers of spherocytes. Small vacuoles may be seen in Romanowsky stained films; on interference phase contrast microscopy these appear as 'pits' or 'craters' but in fact they appear to be autophagic vacuoles.[61] The reticulocyte count is increased. Special stains show small numbers of Heinz bodies. Some large platelets may be noted and the mean platelet volume is higher in relation to the platelet count than in non-splenectomized subjects.

In patients with haematological disorders a greater degree of abnormality is often seen. If there is anaemia which persists postsplenectomy then a marked degree of thrombocytosis is usual. If Heinz bodies are formed (for example because of the presence of an unstable haemoglobin or because an oxidant drug is administered) then large numbers are seen in the peripheral blood in a hyposplenic patient. If there is erythroblast iron overload (for example in sideroblastic anaemia or thalassaemia major) then Pappenheimer bodies are very numerous. If the bone marrow is megaloblastic or dyserythropoietic, Howell–Jolly bodies are particularly large and numerous. In a patient with hereditary

spherocytosis target cells are not usually seen post-splenectomy. The effects of splenectomy on the morphology of other haematological disorders are discussed under the specific conditions.

THE BLOOD FILM OF THE NEONATE

The blood film of a healthy neonate shows hyposplenic features. There are Howell–Jolly bodies, acanthocytes and spherocytes; spherocytes are, however, more numerous than in a hyposplenic adult. In premature babies (see below) hyposplenic features are much more marked (Fig. 3.100) and may persist for the first few months of life. The WBC, neutrophil count, monocyte count and lymphocyte count are much higher in the neonate than in the older child or adult. Nucleated red blood cells may be very numerous, and band forms, metamyelocytes and myelocytes are not uncommon.

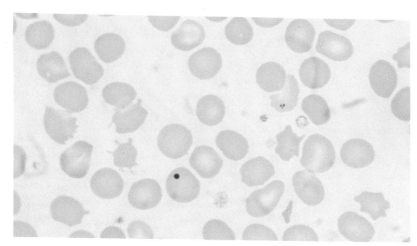

Fig.3.99 *A postsplenectomy blood film in a previously haematologically normal subject; the film shows acanthocytes, a Howell–Jolly body, Pappenheimer bodies and a schistocyte.* × 960.

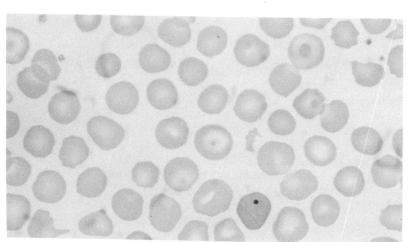

Fig.3.100 *Blood film from a premature but healthy infant, showing macrocytosis (relative to the blood film of an adult), a Howell–Jolly body in a polychromatic cell, target cells and a schistocyte.* × 960.

The haemoglobin concentration, RBC and PCV are higher than at any other time after birth, and the consequent increased viscosity of the blood leads to poor spreading with the blood film appearing 'packed'. This physiological polycythaemia also leads to the ESR being very low. Red cell size is very large in comparison with infants, children or adults. The reticulocyte count is high during the first three days after birth.

Physiological changes in haematological parameters occur in the first days and weeks of life. There is an initial rise, on average of about 60 percent of initial levels, in the WBC and neutrophil count with peak levels being reached at about 12 hours after birth.[142] By 72 hours levels have fallen back to below the level at birth. The lymphocyte count falls to reach its lowest level at about 72 hours and then rises again.[142] By the end of the first week the number of neutrophils has usually fallen below the number of lymphocytes. If there has been late clamping of the umbilical cord there is also a rise in the haemoglobin concentration, PCV and RBC due to 'autotransfusion' from the placenta followed by reduction of the plasma volume. Nucleated red blood cells usually disappear from the blood by about the fourth day in healthy term babies and by the end of the first week most of the myelocytes and metamyelocytes have also disappeared. Band forms are more numerous during the first few days than thereafter, a plateau level being reached by the fifth day.

Premature babies have a lower haemoglobin concentration and a higher MCV and MCH than term babies. They also have greater numbers of NRBC and of metamyelocytes, myelocytes, promyelocytes and blasts. Their neutrophil counts are reduced but reach the levels of term babies by about a week.[24] Lymphocyte counts are lower at birth, reaching the same levels as full term babies by about 6 weeks.[142] Premature babies commonly develop eosinophilia between the second and third weeks after birth.[44]

Infected neonates may be neutropenic rather than having a neutrophilia; this is consequent on increased egress of neutrophils to the tissues with depletion of the relatively small bone marrow granulocyte reserve. An increased proportion of band forms has been found to be more helpful than neutrophilia in identifying infected infants. However, the proportion of bands as well as the total WBC may be increased by crying.[19] The neutrophil count of neonates is increased not only sometimes in infection but also following hypoxia or stressful labour, intrapartum oxytocin, maternal fever, or seizures or hypoglycaemia in the neonate.[84]

Normal ranges for haematological parameters in the neonate are given on page 154.

EFFECTS OF STORAGE AND EXCESS EDTA ON HAEMATOLOGICAL PARAMETERS AND BLOOD CELL MORPHOLOGY

Prolonged storage of blood anticoagulated with EDTA causes crenation or echinocytic change of red blood cells (Fig.3.101a), degeneration of neutrophils (Fig.3.101a) and lobulation of some lymphocyte nuclei (Fig.3.101b). Excess EDTA may itself cause crenation of red cells, and the development of storage changes in red cells is accelerated. Degenerating neutrophils may be similar to necrobiotic neutrophils formed *in vivo* (see Fig.3.31) or they may be completely amorphous necrotic cells. If there is a prolonged delay in blood reaching the laboratory, for example three days or more, most of the neutrophils will have degenerated and the total WBC will have fallen in consequence. If an inexperienced laboratory worker does not recognize the storage artefact and attempts to perform a differential count a factitious neutropenia and lymphocytosis may be recorded. Inexperienced observers may also misclassify neutrophils with a single rounded nuclear mass as NRBC. Storage leads to a rapid increase in platelet size, as measured by the impedance method and a rapid decrease of platelet size as measured by a light-scattering method (page 136). Prolonged storage leads to a moderate increase in size of the red blood cells as measured by the impedance method. With the three-part differential count of later models of the Coulter counter storage leads first to a factitious elevation of the mononuclear count and then to a rejection of the count. On Technicon instruments the fall of mean peroxidase activity which occurs on storage causes a misleading high peroxidase alarm (see page 111).

PARASITES IN THE BLOOD FILM

Some parasites, such as malarial parasites and babesiae, are predominantly blood parasites, while others, such as filariae, have part of their life cycle in the blood. Parasites which may be detected by examination of the blood are given in Fig.3.102.

MALARIA AND BABESIOSIS

Although malarial parasites may be detectable in May–Grunwald–Giemsa stained blood films, their detection and identification is facilitated by Giemsa staining at a higher pH (see page 10). A thick film is preferable for detection of parasites and a thin film for identification of the species. A thick film should be examined for at least 5 minutes before being considered negative. If only a thin film is available it should be examined for at least 15 minutes, or until 100–200 high power fields have been examined, before being considered negative. Partially immune subjects are particularly likely to have a low parasite count so that a prolonged search may be required for parasite detection. In patients with a strong suspicion of malaria whose initial blood films are negative repeated blood examinations may be needed. *Plasmodium falciparum* is associated with the highest parasite counts with often 10–40 percent of red cells being parasitized; paradoxically, patients may be seriously ill with no parasites being detectable on initial blood examination. This is consequent on parasitized red cells being sequestered in tissues. Useful features in distinguishing between the four species of *Plasmodium* that are human parasites and characteristic morphological features are shown in Figs 3.103–3.107. Associated abnormalities which may be noted in the blood films of patients with malaria are anaemia, thrombocytopenia, phagocytosis of parasitized and nonparasitized red cells by monocytes, malarial pigment in monocytes and occasionally in neutrophils (see Fig.3.29), and atypical lymphocytes.

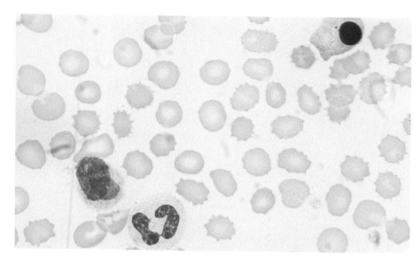

Fig.3.101 *Blood films showing storage artefacts:*
(a) *crenation, a disintegrated cell and a neutrophil with a rounded pyknotic nucleus, × 960*

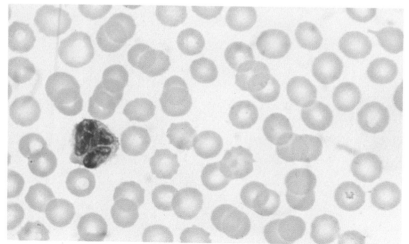

(b) *mild crenation of red cells and lobulation of a lymphocyte nucleus. × 960.*

PARASITES WHICH MAY BE DETECTED IN BLOOD FILMS		
PROTOZOANS		
Parasite	**Disease or common name**	**Usual distribution**
SPOROZOANS		
Plasmodium falciparum	malignant tertian malaria	widespread in tropics and subtropics, particularly in Africa
Plasmodium vivax	benign tertian malaria	widespread in tropics and occurs also in some parts of the temperate zones; not West or Central Africa
Plasmodium malariae	quartan malaria	scattered in the tropics
Plasmodium ovale	benign tertian malaria	tropical West Africa; scattered foci elsewhere including tropical Asia, New Guinea and the Western Pacific
Babesia microti and other species of *Babesiae*	babesiosis	New England, Europe
HAEMOFLAGELLATES		
Trypanosoma rhodesiense	sleeping sickness	East Africa
Trypanosoma gambiense	sleeping sickness	tropical West and Central Africa
Trypansoma cruzi	South American trypanosomiasis or Chagas' disease	wide area of Central and south America
Trypanosoma rangeli	non-pathogenic	Central and South America
Leishmania donovani	visceral leishmaniasis or Kala-Azar	India, China, Central Asia, Central and Northern Africa, the Mediterranean littoral, Central and South America
NEMATODES (OF FAMILY FILARIIDAE)		
Wuchereria bancrofti	filariasis — end stage of disease may be elephantiasis	widespread in tropics and subtropics, particularly Asia, New Guinea, Polynesia, Africa, and Central and South America
Brugia malayi	filariasis — end stage of disease may be elephantiasis	India, South East Asia
Loa loa	eye worm or Calabar swellings	African equatorial rainforest and its fringes
Dipetalonema perstans	persistent filariasis — usually nonpathogenic	tropical Africa, occasionally Central and South America
Mansonella ozzardi	Ozzard's filariasis — usually nonpathogenic	Central and South America

Fig.3.102 *Parasites which may be detected in a blood film, the diseases they cause, and their geographic distribution.*

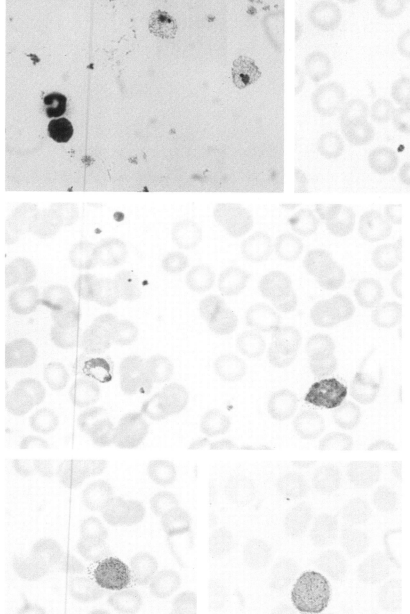
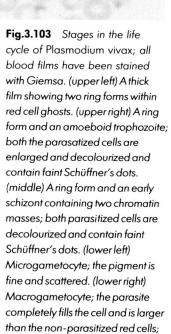

Fig.3.103 *Stages in the life cycle of Plasmodium vivax; all blood films have been stained with Giemsa. (upper left) A thick film showing two ring forms within red cell ghosts. (upper right) A ring form and an amoeboid trophozoite; both the parasatized cells are enlarged and decolourized and contain faint Schüffner's dots. (middle) A ring form and an early schizont containing two chromatin masses; both parasitized cells are decolourized and contain faint Schüffner's dots. (lower left) Microgametocyte; the pigment is fine and scattered. (lower right) Macrogametocyte; the parasite completely fills the cell and is larger than the non-parasitized red cells; the pigment is fine and scattered. × 960.*

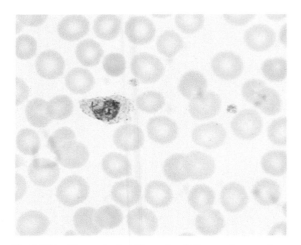

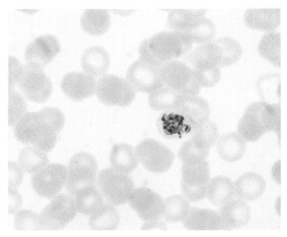

Fig.3.104 *Stages in the life cycle of Plasmodium ovale; all blood films have been stained with Giemsa. (left) A late trophozoite in a red cell which is enlarged, oval and decolourized, and has irregular (fimbriated) margins;* pigment is coarser and darker than in Plasmodium vivax, the parasite is more compact and Schüffner's dots are more prominent. (right) A schizont containing eight merozoites; coarse pigment is clustered centrally. × 960.

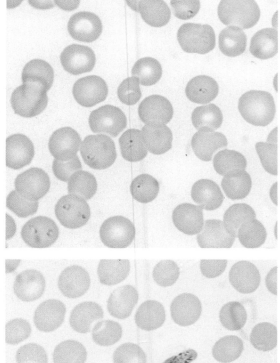

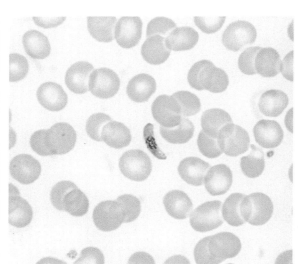

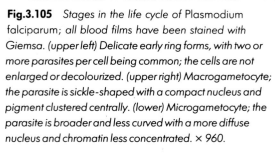

Fig.3.105 *Stages in the life cycle of Plasmodium falciparum; all blood films have been stained with Giemsa. (upper left) Delicate early ring forms, with two or more parasites per cell being common; the cells are not enlarged or decolourized. (upper right) Macrogametocyte; the parasite is sickle-shaped with a compact nucleus and pigment clustered centrally. (lower) Microgametocyte; the parasite is broader and less curved with a more diffuse nucleus and chromatin less concentrated. × 960.*

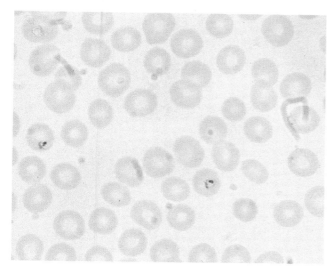

Fig.3.106 *Stages in the life cycle of Plasmodium malariae; all films have been stained with Giemsa.*
(a) *Early ring forms which are small but less delicate than those of Plasmodium falciparum and are found in red cells which are not enlarged or decolourized; one of the parasites has the chromatin dot within the ring.*

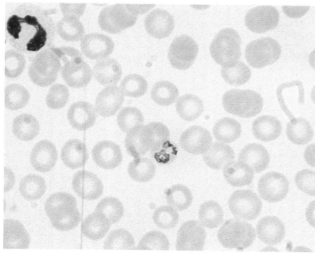

(b) *Amoeboid trophozoite with coarse dark brown pigment; the cell is not enlarged or decolourized.*

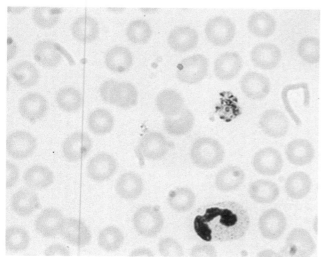

(c) *Schizont with about seven merozoites in a daisy-head arrangement with central coarse brown pigment.* × 960.

	Cell	Early Trophozoite	Late Trophozoite
P. vivax	enlarged, decolourized, multiple infection of red cells fairly common, Schuffner's dots	cells enlarged and pale or pink; a few Schuffner's dots	more numerous Schuffner's dots; amoeboid trophozoite; yellowish brown, fine pigment in cytoplasm of parasite
P. ovale	somewhat enlarged, often oval, ragged edges, decolourized, more marked Schuffner's dots which appear earlier than in P. vivax	cells somewhat enlarged, fimbriated ends; rings similar to vivax, numerous Schuffner's dots	parasites less irregular than vivax; pigment darker and coarser brown, Schuffner's dots prominent
P. falciparum	normal range of sizes, multiple infection of red cells common, 10–40% of cells may be parasitized	shoulder form red cells may be irregular or crenated; fine rings; double chromatin dots common, rare Maurer's dots or clefts	not usually seen in blood (8–32 merozoites; dark brown coarse peripheral clumps of pigment)
P. malariae	small to normal size, multiple infection of red cells rare, lowest percentage of cells parasitized	smaller, more compact rings than vivax; chromatin dot may be inside ring; rarely Ziemann's dots	amoeboid form more compact than vivax, dark brown pigment; cells rarely stippled, pigment is heavy

Fig. 3.107 *Features which are useful in distinguishing between the different species of malarial parasite.*

Early Schizont	Late Schizont	Gametocyte	
		macrogametocyte	**microgametocyte**
  irregular, amoeboid; yellowish brown fine pigment	 12–24 merozoites, 1–2 clumps of peripheral pigment	 nucleus eccentric, deep red larger than normal red cell, round or ovoid, compact nucleus, deep-blue cytoplasm, pigment scattered	 central nucleus or eccentric lighter red larger than normal red cell, round to ovoid; more diffuse nucleus; cytoplasm less blue, may be pink; pigment fine and scattered
  round, compact; pigment heavier and coarser than vivax, darkish brown	 6–12 (usually 8) merozoites, central pigment, merozoites arranged irregularly — like a bunch of grapes	 similar to vivax, somewhat smaller, pigment coarser and blacker, scattered	 similar to vivax but smaller; paler staining than macrogametocyte
not usually seen in blood (amoeboid pigment scattered, light to very dark brown clumps)	not usually seen in blood (oval or round)	 nucleus compact deep red sickle-shaped causing deformation of red cell; blue cytoplasm; compact nucleus, central pigment	 nucleus more diffuse, lighter red less pointed and sickle-shaped; lighter and pinker staining; nucleus more diffuse and pigment more scattered than in macrogametocyte
  compact, round; coarse pigment — dark brown to black	 6–12 (usually 8–10) merozoites in rosette or daisy head formation; central, coarse dark brown pigment	 similar to vivax but smaller; pigment coarse and dark, concentrated in centre and periphery	 similar to vivax but smaller

Babesia is a rare parasite of man and can easily be confused with the malarial parasite. The trophozoites are small rings, similar to those of *P. falciparum*, 1–5 μm in diameter with one or two dark chromatin dots and scanty cytoplasm. Sometimes they are pyriform (pear-shaped) and either paired or with the pointed ends of four parasites being in contact to give a Maltese cross formation (Fig.3.108). Red cells are not enlarged, no pigment is present and no schizonts or gametocytes are seen. Babesiosis occurs particularly, but not exclusively, in hyposplenic subjects. Up to 25 percent of red cells are parasitized, or more in hyposplenic subjects. The method of detection is by thick and thin films, as for malaria. Babesiosis should be particularly considered in

hyposplenic subjects, and when parasites resembling *Plasmodium* species are seen in subjects who have not been in a malaria zone.

HAEMOFLAGELLATES

Trypanosomes may be detected in the peripheral blood as motile, extracellular parasites. They have a slender body and move by means of a flagellum extending from the kinetoplast at the rear end of the parasite to the front end where the flagellum is free (Fig.3.109); the flagellum is joined to the body by an undulating membrane. The parasites may be seen moving in a wet preparation when a drop of anticoagulated blood is placed on

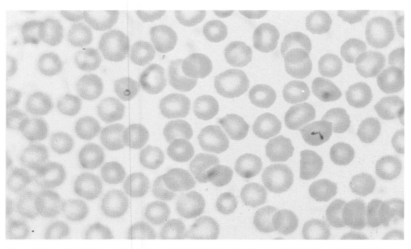

Fig.3.108 *Blood film from a splenectomized monkey parasitized by* Babesia microti. **(a)** *A single ring form and a pair of pyriform parasites.*

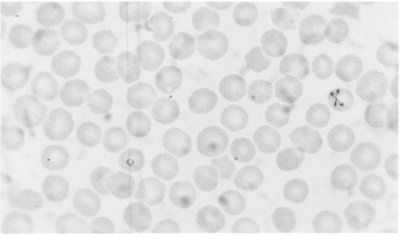

(b) *Four pyriform parasites in a tetrad or Maltese cross formation and a single ring form.* × 960.

MORPHOLOGICAL FEATURES OF HAEMOFLAGELLATES IN PERIPHERAL BLOOD

Trypanosomia rhodesiense and Trypanosoma gambiense

the two species are morphologically identical to each other; extracellular; 8–30μm in length; polymorphic-ranging from long and slender with a free flagellum to short and blunt with an abbreviated flagellum; serpentine; small kinetoplast; flagellated pointed front end; blunt back end

Trypanosomia cruzi

extracellular; 20–25 μm in length; more uniform in morphology than the African species with a larger kinetoplast and less convolution of the undulating membrane; S– or U–shaped; sometimes sharp at both ends

Trypanosomia rangeli

extracellular; longer and thinner than T. cruzi with a smaller kinetoplast and more convolution of the undulating membrane; nucleus somewhat anterior whereas that of T. cruzi is central

Leishmania donovani

parasite within monocytes; fairly uniform in size; approximately 2–6 × 1–3 μm; contains a nucleus and a rod–shaped kinetoplast

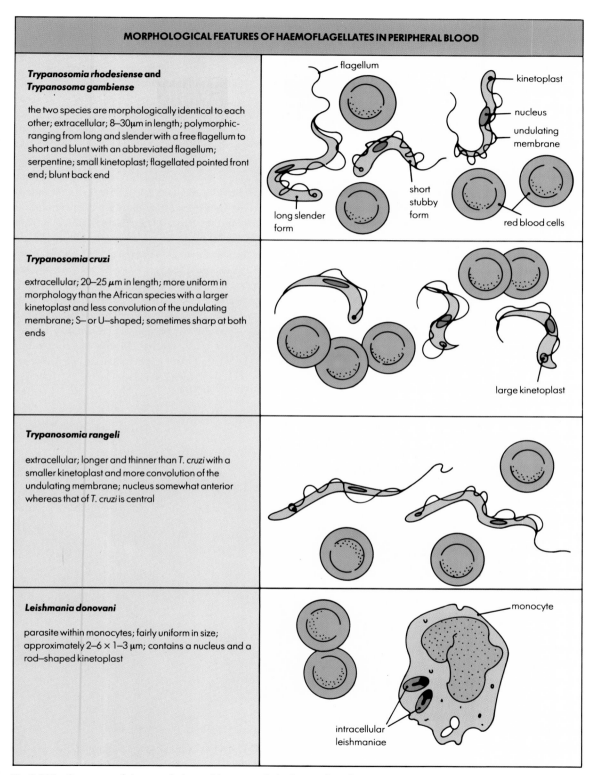

Fig.3.109 *Summary of the morphological features of the haemoflagellates.*

a slide, beneath a coverslip, for microscopic examination. They may also be detected in fixed preparations such as thick or thin films or buffy coat films. When parasites are scanty they are more readily detected by examining the sediment of 10–20 ml of haemolysed blood. *Trypanosoma rhodesiense* and *T. gambiense* (Fig.3.110) are morphologically identical. They are distinguished by their different geographical distributions (Fig.3.102). Examination of the peripheral blood is more likely to be useful in ·he case of *T. rhodesiense*. Concentration techniques may be needed with *T. gambiense*, or parasites may be undetectable in the blood, lymph node puncture being required for diagnosis.

T. cruzi (Fig.3.111) differs morphologically from the African parasites. It is rarely detected by direct examination of the blood, concentration procedures being more often required. It can be distinguished on morphological grounds from the nonpathogenic *T. rangeli* which has a similar geographic distribution (Fig.3.109). *Leishmania donovani*, the causative organism of kala azar, may be detected in peripheral blood monocytes in thick or thin films or buffy coat preparations (see Fig.3.53a,b). The detection rate is higher if bone marrow aspiration or splenic puncture is employed, but

examination of the peripheral blood may avoid the necessity for other more invasive procedures. Associated features which may be noted in patients with kala azar are leucopenia, neutropenia, anaemia and increased rouleaux formation.

FILARIAE

In filariasis (Fig.3.102) adult worms reside in tissues and release microfilariae into the blood stream. Microfilariae are detectable during the acute phase of the disease, but are not detectable in patients with chronic tissue damage but without active disease. As the microfilariae are motile, examination of a wet preparation is often useful; they may also be detected in thick and thin films. Repeated blood examination may be needed and blood specimens must be obtained at a time appropriate for the species being sought: *Wuchereria bancrofti* and *Brugia malayi* release their microfilariae at night, whereas those of *Loa loa* are released during the day; *Mansonella ozzardi* is nonperiodic. *Dipetalonema perstans* is usually nonperiodic but release may be nocturnal or, less often, diurnal. Morphological features useful in distinguishing microfilariae of different species are shown in Figs 3.112–3.114.

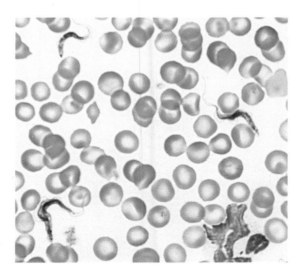

Fig.3.110 *Trypanosoma gambiense; the parasites are serpentine with a small kinetoplast.* × 384.

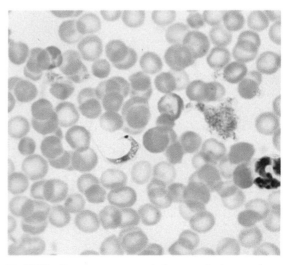

Fig.3.111 *Trypanosoma cruzi; the parasite is curved but not usually serpentine, and has a large kinetoplast.* × 384.

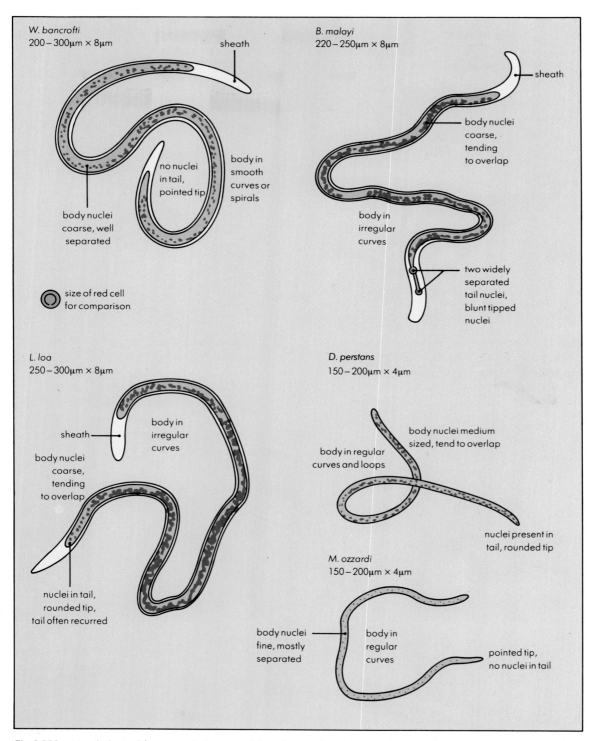

Fig.3.112 *Morphological features which are useful in distinguishing between the microfilariae of the different species of filariae.*

Microfilariae moving through tissues are responsible for the syndrome known as tropical eosinophilia in which respiratory symptoms are associated with eosinophilia, increased rouleaux formation and an elevated erythrocyte sedimentation rate. Microfilariae are not usually detectable in the peripheral blood of patients with tropical eosinophilia.

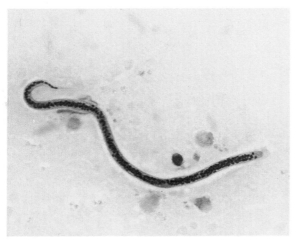

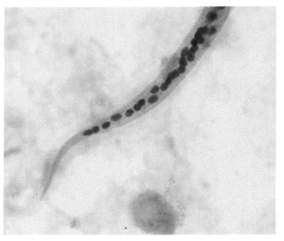

Fig.3.113 *Microfiliariae of Wuchereria bancrofti. (a) In a thick blood film, magnification × 380; the negative impression of the sheath can be faintly seen.*

(b) In a thick blood film, magnification × 960; the nuclei do not extend to the end of the tail.

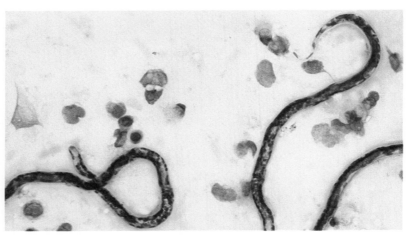

Fig.3.114 *Microfilariae of Loa Loa. (a) In a thick film, magnification × 380; the nuclei extend to the end of the tail.*

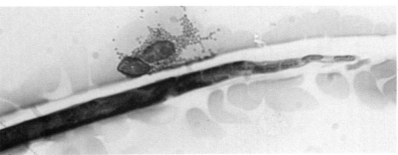

(b) In a thin blood film, magnification × 960; the nuclei extend to the end of the tail and the negative impression of the sheath is clearly seen.

References

1. Abernathy MR (1966) Döhle bodies associated with uncomplicated pregnancy. *Blood*, **27**, 380–385.

2. Akenzua GT, Hui YT, Milner R & Zipursky A (1974) Neutrophils and band counts in the diagnosis of neonatal infections. *Pediatrics*, **54**, 38–42.

3. Archer RK, Engisch HJC, Gaha T & Ruxton J (1971) The eosinophil leucocyte in the blood and bone marrow of patients with Down's anomaly. *British Journal of Haematology*, **21**, 271–276.

4. Ardeman S, Chanarin I & Frankland AW (1963) The Pelger–Huët anomaly, *Blood*, **22**, 472–476.

5. Austen RF & Desforges JF (1969) Hereditary elliptocytosis: an unusual presentation of hemolysis in the newborn associated with transient morphological abnormalities. *Pediatrics*, **44**, 196–200.

6. Bain BJ, Catovsky D, O'Brien M, Spiers ASD & Richards HGH (1977) Megakaryoblastic transformation of chronic granulocytic leukaemia. *Journal of Clinical Pathology*, **30**, 235–242.

7. Bain BJ & Wickramasinghe SNW (1974) unpublished observations.

8. Bassen FA & Korzweig AL (1950) Malformation of the erythrocytes in a case of atypical retinitis pigmentosa. *Blood*, **5**, 381–387.

9. Bessis M, Translated by Weed RI (1973) *Living blood cells and their ultrastructure.* Berlin: Springer-Verlag.

10. Beutler E, West C, Tavassoli M & Grahn E (1980) The Woronets Trait: a new familial erythrocyte anomaly. *Blood Cells*, **6**, 281–287.

11. Bird AR, Wood K, Leisegang F, Mathew CG, Ellis P, Hartley PS & Karabus CD (1984) Hemoglobin E variants: a clinical, haematolgical and biosynthetic study of four South African families. *Acta Haematologica*, **72**, 135–137.

12. Bouroncle BA (1966) Sternberg–Reed cells in the peripheral blood of patients with Hodgkin's disease. *Blood*, **27**, 544–556.

13. Brecher G & Bessis M (1972) Present status of spiculated red cells and their relation to the discocyte – echinocyte transformation: a critical review. *Blood*, **40**, 333–344.

14. Brunning RD (1970) Morphological alterations in nucleated blood and marrow cells in genetic disorders, *Human Pathology*, **1**, 99–124.

15. Bunn HF (1987) Subunit assembly of hemoglobin: an important determinant of hematologic phenotype. *Blood*, **69** 1–6.

16. Cauchi MN & Smith MB (1981) Quantitative aspects of red cell size variation during pregnancy. *Clinical and Laboratory Haematology*, **4**, 149–154.

17. Chanarin I (1979) *Megaloblastic Anaemias*, 2nd edn. St. Louis: CV Mosby Co.

18. Chomet B, Kirslen MM, Schaeffer G & Mudrik P (1953) The finding of the L.E. (lupus erythematosus) cells in smears of untreated freshly drawn blood. *Blood*, **8**, 1107–1109.

19. Christensen RD & Rothstein G (1978) Pitfalls in the interpretation of leukocyte counts of newborn infants. *American Journal of Clinical Pathology*, **72**, 608–611.

20. Christensen RD, Rothstein G, Anstall HB & Bybee B (1981) Granulocyte transfusions in neonates with bacterial infection, neutropenia and depletion of mature marrow neutrophils. *Pediatrics*, **70**, 1–6.

21. Christensen WN, Ultmann JE & Mohos SC (1956) Disseminated neuroblastoma in an adult presenting the picture of thrombocytopenic purpura. *Blood*, **11**, 273–278.

22. Cooke WE (1927) The macropolycyte. *British Medical Journal*, **i**, 12–13.

23. Coser P, Quaglino D, de Pasquale A, Colombetti V & Prinoth O (1980) Cytobiological and clinical aspects of tissue mast cell leukaemia. *British Journal of Haematology*, **45**, 5–12.

24. Coulombel L, Dehan M, Tchernia G, Hill C & Vial M (1979) The number of polymorphonuclear leukocytes in relation to gestational age in the newborn. *Acta Pediatrica Scandinavica*, **68**, 709–711.

25. Dacie JV (1985) *The haemolytic anaemias. Volume 1. The hereditary haemolytic anaemias. Second edition* Edinburgh: Churchill Livingstone.

26. Davidson RJ & McPhie JL (1980) Cytoplasmic vacuolation of peripheral blood cells in acute alcoholism. *Journal of Clinical Pathology*, **33**, 1193–1196.

27. Davidson WM (1968) Inherited variations in leukocytes. *Seminars in Haematology*, **5**, 255–274.

28. Davidson WM, Fowler JF & Smith DR (1958) Sexing the neutrophil leucocytes in natural and artificial chimaeras. *British Journal of Haematology*, **4**, 231–238.

29. Davidson WM & Smith DR (1954) A morphological sex difference in the polymorphonuclear neutrophil leucocytes. *British Medical Journal*, **ii**, 6–9.

30. Deiss A & Kurth D (1970) Circulating reticulocytes in normal adults as determined by the new methylene blue method. *American Journal of Clincial Pathology*, **53**, 481–484.

31. Douglas SD, Blume RS & Wolff SM (1969) Fine structural studies of leukocytes from patients and heterozygotes with the Chédiak–Higashi syndrome. *Blood*, **33**, 527–540.

32. Eastham RD & Jancar J (1970) Macrocytosis in Down's syndrome and during long-term anticonvulsant therapy. *Journal of Clinical Pathology*, **23**, 296–298.

33. Edwin E (1967) The segmentation of polymorphonuclear neutrophils. *Acta Medica Scandinavica*, **182**, 401–410.

34. Efrati P & Rozenszajn L (1960) The morphology of buffy coats in normal human adults. *Blood*, **15**, 1012–1019.

35. Eichner ER (1984) Spider bite hemolytic anemia: positive Coombs' test, erythrophagocytosis and leukoerythroblastic smear. *American Journal of Clinical Pathology*, **81**, 683–687.

36. Eichner ER (1984) Erythroid karyorrhexis in the peripheral blood smears in severe arsenic poisoning: a comparison with lead poisoning. *American Journal of Clinical Pathology*, **81**, 533–537.

37. Epstein CJ, Sahud MA, Piel CF, Goodman JR, Bernfield MR, Kushner JH & Ablin AR (1972) Hereditary macrothrombocytopathia, nephritis and deafness. *American Journal of Medicine*, **52**, 299–310.

38. Estes JW (1968) Platelet size and function in the heritable disorders of connective tissue. *Annals of Internal Medicine*, **68**, 1237–1249.

39. Estes JW, Morley TJ, Levine IM & Emerson CP (1968) A new hereditary acanthocytosis syndrome. *American Journal of Medicine*, **42**, 868–881.

40. Fairbanks VF, Gilchrist GS, Brimhall B, Gereb JA & Goldston EC (1979) Hemoglobin E trait reexamined: a cause of microcytosis and erythrocytosis. *Blood*, **53**, 109–115.

41. Fajardo LF & Tallent C (1979) Malaria parasites within human platelets. *Journal of the American Medical Association*, **229**, 1205–1207.

42. Gale PF, Parkin JL, Quie PG, Pettitt RE, Nelson RP & Brunning RD (1986) Leukocyte granulation abnormality associated with normal neutrophil function and neurological abnormality. *American Journal of Clinical Pathology*, **86**, 33–49.

43. Gallivan MVE & Lokick JJ (1984) Carcinocythemia (carcinoma cell leukemia). *Cancer*, **53**, 1100–1102.

44. Gibson EL, Vaucher Y & Corrigan JJ (1979) Eosinophilia in premature infants: relationship to weight gain. *Journal of Pediatrics*, **95**, 99–101.

45. Giles C (1981) The platelet count and mean platelet volume. *British Journal of Haematology*, **48**, 31–38.

46. Girolami A, Fabris F, Caronato A & Randi ML (1980) Increased numbers of pseudodrumsticks in neutrophils and large platelets. A new congenital leukocyte and platelet morphological abnormality. *Acta Haematologica*, **64**, 324–330.

47. Goudsmit R, van Leeuwen AM & James J (1971) Döhle bodies and acute myeloblastic leukaemia in one family: a new familial disorder? *British Journal of Haematology*, **20**, 557–561.

48. Groover RV, Burke EC, Gordon H & Berdon WE (1972) The genetic mucopolysaccharidoses. *Seminars in Haematology*, **9**, 371–402.

49. Guibaud S, Plumet-Leger A & Frobert Y (1983) Transient neutrophil aggregation in a patient with infectious mononucleosis. *American Journal of Clincial Pathology*, **80**, 883–884.

50. Gustke SS, Becker GA, Garancis JC, Geimer NF & Pisciotta RV (1970) Chromatin clumping in mature leukocytes: a hitherto unrecognized abnormality. *Blood*, **35**, 637–658.

51. Hamilton RW, Shaikh BS, Ottie JN, Storch AE, Saleem A & White JG (1980) Platelet function, ultrastructure and survival in the May–Hegglin anomaly. *American Journal of Clinical Pathology*, **74**, 663–668.

52. Hann IM, Rankin A, Lake BD & Pritchard J (1983) *Colour Atlas of Paediatric Haematology*. Oxford: Oxford University Press.

53. Hansen M & Pedersen NT (1978) Circulating megakaryocytes in blood from the antecubital vein in healthy, adult humans. *Scandinavian Journal of Haematology*, **20**, 371–376.

54. Hansen M & Pedersen NT (1979) Circulating megakaryocytes in patients with pulmonary inflammation and in patients subjected to cholecystectomy. *Scandinavian Journal of Haematology*, **23**, 211–216.

55. Harlan WR, Shaw WA & Zelkowitz M (1976) Echinocytes and acquired deficiency of plasma lipoproteins in burned patients. *Archives of Internal Medicine*, **136**, 71–76.

56. Helman N & Rubenstin LS (1975) The effects of age, sex, and smoking on erythrocytes and leukocytes. *American Journal of Clinical Pathology*, **63**, 33–44.

57. Hernandez JA, Alred SW, Bruce JR, Vanatta PR, Mattingly TL & Sheehan WW (1980) 'Botryoid' nuclei in neutrophils of patients with heat stroke. *Lancet*, **ii**, 642 (letter).

58. Hernandez JA & Steane SM (1984) Erythrophagocytosis by segmented neutrophils in paroxysmal cold hemoglobinuria. *American Journal of Clinical Pathology*, **81**, 787–789.

59. Hicsönmez G & Ozkaynak F (1984) Diagnosis of heterozygous states for Bernard–Soulier disease. *Acta Haematologica*, **71**, 285–286.

60. Hillman RS & Finch CA (1985) *Red Cell Manual*, 5th edn. Philadelphia: F.A. Davis Company.

61. Holroyde CP & Gardner FH (1970) Acquisition of autophagic vacuoles by human erythrocytes. Physiological role of the spleen. *Blood*, **36**, 566–575.

62. How J, Davidson RJL & Bewsher PD (1979) Red cell changes in hyperthyroidism. *Scandinavian Journal of Haematology*, **23**, 323–328.

63. Huehns ER, Luetzner M & Hecht F (1964) Nuclear abnormalities of the neutrophils in D_1 (13-15)-trisomy syndrome. *Lancet*, **i**, 589–590.

64. Itoga T & Laszlo J (1962) Döhle bodies and other granulocytic alterations during chemotherapy with cyclophosphamide. *Blood*, **20**, 668–674.

65. Jenis MEH, Takeuchi A, Dillon DE, Ruymann FB & Rivkin S (1971) The May–Hegglin anomaly: ultrastructure of the granulocyte inclusion. *American Journal of Clinical Pathology*, **55**, 187–196.

66. Jobe MG & Koepke JA (1966) Histoplasmosis in peripheral blood. *American Journal of Clinical Pathology*, **45**, 158–159.

67. Jordans GHW (1953) The familial occurrence of fat containing vacuoles in the leucocytes in two brothers suffering from dystrophia musculorum progressiva. *Acta Medica Scandinavica*, **145**, 419–423.

68. Kahoh T, Saigo K & Yamagishi M (1986) Neutrophils with ring-shaped nuclei in chronic neutrophilic leukaemia. *American Journal of Clinical Pathology*, **86**, 748–751.

69. Kapff CT & Jandl JH (1981) *Blood: Atlas and Sourcebook of Hematology*. Boston: Little Brown & Co.

70. Kaplan E, Zuelzer WW & Neal JV (1953) Further studies on haemoglobin C. *Blood*, **8**, 735–746.

71. Kay NE, Nelson DA & Gotleib AJ (1973) Eosinophil Pelger–Huët anomaly with myeloproliferative disorder. *American Journal of Clinical Pathology*, **60**, 663–668.

72. Klein A, Hussar AE & Bornstein S (1955) Pelger–Huët anomaly of the leukocytes. *New England Journal of Medicine*, **253**, 1057–1062.

73. Kolodny EH (1972) Clinical and biochemical genetics of the lipidoses. *Seminars in Haematology*, **9**, 251–271.

74. Krause JR (1979) Carcinocythemia. *Archives of Pathology and Laboratory Medicine*, **103**, 98 (letter).

75. Kukerski TT (1977) Intraleukocyte spore formation and leukocyte vacuolization during *Clostridium perfringens* septicaemia. *American Journal of Clinical Pathology*, **68**, 794–796.

76. Langenhuijsen MMAC (1984) Neutrophils with ring shaped nuclei in myeloproliferative disorders. *British Journal of Haematology*, **58**, 227–230.

77. Larrick JW & Hyman ES (1984) Acquired iron deficiency anaemia caused by an antibody against the transferrin receptor. *New England Journal of Medicine*, **311**, 214–218.

78. Lock SP, Smith RS & Hardisty RM (1961) Stomatocytosis: a hereditary red cell anomaly associated with haemolytic anaemia. *British Journal of Haematology*, **7**, 303–314.

79. McBride JA & Jacob HS (1970) Abnormal kinetics of red cell membrane cholesterol and acanthocytes: studies in genetic and experimental abetalipoproteinaemia and in spur cell anaemia. *British Journal of Haematology*, **18**, 383–397.

80. McGrath KM, Zalcberg JR, Slonin J & Wiley JS (1982) Intralipid-induced haemolysis. *British Journal of Haematology*, **50**, 376–378.

81. McGrath KM, Collecutt MF, Gordon A, Sawers RJ & Faragher BS (1984) Dehydrated hereditary stomatocytosis — a report of two families and a review of the literature. *Pathology*, **16**, 146–150.

82. Maggio A, Gagliano F & Siciliano S (1984) Hemoglobin phenotype and mean erythrocyte volume in Sicilian people. *Acta Haematologica*, **71**, 214 (letter).

83. Mallory DM, Rosenfield RE, Wong KY, Heller C, Rubinstein P, Allen FH, Walker ME & Lewis M (1976) Rh$_{mod}$, a second kindred (Craig). *Vox Sanguinis*, **30**, 430–440.

84. Manroe BL, Weinberg AG, Rosenfeld CR & Browne R (1979) The neonatal blood count in health and disease I Reference values for neutrophilic cells. *Journal of Pediatrics*, **95**, 89–98.

85. Mant MJ, Doery JCG, Gauldie J & Sims H (1975) Pseudothrombocytopenia due to platelet aggregation and degranulation in blood collected in EDTA. *Scandinavian Journal of Haematology*, **15**, 161–170.

86. Mathy KA & Koepke JA (1974) The clinical usefulness of segmented vs stab neutrophil criteria for differential leukocyte counts. *American Journal of Clinical Pathology*, **61**, 947–958.

87. Melamed MR, Cliffton EE & Seal SH (1962) Cancer cells in the peripheral venous blood. A quantitative study of cells of problematic origin. *American Journal of Clinical Pathology*, **37**, 381–388.

88. Miale JB (1982) *Laboratory Medicine: Hematology*, 6th edn. St. Louis: C.V. Mosby.

89. Miller DR, Rickles FR, Lichtman MA, La Celle PL, Bates J & Weed RI (1971) A new variant of hereditary hemolytic anaemia with stomatocytosis and erythrocyte cation abnormality. *Blood*, **38**, 184–204.

90. Mittwoch U (1963) The incidence of drumsticks in patients with three X chromosomes. *Cytogenetics*, **2**, 24–33.

91. Moore CM & Weinger RS (1980) Pseudo-drumsticks in granulocytes of a male with a Yqh+ polymorphism. *American Journal of Haematology*, **8**, 411–414.

92. Murthy MSN & Emmerich von H (1958) The occurrence of the sex chromatin in white blood cells of young adults. *American Journal of Clinical Pathology*, **30**, 216–223.

93. Neftel KA & Müller OM (1981) Heat-induced radial segmentation of leucocyte nuclei: a non-specific phenomenon accompanying inflammatory and necrotizing disease. *British Journal of Haematology*, **48**, 377–382.

94. Neilsen JA & Strunk KW (1968) Homozygous hereditary elliptocytosis as the cause of haemolytic anaemia in infancy. *Scandinavian Journal of Haematology*, **5**, 486–495.

95. Newberger PE, Robinson JM, Pryzansky KB, Rosoff PM, Greenberger JS & Tauber AI (1983) Human neutrophil dysfunction with giant granules and defective activation of the respiratory burst. *Blood*, **61**, 1247–1257.

96. Nosanchuk J, Terzian J & Posso M (1987) Circulating mucopolysaccharide (mucin) in two adults with metastatic adenocarcinoma. *Archives of Pathology and Laboratory Medicine*, **111**, 545–548.

97. Numez C, Abboud SL, Lemon NC & Kemp JA (1983) Ovarian rhabdomyosarcoma presenting as leukemia. *Cancer*, **52**, 297–300.

98. Oski FA & Barness LA (1967) A previously unrecognized cause of hemolytic anemia in the premature infant. *Journal of Pediatrics*, **70**, 211–220.

99. Parmley RT, Zzeng DY, Baehner RL & Boxer LA (1983) Abnormal distribution of complex carbohydrates in neutrophils of a patient with lactoferrin deficiency. *Blood*, **62**, 538–548.

100. Pederson NT & Cohn J (1981) Intact megakaryocytes in the venous blood as a marker of thrombopoiesis. *Scandinavian Journal of Haematology*, **27**, 57–63.

101. Pederson NT & Laursen B (1983) Megakaryocytes in cubital vein blood in patients with chronic myeloproliferative disorders. *Scandinavian Journal of Haematology*, **30**, 50–58.

102. Pederson NT & Petersen S (1980) Megakaryocytes in the fetal circulation and in cubital vein blood in the mother before and after delivery. *Scandinavian Journal of Haematology*, **25**, 5–11.

103. Perotta AL & Finch CA (1972) The polychromatophilic erythrocyte. *American Journal of Clinical Pathology*, **57**, 471–477.

104. Peterson LC, Rao KV, Crosson JT & White JG (1985) Fechtner syndrome — a variant of Alport's syndrome with leukocyte inclusions and macrothrombocytopenia. *Blood*, **65**, 397–406.

105. Plum CM, Warburg M & Danielsen J (1978) Defective maturation of granulocytes, retinal cysts and multiple skeletal malformations in a mentally retarded girl. *Acta Haematologica*, **59**, 53–63.

106. Pollak ER, Miller HJ & Vye MV (1981) Medulloblastoma presenting as leukemia. *American Journal of Clinical Pathology*, **76**, 98–103.

107. Porter KG, McMaster D, Elmes ME & Love AHG (1977) Anaemia and low serum copper during zinc deficiency. *Lancet*, **ii**, 774.

108. Powell HC & Wolf PL (1976) Neutrophilic leukocyte inclusions in colchicine intoxication. *Archives of Pathology and Laboratory Medicine*, **100**, 136–138.

109. Pryor DS & Pitney WR (1967) Hereditary elliptocytosis: a report of two families from New Guinea. *British Journal of Haematology*, **10**, 468–476.

110. Presentey BZ (1968) A new anomaly of eosinophil granulocytes. *American Journal of Clinical Pathology*, **49**, 887–890.

111. Raccuglia G (1971) Gray platelet syndrome. A variety of qualitative platelet disorder. *American Journal of Medicine*, **51**, 818–827.

112. Rosenszajn L, Klajman A, Jaffe D & Efrati P (1966) Jordans' anomaly in white blood cells. *Blood*, **28**, 258–265.

113. Rowles PM & Williams ES (1983) Abnormal red cell morphology in venous blood of men climbing at high altitude. *British Medical Journal*, **286**, 1396.

114. Sakai T, Mawatari S, Iwashita H, Goto I & Kuroiwa Y (1981) Choreoacanthocytosis. *Archives of Neurology*, **38**, 335–338.

115. Schofield KP, Stone PCW, Beddall AC & Stuart J (1983) Qualitative cytochemistry of the toxic granulation of neutrophils. *British Journal of Haematology*, **53**, 15–22.

116. Schopfer K & Douglas SD (1976) Fine structural studies of peripheral blood leucocytes from children with kwashiorkor: morphological and functional studies. *British Journal of Haematology*, **32**, 573.

117. Seman G (1959) Sur une anomalie constitutionnelle héréditaire du noyau des polynucléaires neutrophiles. *Revue d'Hématologie*, **14**, 409–412.

118. Sen Gupta PC, Ghosal SP, Mukherjee AK & Maity TR (1983) Bilirubin crystals in neutrophils of jaundiced neonates and infants. *Acta Haematologica*, **70**, 69–70.

119. Shanberge JN (1954) Accidental occurrence of endothelial cells in peripheral blood smears. *American Journal of Clinical Pathology*, **25**, 460–464.

120. Sheehan RG & Frenkel EP (1983) Influence of haemoglobin phenotype on the mean erythrocyte volume. *Acta Haematologica*, **69**, 260–265.

121. Sinks LF & Clein CP (1966) The cytogenetics and cell metabolism of circulating Reed–Sternberg cells. *British Journal of Haematology*, **12**, 447–453.

123. Skendzel LP & Hoffman GC (1962) The Pelger anomaly of leukocytes: forty cases in seven families. *American Journal of Clinical Pathology*, **37**, 294–301.

123. Smith H (1967) Unidentified inclusions in haemopoietic cells, congenital atresia of the bile ducts and livedo reticularis in an infant ? a new syndrome. *British Journal of Haematology*, **13**, 695–705.

124. Stavem P, Hjort PF, Vogt E & Van der Hagen CB (1969) Ring-shaped nuclei of granulocytes in a patient with acute erythroleukaemia. *Scandinavian Journal of Haematology*, **6**, 31–32.

125. Stavem P & Kjaerheim A (1977) *In vitro* platelet stain preventing (degranulating) effect of various substances. *Scandinavian Journal of Haematology*, **18**, 170–176.

126. Stavem P, Romslo I, Hovig T, Rostwelt K & Emblem R (1985) Ferrochelatase deficiency of the bone marrow in a syndrome of congenital microcytic anaemia with iron overload of the liver and hyperferraemia. *Scandinavian Journal of Haematology*, **34**, 204–206.

127. Strauss RG, Bove KE, Jones JF, Mauer AM & Fulginite VA (1974) An anomaly of neutrophil morphology with impaired function. *New England Journal of Medicine*, **296**, 478–484.

128. Symmans WA, Shepherd CS, Marsh WL, Oyen R, Shohet SB & Lineham BJ (1979) Hereditary acanthocytosis associated with the McLeod phenotype of the Kell blood group system. *British Journal of Haematology*, **42**, 575–583.

129. Tomonaga M, Matsuura G, Watanabe B, Kamochi Y & Ozono N (1961) Leukocyte drumsticks in chronic granulocytic leukaemia and related disorders. *Blood*, **18**, 581–590.

130. Tracey R & Smith H (1978) An inherited anomaly of human eosinophils and basophils. *Blood Cells*, **4**, 291–300.

131. Tuffy P, Brown AK & Zuelzer WW (1959) Infantile pyknocytosis. A common erythrocyte abnormality in the first trimester. *American Journal of Diseases of Children*, **98**, 227–241.

132. Tulliez M, Testa U, Rochant H, Henri A, Vainchenker W, Toubol J, Breton-Gorius J & Dreyfus B (1982) Reticulocytosis, hypochromia and microcytosis: an unusual presentation of the preleukaemic syndrome. *Blood*, **59**, 293–299.

133. Udden MM, Umeda M, Hirono Y & Marcus DM (1987) New abnormalities in the morphology, cell surface receptors and electrolyte balance in In(Lu) erythrocytes. *Blood*, **69**, 52–57.

134. Valentine WN (1979) Hemolytic anaemia and inborn errors of metabolism. *Blood*, **54**, 549–559.

135. Van Slyck EJ & Rebuck JW (1974) Pseudo-Chediak–Higashi anomaly in acute leukaemia. *American Journal of Clinical Pathology*, **62**, 673–678.

136. Volpé R & Ogryzlo MA (1955) The cryoglobulin inclusion cell. *Blood*, **10**, 493–496.

137. Von Behrens WE (1975) Splenomegaly, macrothrombocytopenia and stomatocytosis in healthy Mediterranean subjects. *Scandinavian Journal of Haematology*, **14**, 258–267.

138. Weil SC & Hrisinko MA (1987) A hybrid eosinophilic–basophilic granulocyte in chronic granulocytic leukaemia. *American Journal of Clinical Pathology*, **87**, 66–70.

139. Weil SC, Holt S, Hrisinko MA, Little L & de Backer N (1985) Melanin inclusions in the peripheral blood leukocytes of a patient with malignant melanoma. *American Journal of Clinical Pathology*, **84**, 679–681.

140. Wilkinson LS, Tang A & Gjedsted A (1983) Marked lymphocytosis suggesting chronic lymphocytic leukemia in three patients with hyposplenism. *American Journal of Medicine*, **75**, 1053–1056.

141. Wolf PL & Koelt J (1980) Hemolytic anaemia in hepatic disease with decreased erythrocyte adenosine triphosphatase. *American Journal of Clinical Pathology*, **73**, 785–788.

142. Xanthou M (1970) Leucocyte blood picture in full-term and premature babies during neonatal period. *Archives of Diseases of Childhood*, **45**, 242–249.

143. Yoo D, Weems H & Lessin LS (1982) Platelet to leukocyte adherence phenomenon. *Acta Haematologica*, **68**, 142–148.

144. Zarkowsky HS, Mohandas N, Speaker CB & Shohet SB (1975) A congenital haemolytic anaemia with thermal sensitivity of the erythrocyte membranes. *British Journal of Haematology*, **29**, 537–543.

4. The differential count

THE MANUAL DIFFERENTIAL COUNT

A differential leucocyte count is the assigning of cells in the blood to their individual categories, this categorization being expressed as a percentage or, when the total leucocyte count is available, as an absolute number. When cells are classified on a stained blood film by a human observer the term 'manual differential count' is used. A manual differential count may be performed on a manually or mechanically spread wedge film or on a blood film prepared by centrifugation. Cells normally present in the peripheral blood may be assigned to five or six categories, depending on whether segmented neutrophils are separated from non-segmented or band forms or are grouped with them. The differential count also includes any abnormal cells which may be present. Nucleated red blood cells (NRBC) may be included as one category in the differential count, or alternatively their numbers may be expressed as the number per 100 white blood cells. Depending on which convention is followed the full blood count will include either a total nucleated cell count (TNCC) or a white cell count (WBC) which is the TNCC corrected for any NRBC which are present.

ACCURACY AND PRECISION OF THE MANUAL DIFFERENTIAL COUNT

In assessing the manual differential count and in comparing it with other methods of differential counting it is necessary to consider the precision and the accuracy of the count. Accuracy is the closeness of an estimate to the true value whereas precision is the reproducibility of an estimate. In the case of the differential count accuracy means that the count produced represents the true distribution of the cell types in the blood sample. The concept of accuracy can also be applied to the identification of an individual cell or class of cell. A manual differential count is, in general, accurate but relatively imprecise.

Accuracy

Since the visual identification of a cell under the microscope is the basis of the differential count this method provides the standard by which the accuracy of other methods is assessed. A manual differential count performed on an adequate number of cells on a well spread blood film by a single experienced observer may be regarded as a reasonably accurate count. The consensus view of a number of experienced observers using a number of blood films may have a higher degree of accuracy and may therefore be preferred. There are two causes of inaccuracy in manual differential counts, maldistribution of cells and misidentification of cells.

Maldistribution

Some maldistribution of different cell types occurs in a wedge-spread film. The tail of the film contains more neutrophils and fewer lymphocytes, whereas monocytes are fairly evenly distributed along the length of the film.[30] The distribution of the different cell types is more even and consistent in a film prepared by centrifugation. If a wedge film is too thin, for example when spreading has been too slow, then the maldistribution of cells is much greater. The use of spreaders with rough edges also causes considerable maldistribution of cells. When white cell aggregation occurs the distribution of cells is so irregular that an accurate differential count is impossible. When large immature cells (blasts, promyelocytes and myelocytes) are present they are found preferentially distributed on the edge of the film rather than in the centre, and distally rather than proximally;[9] conversely lymphocytes, basophils, neutrophils, and metamyelocytes are found preferentially proximally and centrally in relation to the immature cells.[9] Maldistribution of the different cell types could affect not only the accuracy of the differential count but, if different parts of the film were counted on different occasions, then also the precision. In practice maldistribution is not great in a carefully prepared blood film and the accuracy of the count is not much affected. Counting along the length of a blood film shows good agreement with counting a slide prepared by centrifugation.[30] Preparation of a blood film by centrifugation gives at best a 10 percent improvement in precision in comparison with a wedge-spread film.[16] Various methods of tracking over a slide have been recommended in an attempt to compensate for maldistribution of cells. The method shown in Fig. 4.1a compensates for maldistribution between body and tail but not for maldistribution between the centre and the edge, whereas the 'battlement' method shown in Fig. 4.1b tends to do the reverse, since the customary 100 cell differential count will not cover a very large proportion of the length of the blood film. A modified battlement track (Fig. 4.1c) is a compromise between the two methods.

Misidentification

Inaccuracy due to misidentification of cells by a human observer is usually not great when differential counts are performed on high quality blood films by experienced laboratory workers. An exception is the differentiation between band forms and mature neutrophils. Inaccurate identification of a cell commonly also leads to imprecision since a cell which is difficult to classify is often classified inconsistently. Interlaboratory surveys have repeatedly shown that there are systematic differences between laboratories as to the percentage of cells which are classified as band forms reflecting the application of different criteria, and there is also some considerable imprecision in the band count in individual laboratories indicating the difficulty of applying the criteria consistently. The distinction between a monocyte and a large lymphocyte can also occasionally cause problems; the precision of the manual monocyte count is poorer than would be anticipated from the number of cells counted suggesting that a proportion are identified inaccurately. Basophils may be misclassified as neutrophils if they are degranulated

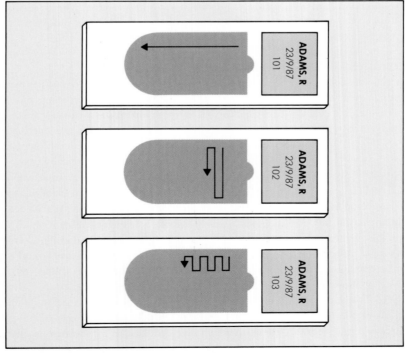

Fig. 4.1 Blood films showing tracking patterns used in differential counting:

(a) tracking along the length of the film;

(b) battlement method;

(c) modified battlement method; two fields are counted close to the edge along the length of the film, then four fields in from the edge, then two fields parallel to the edge and so on.

or poorly stained. Marked storage artefact in a film renders the differential count very inaccurate; specifically, degenerating neutrophils may be misclassified as NRBC and preferential disintegration of neutrophils may cause a factitious elevation of the lymphocyte count. Inaccuracy can be introduced into a differential count if smear cells are present in appreciable numbers and if they are not included in the differential count. If the smear cells are, for example, lymphocytes then the percentage and absolute number of lymphocytes will be falsely low and the percentage and absolute number of all other cell types will be falsely elevated. Smear cells whose nature can be determined should be counted with the cells from which they originate. Smear cells the nature of which is not clear should be counted as a separate category or the percentage and absolute numbers of cells of other classes will be falsely elevated. If an accurate differential count is important but is prevented by a large proportion of smear cells which cannot be identified then a further blood film should be made after adding albumin to the blood.

Precision

The reproducibility of a count or its precision can be expressed as either the standard deviation (SD) or the coefficient of variation (CV) of replicate counts. Although a manual differential count is generally accurate its precision is rather poor.[28] This is consequent on the small number of cells which are usually counted. When replicate counts are made of the percentage of cells of a given type among randomly distributed cells the SD of the count is related to the square root of the number of cells counted. Specifically the SD of the proportion, θ, of a given type of cell is equal to:[12]

$$\sqrt{\frac{\theta(1-\theta)}{n}}$$

the 95 percent confidence limits of the proportion, that is the limits within which 95 percent of replicate counts would be expected to fall, are equal to $\theta \pm 1.96$ SD. The confidence limits of a given percentage of cells when 100 or more cells are counted is shown in Fig. 4.2. It will be seen that the confidence limits are wide. For example the 95 percent confidence limits of an eosinophil count of 10 percent on a 100-cell differential count are 4–18 percent. The precision of the absolute count of any given cell type cannot be any better than the precision of the percentage, but if it is calculated from an

automated WBC, which itself is quite a precise measurement, then it is not a great deal worse. The imprecision of a manual differential count is greatest for those cells which are present in the smallest numbers, particularly the basophils. If it is diagnostically important to know whether or not a basophilia exists then it is necessary to improve precision, either by performing an absolute basophil count in a haemocytometer or by counting many more than the usual 100 cells (for example 200 or 500). Similarly, if neutrophils constitute only a small proportion of white cells (as, for example, in chronic lymphocytic leukaemia) it is again necessary to count a larger number of cells to improve precision and determine whether neutropenia is present. Although precision would be improved by routinely counting more cells it is not feasible in a diagnostic laboratory to routinely count more than 100 or at the most 200 cells. The poor precision of the count of the cells present in the lowest proportions means that the reference limits for manual basophil and eosinophil counts include zero and it is therefore impossible on the basis of a 100-cell differential count to say that a patient has basopenia or eosinopenia.

REFERENCE METHOD

No internationally agreed reference method exists for the differential leucocyte count, but a proposed reference method has been published by the USA National Committee for Clinical Laboratory Standards.[19] It uses a Romanowsky-stained manually-spread blood film of K_3EDTA-anticoagulated blood. Two hundred cells are counted per slide using a 'battlement' track for finding white cells for identification (see Fig. 4.1b). When a reference count is required for comparison with a test method the consensus of 200-cell counts performed by each of four observers is used (that is, an 800-cell differential count is produced).

THE AUTOMATED DIFFERENTIAL COUNT

Manual differential counts are labour-intensive and therefore expensive investigations. This has led to the development of automated differential counters. As discussed above, the manual count is also very imprecise and some of the automated counters which have been developed have improved precision very considerably by counting very large numbers of cells.

One possibility is to automate only the finding of the cell on the slide, leaving the human observer to identify it. This increases the speed at which differential counts can be performed but most laboratory workers do not consider it a very useful advance. This was the principle of the Honeywell ACS 1000.

Observed percentage of cell	Total number of cells, n				
	100	200	500	1000	10 000
0	0–4	0–2	0–1	0–1	0–0.04
1	0–6	0–4	0–3	0–2	0.8–1.2
2	0–8	0–6	0–4	1–4	1.7–2.3
3	0–9	1–7	1–5	2–5	2.7–3.3
4	1–10	1–8	2–7	2–6	3.6–4.4
5	1–12	2–10	3–8	3–7	4.6–5.4
6	2–13	3–11	4–9	4–8	5.5–6.5
7	2–14	3–12	4–10	5–9	6.5–7.5
8	3–16	4–13	5–11	6–10	7.4–8.6
9	4–17	5–15	6–12	7–11	8.4–9.6
10	4–18	6–16	7–14	8–13	9.4–10.6
15	8–24	10–21	12–19	12–18	14.6–15.4
20	12–30	14–27	16–24	17–23	19.6–20.4
25	16–35	19–32	21–30	22–28	24.6–25.4
30	21–40	23–37	26–35	27–33	29.5–30.5
35	25–46	28–43	30–40	32–39	34.5–35.5
40	30–51	33–48	35–45	36–44	39.5–40.5
45	35–56	38–53	40–50	41–49	44.5–45.5
50	39–61	42–58	45–55	46–54	49.5–50.5

Fig. 4.2 Ninety-five percent confidence limits of the observed percentage of cells when the total number of cells counted (n) varies from 100 to 10000. Ranges for n = 100 to n = 1000 are derived from ref. 28.

Automated differential counters which both identify and classify cells fall into two main classes. Image-recognition instruments simulate the activity of the human eye and brain and classify cells on the basis of their size, shape and staining properties on a conventionally stained blood film. They classify relatively small numbers of cells. Flow-cytometry methods classify large numbers of cells flowing in suspension. Classification may be based on (i) size and cytochemical reactions (flow-cytochemistry), (ii) volume of cells or cell residues as measured by aperture impedance technology and (iii) light-scattering properties which depend on size and certain other characteristics of the cell or cell residue. Image-recognition methods do not substantially improve on the precision of manual differential counts and may also be inaccurate. Flow-cytochemical and other flow cytometrical methods vary in their accuracy but all substantially improve on the precision of the manual differential count. Image-recognition methods initially proved more acceptable to haematologists because they reproduced familiar techniques of cell identification and generally allowed individual cells to be reviewed by the instrument operator. However it seems likely that in the long term methods based on cytochemistry or size-classification will prove more useful.

Automated differential counters often produce extra parameters which supplement the differential count. Some of these seek to give information equivalent to that which may be obtained from examining a blood film whereas others provide information of a new type. Automated counters also incorporate 'flags' or 'alarms' which indicate an abnormal blood sample.

IMAGE-RECOGNITION INSTRUMENTS

Image-recognition instruments classify cells on a stained blood film. Consistent stains are required or accuracy is reduced. Slides must be well spread. Some instruments require a slide prepared by centrifugation. Others will accept a wedge-spread film prepared with an automated spreader, or even a manually spread wedge film. Cells are classified by a computer programme which assesses features such as size, shape, nuclear configuration and staining characteristics. The best established instrument, the Hematrak (Geometric Data Corporation), analyses cells using light of three colours — red, blue and green. Image-recognition is a relatively slow process and therefore with most instruments it is not feasible to classify more than 100, or at the most 200, cells; the precision of the count is thus little better than that of the usual manual differential count. Most instruments have the ability to recall abnormal cells for review by the human observer. They may also make some assessment of red cell morphology or platelet numbers. Image-recognition instruments currently in use include various models of the Hematrak, the Diff3/50 (Coulter Electronics Inc.) and several instruments manufactured in Japan. However since no further image-recognition instruments are being manufactured outside Japan it is likely that within a few years this technology will no longer be employed in Europe or the USA.

FLOW-CYTOCHEMICAL DIFFERENTIAL INSTRUMENTS

The Technicon Corporation have produced a sequence of three automated differential leucocyte counters, two of which are part of an automated full blood counter (Fig. 4.3). The differential counting components of the three instruments are based on similar principles; classification of cells is by a combination of cell size and cytochemical reactions. These instruments generally classify large numbers of cells so that precision is high (Fig. 4.2). The Hemalog D usually classifies 10 000 cells and even when leucopenia is present 1000. The two later instruments classify a comparable number of cells, the precise number being determined by the WBC.

The technology used in the Hemalog D and the automated differential counting component of the H 6000 are very similar (Fig.4.3), though the Hemalog D has three white cell channels and the H 6000 has two. In both, a peroxidase channel identifies neutrophils and eosinophils by a reaction product, respectively grey or black, made with 4-chloro-1-naphthol as a substrate. A scattergram is produced showing forward light scatter plotted against light absorption, these parameters being generally equivalent to cell size and peroxidase activity respectively; thresholds, some of which are fixed and some of which move in response to the characteristics of the blood sample, divide the scattergram into boxes containing clusters of cells of a certain type (Fig. 4.4a). As the neutrophils of different individuals vary in their peroxidase activity and as variation also occurs with time from venesection, the thresholds on either side of the neutrophil cluster move to enclose the cluster. The thresholds are set a fixed distance on either side of the modal light absorption. If the left-hand (lower) threshold, M_T, is forced to move as far as the fixed low absorbance threshold, A_L (Fig. 4.4a), in order to enclose the neutrophil cluster then a low peroxidase alarm

	Hemalog D	H 6000	H.1
Neutrophil	moderately strong peroxidase activity at pH 3.2	moderately strong peroxidase activity at pH 7.3	moderately strong peroxidase activity at pH 7.3
Eosinophil	strong peroxidase activity at pH 3.2	strong peroxidase activity at pH 7.3	strong peroxidase activity at pH 7.3
Lymphocyte	small cells with no peroxidase activity	small cells with no peroxidase activity	small cells with no peroxidase activity
Monocyte	large cells with esterase activity	large cells with weak peroxidase activity at pH 7.3	large cells with weak peroxidase activity at pH 7.3
Basophil	binding of alcian blue or astra blue to granules	binding of alcian blue or astra blue to granules	resistance of cytoplasm to stripping

PEROXIDASE CHANNEL	ESTERASE CHANNEL	BASOPHIL CHANNEL

Fig. 4.3 *Principles of the automated differential count of three instruments manufactured by Technicon International.*

(LPX) is produced. The eosinophil cluster is recognized by the high peroxidase content and apparent small size of the cells. The apparent size is an artefact of the measuring system. The intense black colour consequent on strong peroxidase activity leads to increased light absorption; the reduced forward scatter of light makes cells appear smaller than their true size. In the peroxidase channel monocytes and basophils appear in the same area, to the left of the neutrophils. To the left of

the monocyte/basophil box are large unstained (that is, peroxidase negative) cells (LUC), of which there are only a few percent in normal blood. Lymphocytes appear as small, unstained cells. Cell debris, platelets and nucleated red cells appear in the debris box, though NRBC may stretch up into the lymphocyte and even the LUC boxes.

In the Hemalog D monocytes and basophils are counted in two further channels, monocytes by an

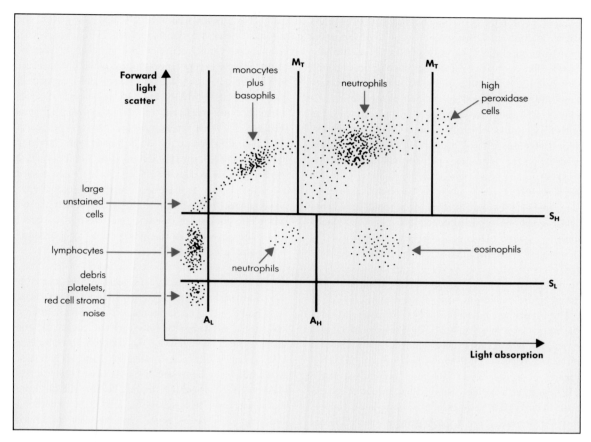

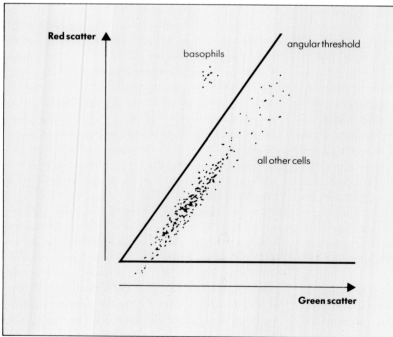

Fig. 4.4 (a) Scattergram of forward light scatter plotted against light absorption in the peroxidase channel of a Technicon H 6000 counter. Forward light scatter is largely determined by cell size and light absorption is largely determined by peroxidase activity. A_L and A_H are respectively low and high thresholds for absorption. S_L and S_H are respectively low and high thresholds for scatter. M_T are moving thresholds. (b) Scattergram of red scatter plotted against green scatter in the basophil channel of the Technicon H 6000.

esterase reaction using α-naphthyl butyrate as the substrate, and basophils by the ability of their heparin-containing granules to bind to various dyes. Initially Alcian Blue was used for basophil identification and subsequently Astra Blue. In the basophil channel, forward scatter in red and green light is measured; unstained cells scatter red and green light equally whereas basophil granules which have bound the blue dye exhibit predominately red scatter (Fig. 4.4b). Abnormal basophils, for example in chronic granulocytic leukaemia, may have reduced ability to bind to the dye and therefore they may not all be correctly classified.[15]

In the H 6000, conditions for the peroxidase reaction have been altered by using dextrose enhancement and a slightly alkaline pH in contrast to the low pH of the Hemalog D. This has allowed monocytes to be detected by their peroxidase activity and the esterase channel has been omitted. As for the Hemalog D, basophils are detected by their ability to bind Alcian or Astra Blue.

The Hemalog D and the H 6000 produce various alarms or 'flags' (see Fig. 4.5). The presence of a flag is an indication to examine a blood film for an explanation of the abnormality. The low peroxidase alarm (LPX) has already been described. The high peroxidase alarm (HPX) indicates an increase of cells with high peroxidase activity falling outside the right-hand (upper) mobile threshold, M_T, of the neutrophil box. This can be consequent on a true increase of cells with high peroxidase activity, or on a decrease of mean peroxidase activity causing the mobile thresholds to move to the left so that cells with normal peroxidase activity fall above the upper threshold; this latter effect is responsible for the HPX alarm which may be seen with old blood. A low rate (LR) alarm indicates a reduced number of peroxidase-positive cells or a heterogenous distribution. An increased number of LUC should be regarded as an alarm. In the case of the Hemalog D the sum of the monocytes and basophils should equal the number of cells in the basophil-monocyte box of the peroxidase channel. Any difference is indicated as a remainder (REM) and a high negative or positive remainder serves as an alarm (Fig. 4.5). The precise figures to be accepted as alarms vary with the age of the subject. For example, healthy children have more LUC than adults[8] and HPX and LR alarms are also seen more frequently in children.

A lymphocyte percentage higher than the neutrophil percentage or an apparent lymphocytosis should be regarded as an alarm. Haemoglobin C trait, haemoglobin C disease and double heterozygosity for haemoglobins S and C commonly lead to failure of lysis of cells in the peroxidase channel, non-lysed cells being classified as lymphocytes and leading to the unusual differential count;[4] rarely this occurs with cord blood and in sickle cell anaemia (SS), S/β thalassaemia, haemoglobin S trait, haemoglobin E trait, haemoglobin E disease, haemoglobin D trait, and in other rare haemoglobinopathies.[4,25] With the Hemalog D this phenomenon was also very common with blood from uraemic patients[1] but with the H 6000 this is only occasionally a problem. When it occurs, LUC may be increased as well as lymphocytes. It has been suggested that hypoproteinaemia might also cause this phenomenon[29] but as the two patients in question had recently had renal transplants it is possible that it was the effect of uraemia which was being observed.

On the H 6000 abnormal cells of various types may appear in the LUC category; such cells include the atypical mononuclears of infectious mononucleosis, blast cells, hairy cells and lymphoma cells. However, abnormal cells may appear in various parts of the scattergram.[11] Myeloblasts may fall into lymphocyte, LUC, monocyte/basophil, neutrophil and HPX boxes, depending on their size and the intensity of their peroxidase reaction. Monoblasts mainly fall into the LUC and monocyte/basophil boxes with a few in the neutrophil and lymphocyte boxes. Some hypergranular promyelocytes fall into the eosinophil box. Lymphoblasts fall into both the lymphocyte and LUC boxes, as do hairy cells. Although abnormal cells may be misclassified with normal cells such blood counts are usually flagged in some way. The associated abnormal scattergram may be of use in the classification of leukaemia.

If an H 6000 is not correctly adjusted the eosinophil count can vary with the haemoglobin concentration; with increasing levels of Hb some eosinophils are misclassified as neutrophils.[14] The basophil count is falsely elevated if a specimen is contaminated with heparin. This is not surprising since the count depends on the binding of Alcian or Astra Blue to the heparin in basophil granules.

The differential count of the H.1 uses new technology for basophil counting which also allows the flagging of suspected blast cells, immature granulocytes, atypical lymphocytes and NRBC.[27] The principles of classification of cells by size and peroxidase activity are similar to those of the earlier instruments, but cells are now analysed as clusters, the position of which is compared with the usual positions of clusters of normal cells. The H.1 has two fixed linear thresholds bounding the

POSSIBLE SIGNIFICANCE OF 'FLAGS' ON THE TECHNICON HEMALOG D AND H 6000 COUNTERS[15,21,29]	
Low peroxidase (LPX)	**Low rate (LR)**
hereditary myeloperoxidase deficiency (partial or complete)	neutropenia
acute myeloid leukaemia	relative neutropenia (e.g. CLL or the inverted differential count of children)
chronic myeloid leukaemia	myeloperoxidase deficiency
myelodysplastic syndromes	**Large unstained cells (LUC) increased**
acute lymphoblastic leukaemia	
chronic lymphocytic leukaemia	large lymphocytes
iron deficiency[14]	lymphocytosis
High peroxidase (HPX)	atypical lymphocytes (e.g. infectious mononucleosis)
	non-Hodgkin's lymphoma
increase of band cells or immature cells of the granulocyte series	chronic lymphocytic leukaemia
old blood (due to a fall of the average peroxidase activity)	prolymphocytic leukaemia
myeloperoxidase deficiency	acute lymphoblastic leukaemia
neutropenia	Sézary syndrome
chronic myeloid leukaemia with neutrophilia	hairy cell leukaemia
acute myeloid leukaemia	plasma cell leukaemia
high eosinophil count	nucleated red blood cells
high monocyte count	peroxidase deficient neutrophils
acquired immune deficiency syndrome (AIDS)[10]	peroxidase deficient monocytes
acute lymphoblastic leukaemia (occasionally)	acute myeloid leukaemia (particularly acute monocytic and myelomonocytic leukaemias)
chronic lymphocytic leukaemia (occasionally)	chronic myeloid leukaemia
platelet satellitism[17]	uraemia
increased platelet count (occasionally)[17]	
cold agglutinins[24]	(continued over page)

Fig. 4.5 *Possible significance of 'alarms' and abnormalities indicated by the Technicon Hemalog D and H 6000 counters.*

Positive remainder — (Hemalog D only) monocytes plus basophils < monocytes plus basophils in the peroxidase channel	Negative remainder — (Hemalog D only) monocytes plus basophils > monocytes plus basophils in the peroxidase channel
low-peroxidase neutrophils classified as monocytes low-esterase monocytes not classified as monocytes (may occur in healthy subjects, in myelomonocytic leukaemia, with ageing of some blood samples, and following exposure to organophosphate insecticides[18])	esterase-positive but peroxidase negative monocytes scored as LUC high eosinophil count (>15 percent) high-esterase neutrophils scored as monocytes high monocyte count high-peroxidase monocytes scored as neutrophils
Increased lymphocytes	
true lymphocytosis acute lymphoblastic leukaemia acute myeloid leukaemia (occasionally) chronic myeloid leukaemia NRBC * uraemia (particularly with Hemalog D) * haemoglobin C trait and disease * double heterozygosity for haemoglobins S and C * sickle cell trait (rarely) * sickle cell anaemia (rarely) * haemoglobin S/β thalassaemia * other abnormal haemoglobins (rarely) * cord blood (rarely)	**Increased basophils**
	true basophilia heparin contamination
	Increased eosinophils
	true eosinophilia hypergranular promyelocytic leukaemia[21]
	Increased neutrophils in lower neutrophil box
	acute myeloid leukaemia

* consequent on non-lysis of red cells

Fig. 4.5 (continued) Possible significance of 'alarms' and abnormalities indicated by the Technicon Hemalog D and H 6000 counters.

lymphocyte box and the noise box on the absorption axis but other thresholds are mobile and may be curvilinear; earlier instruments had only linear thresholds, either fixed or mobile (Fig. 4.6a). The peroxidase channel continues to employ white light. The basophil channel employs a laser and analyses cells which have been stripped of their cytoplasm by a lytic agent. Basophils are resistant to this treatment and therefore appear as large cells causing a lot of forward light scatter (Fig. 4.6b). The small cell residues representing cells other than basophils are further analysed by their high angle light scatter (light absorption) which is a function of

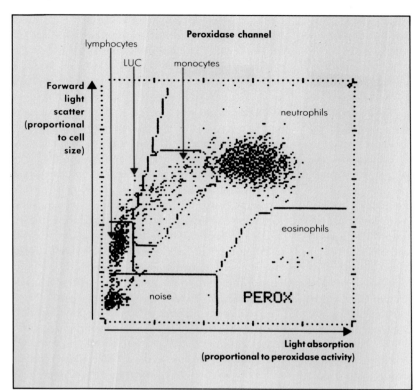

Fig. 4.6

(a) *Scattergram of forward light scatter (proportional to cell size) plotted against light absorption (proportional to peroxidase activity) in the peroxidase channel of a Technicon H.1 counter.*

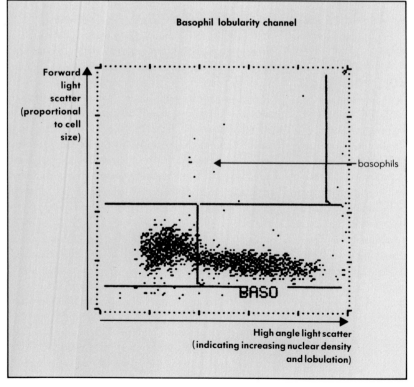

(b) *Scattergram of forward light scatter (proportional to size of cell residue) plotted against high angle light scatter in the basophil channel of a Technicon H.1 counter.*

chromatin density and the degree of lobulation of the nucleus. A mobile threshold searches for a valley and divides residues into two main clumps; to the left of the threshold are lymphocytes, monocytes and immature cells of the granulocyte series, while to the right are neutrophil and eosinophil polymorphs, band cells and NRBC. The suspicion of NRBC is indicated by the instrument when there are excess cells in the neutrophil/eosinophil area of the basophil channel in comparison with the sum of neutrophils and eosinophils in the peroxidase channel. Conversely fewer cells in the neutrophil/eosinophil area of the basophil channel than are expected from the peroxidase channel may indicate that there are immature cells of the granulocytic series which are peroxidase positive but are non-lobulated and are therefore to the left of the valley in the basophil channel. Blast cells appear to the left of the lymphocyte/monocyte cluster in the basophil channel and their suspected presence can therefore be flagged. An increase of LUC without there being any evidence of blasts in the basophil channel leads to a 'suspect atypical lymphocytes' flag. A lobularity index, dependent on the high angle light scatter of a more lobulated nucleus, is derived in the basophil channel; it is expressed as the ratio of the modal channel of the granulocyte cluster to the modal channel of the mononuclear cluster and is thought to reflect left and possibly right shift. 'Flags' which may be produced by the H.1 counter are summarized in Fig. 4.7.

INSTRUMENTS BASED ON CELL SIZING

Several instruments have been designed which classify cells on the basis of cell size after exposure to specified reagents. Such an assessment may be by aperture impedance or light-scatter technology. Information on size may be supplemented by measurements which are determined by the internal structure of the cell. These methods usually produce a limited classification of leucocytes or a 'screening differential count' with cells divided into two or three categories. Current Coulter instruments use cell size as measured by aperture impedance technology whereas Ortho instruments have a classification which is based on two measurements — low-angle light scatter, which is largely determined by cell size, and high-angle light scatter, which is mainly determined by the internal structure of the cell, particularly by granularity.

Coulter instrumentation

The Coulter S Plus IV and related instruments initially produced a two-part differential count (lymphocytes and non-lymphocytes or myeloid cells) on the basis of the size of the cell residues following partial lysis of the cytoplasm. Subsequently the lytic system was modified so that cell residues could be separated into three categories on the basis of size: lymphocytes, mononuclear cells and granulocytes (see Fig. 2.10). The term mononuclear cell is used here to include monocytes plus certain abnormal cells. The instrument uses floating thresholds to search for the valleys between the different populations. Cells are classified as lymphocytes if their residues fall between 35 and approximately 90 fl, as mononuclear cells if they fall between approximately 90 and approximately 160 fl, and as granulocytes if they fall between approximately 160 and approximately 450 fl. The instrument lymphocyte count has been found to correlate well with lymphocyte counts derived from manual differential counts, although a small proportion of lymphocytes are classified with mononuclear cells.[2,5] The instrument 'granulocyte' count has been found to correlate well with both the neutrophil count and the granulocyte (neutrophil plus eosinophil plus basophil) count derived from manual differential counts, although evidence has been produced that some eosinophils are classified as mononuclear cells rather than as granulocytes[2,5,13] and that basophils fall into the mononuclear rather than the granulocyte category.[5,7]

The mononuclear category is more problematical. The manufacturer has reported a moderately good correlation of the mononuclear cell count with a manual monocyte count, with the correlation coefficient being 0.7[6] but in another publication of the manufacturer a correlation coefficient of only 0.54 was reported.[26] Even a correlation coefficient of 0.7 would mean that only half the variation in a manual monocyte count was explained by variation in the instrument mononuclear count ($r^2 = 0.49$) and the results of the second comparison would mean that only 29 percent of the variation was explained ($r^2 = 0.295$). In other comparisons the correlation coefficient has not been as high as 0.7. Nelson et al.[20] found a correlation of 0.6 with a 200- or 300-cell differential count even after outliers and instrument mononuclear counts of greater than $1.5 \times 10^9/l$ had been excluded. Bain[2] found the correlation between the mononuclear cell count and the monocyte count derived from a 500-cell manual count to vary between $r = 0.31$ and $r = 0.40$. Clarke et al.[5] found only 6 percent of the variation of an H 6000 monocyte count was explained by variation in the S Plus IV monocyte count ($r = 0.246$); since both automated methods

POSSIBLE SIGNIFICANCE OF 'FLAGS' OR ABNORMAL OBSERVATIONS PRODUCED BY THE TECHNICON H.1 COUNTER	
Flag	**Possible significance**
reduction of mean peroxidase index (MPXI) of neutrophils	hereditary or acquired myeloperoxidase deficiency degranulation of neutrophils in infection
increase of large unstained cells (LUC)	presence of blasts, atypical lymphocytes
suspect atypical lymphocytes	LUC increased with no blasts being detectable in the basophil channel
increased debris (peroxidase channel)	NRBC
band in the peroxidase display parallel to the normal lymphocyte band	malarial parasites giant platelets platelet aggregates
neutrophils plus eosinophils in basophil channel > neutrophils plus eosinophils in the peroxidase channel (suspect NRBC flag)	NRBC myeloperoxidase deficiency
neutrophils plus eosinophils in the basophil channel < neutrophils plus eosinophils in the peroxidase channel (suspect IMM GRAN flag)	immature granulocytes Pelger–Hüet anomaly
cells to the left of the lymphocyte/monocyte cluster in the basophil channel (suspect blasts flag)	blast cells
increased basophils	true basophilia blast cells lymphoma cells atypical lymphocytes
decreased lobularity index (LI)	left shift of neutrophils
suspect left shift flag	immature granulocytes samples from obstetric patients samples greater than 18 hours old
discrepancy between WBC in peroxidase channel and basophil channel (indicated by asterisk on WBC)	non-lysis of red cells

Fig. 4.7 *Possible significance of 'alarms' and abnormalities on the Technicon H.1 counter.*

are considerably more precise than a manual differential count this poor correlation indicates a considerable difference between the results of the two methods of classification. The poor correlation between manual monocyte and S Plus IV mononuclear cell counts is probably attributable to the following observations: (i) not all monocytes are classified as mononuclear cells, some being classified as lymphocytes and some as granulocytes;[2] (ii) cells which are not monocytes are classified as mononuclear cells; these include some of the lymphocytes,[2,5] some of the eosinophils,[2,5,13] some of the basophils[23] and some of the neutrophils.[2] Certain abnormal cells will also be classified as mononuclear cells; these include some blasts, some plasma cells, some hairy cells, some lymphoma cells and some atypical mononuclear cells or reactive lymphocytes. The precision of the mononuclear percentage is also worse than would be expected for the number of cells counted; this may be partly consequent on granulocytes being classified as mononuclear cells as time from venesection

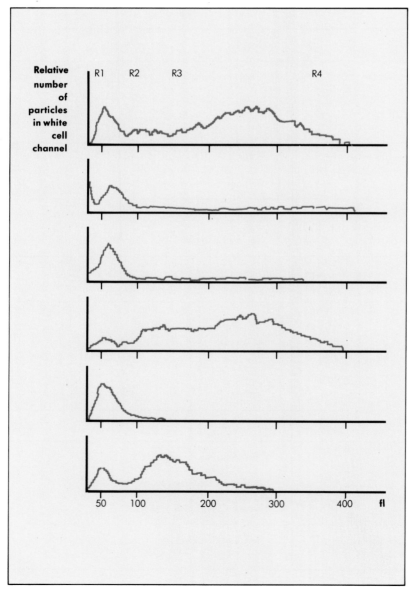

Fig. 4.8 White cell histograms from a Coulter S Plus IV counter: (a) normal histogram indicating the area of the histogram where an abnormality is indicated by R1 to R4 flags; (b) histogram which showed backlighting of the total WBC and absolute lymphocyte, mononuclear cell and granulocyte counts as a consequence of the presence of Plasmodium vivax parasites; (c) histogram which showed an R1 flag together with backlighting of the 'WBC' and absolute granulocyte, mononuclear cell and granulocyte counts consequent on the presence of NRBC which constituted 70 percent of the TNCC; (d) histogram which showed backlighting of an increased mononuclear cell percentage and absolute count which was attributable to monocytosis: (e) histogram which showed an R2 flag consequent on the presence of a small percentage of hairy cells which have expanded the lymphocyte component of the histogram to the right; (f) histogram which showed an R3 flag consequent on ageing of the blood sample which has caused movement of the granulocyte component of the histogram to the left so that it merges with the mononuclear cell component, obliterating the trough between them.

increases, even within 6 hours according to some but not all observers.[2] It may reasonably be concluded that a high mononuclear cell count is likely to indicate either an abnormality of the blood or old blood but little significance should be attached to the exact value of the mononuclear cells.

The S Plus IV and related instruments have a system of flagging which indicates that a histogram does not conform to what is expected. The area of the histogram where an abnormality lies is indicated by specific flags as shown in Fig. 4.8. Haematological abnormalities which are known to cause flagging of the histogram are summarized in Fig. 4.9. The full differential count will not be computed if a histogram is flagged. A mononuclear cell count of greater than 1.5×10^9/l is backlit, this also acting as a flag. Following recent modifications to the S Plus IV and related instruments suspected basophilia and suspected eosinophilia are also flagged.

A number of instruments produced by other manufacturers but using principles similar to those of Coulter counters also perform a two or three category differential count. Included among these are the Toa-Sysmex E 5000 and the Sequoia-Turner Cell Dyne 2000.

Ortho instruments

The Ortho ELT 15, ELT 1500 and upgraded earlier instruments use scattering of a laser beam to produce a limited differential count based on both cell size and cell content. Light scattered at a small forward angle represents mainly light refracted by the surface of the cell and is proportional to cell size, whereas light reflected at 90 degrees is due primarily to refraction and to reflection from structures inside the cell (such as the nucleus and any granules) and therefore depends on the nature of the cell. A plot of forward scatter against right angle scatter allows cells to be divided into granulocytes, lymphocytes and mononuclear cells. The two-dimensional scattergram is converted mathematically into a histogram (see Fig. 2.11). Thresholds which separate the different clusters of cells are mobile. The granulocyte category is said to include neutrophils, eosinophils and basophils. Comparisons of automated differential counts with manual counts have generally found a good correlation for granulocyte and lymphocyte counts. Mean instrument monocyte counts have generally been a few percent higher than manual monocyte counts performed on wedge-spread blood films. The histogram may be rejected when abnormal cells are present, this acting as a flag. Ortho instruments are able to produce a differential count on blood up to 24 hours old.

ABNORMALITIES OF THE BLOOD WHICH MAY CAUSE FLAGS ON THE COULTER S PLUS SERIES OF COUNTERS

Backlighting of WBC
excess of particles < 35 fl (as for R1)

Backlighting of mononuclear cells > 1.5×10^9/l
monocytosis
chronic lymphocytic leukaemia
infectious mononucleosis
eosinophilia
presence of blast cells

Above range + + + +
WBC > 99.9×10^9/l

Incomplete computation . . . .
WBC above range so differential counts not computed

Vote out - - - -
discrepancy between apertures

R1 flag
platelet clumps
large platelets
nucleated red blood cells
malarial parasites
non-lysed red cells
(e.g. due to the presence of a cold agglutinin)
fibrin strands
cryoprotein

R2 flag
lymphocytes of infants
reactive lymphocytes (including infectious mononucleosis)
lymphoma cells
hairy cells
plasma cells
blast cells
monocytosis
eosinophilia
basophilia[23]
ageing of blood

R3 flag
neutrophilia
immature granulocytes
blast cells
eosinophilia
monocytosis
processing a sample within 30 minutes of blood collection[13]
ageing of blood

R4
neutrophilia
monocytosis
samples from infants[13]

Fig. 4.9 *Abnormalities of the blood which may cause flagging with the Coulter S Plus series of counters.*

NEW WHITE CELL PARAMETERS

With the introduction of automated differential counters, efforts have been made to produce information which might be equivalent to the observation of left shift, toxic granulation or Döhle bodies on a blood film.

The Hemalog D and the H 6000 produce a high peroxidase (HPX) alarm. Several studies have shown a correlation of HPX with the presence of toxic changes in the blood film[22] and with clinical and microbiological evidence of inflammation or infection in the patient.[3] Correlation with band counts has often been poor, but this is likely to be at least in part due to the very poor precision of a band count. A variety of other abnormalities in addition to infection and inflammation can also cause an HPX alarm (Fig. 4.5). Consequently, although this alarm may be regarded as a valid indication of either an abnormal blood sample or of ageing of the sample, from the point of view of the diagnosis of infection or inflammation false positive alarms are not uncommon. The H.1 produces a value for HPX flag on a research report and also derives a lobularity index (LI) (see page 114) for neutrophils, and flags 'left shift' and 'suspect immature granulocytes'. 'Left shift' is graded + to + + and is generally based on the LI. Immature granulocytes are suspected when there is a discrepancy between the two channels of the instruments (see page 114). The LI has been found to correlate with the HPX, the manual band count and the absolute neutrophil count.[3] Both it and the immature granulocytes flag were found to be useful as indicators of the presence of infection or inflammation;[3] neither was more sensitive than the absolute neutrophil count but both were found superior to a routine band count. Contrary findings were reported in another study in which the band percentage was found to be superior to the various automated white cell parameters in the diagnosis of infection.[31] The left shift and immature granulocyte alarms (Fig. 4.7) are not specific for infection and inflammation.

On the Coulter S Plus series expansion of the neutrophil component of the histogram to the right (Fig. 4.8) and an R3 or R4 flag may be seen when the blood film shows left shift and toxic changes.

References

1. Bain BJ, Scott D & Scott TJ (1980) Automated differential leucocyte counters: an evaluation of the Hemalog D and a comparison with the Hematrak. II. Evaluation of performance on routine blood samples from hospital patients. *Pathology*, **12**, 101–109.
2. Bain BJ (1986) An assessment of the three-population differential count on the Coulter Counter Model S Plus IV. *Clinical and Laboratory Haematology*, **8**, 347–359.
3. Bentley SA, Pegram MD & Ross DW (1987) Diagnosis of infective and inflammatory disorders by flow cytometric analysis of blood neutrophils. *American Journal of Clinical Pathology*, **88**, 177–181.
4. Booth F & Mead SV (1983) Resistance to lysis of erythrocytes containing haemoglobin C — detected in a differential white cell counting system. *Journal of Clinical Pathology*, **36**, 816–818.
5. Clarke PT, Henthorn JS & England JM (1985) Differential white cell counting on the Coulter Counter. *Clinical and Laboratory Haematology*, **7**, 335–351.
6. Coulter Electronics Inc. (1983) *Coulter Counter Model S Plus IV Product Reference manual.*
7. Cox CJ Habermann TM, Payne BA, Klee GG & Pierre RV (1985) Evaluation of the Coulter Counter Model S Plus IV. *American Journal of Clinical Pathology*, **84**, 297–306.
8. Cranendonk E, Abeling NGGM, Bakker A, de Jong ME, van Gennip AH & Behrendt H (1984) Evaluation of the use of the Hemalog D in acute lymphoblastic leukaemia and disseminated non-Hodgkin's lymphoma. *Acta Haematologica*, **71**, 18–24.
9. Davidson E (1958) The distribution of cells in peripheral blood smears. *Journal of Clinical Pathology*, **11**, 410–411.
10. d'Onofrio G, Mancini S, Tamburrini E, Mango G & Ortona L (1987) Giant neutrophils with increased peroxidase activity. Another evidence of dysgranulopoiesis in AIDS. *American Journal of Clinical Pathology*, **87**, 584–591.
11. Drewinko B, Bollinger P, Brailas C, Moyle S, Wyatt J, Simson E, Johnston D & Trujillo JM (1987) Flow cytochemical patterns of white blood cells in human haemopoietic malignancies. *British Journal of Haematology*, **65**, 27–36.
12. England JM & Bain BJ (1976) Total and differential leucocyte count. *British Journal of Haematology*, **33**, 1–7.
13. Griswold DJ & Champagne VD (1985) Evaluation of the Coulter S Plus IV three-part differential in an acute care hospital. *Amercian Journal of Clinical Pathology*, **84**, 49–57.
14. Hewitt J & Reardon DM (1985) Neutrophil mean peroxidase: a biologically interesting parameter with a potential for WBC differential quality control. *Clinical and Laboratory Haematology*, **7**, 33–42.
15. Hinchcliffe RF, Lilleyman JS, Burroughs NF & Swan HT (1981) Use of the Hemalog D automated leucocyte differential counter in the diagnosis and therapy of leukaemia. *Acta Haematologica*, **65**, 79–84.
16. Koepke JA (1977) A delineation of performance criteria for the differentiation of leukocytes. *American Journal of Clinical Pathology*, **68**, 202–206.

17. Larson JH & Pierre RV (1976) Platelet satellitism as a cause of abnormal Hemalog D differential results. *American Journal of Clinical Pathology*, **68**, 758–759.

18. Lee MJ & Waters HC (1977) Inhibition of monocyte esterase activity by organophosphate insecticides. *Blood* **50**, 947–951.

19. NCCLS (1984) *Tentative standard, leukocyte differential counting, H 20-T.* Villanova, Pennsylvania: U.S.A. National Committee for Clinical Laboratory Standards.

20. Nelson L, Charache S, Keyser E & Metzger P (1985) Laboratory Evaluation of the Coulter three-part electronic differential. *American Journal of Clinical Pathology*, **83**, 547–554.

21. Patterson KG, Cawley JC, Goldstone AH, Richards JDM & Janossy D (1980) A comparison of automated cytochemical analysis and conventional methods in the classification of acute leukaemia. *Clinical and Laboratory Haematology*, **2**, 281–291.

22. Peacock JE, Ross DW & Cohen MS (1982) Automated cytochemical staining and inflammation. *American Journal of Clinical Pathology*, **78**, 445–449.

23. Pierre RV (1984) quoted by Griswold DJ & Champagne VD op cit.

24. Pradella M & Rigolin F (1983) The ABC's of HPX. *American Journal of Clinical Pathology*, **80**, 128–129.

25. Rees J, Williamson D & Carrell RW (1985) Detection of abnormal haemoglobins by the Technicon H6000. *British Journal of Haematology*, **59**, 734–736.

26. Richardson-Jones A, Hellman R & Twedt D (1985) *The Coulter Counter trimodal leukocyte analyser.* International publication of Coulter Corporation.

27. Ross DW & Bentley SA (1986) Evaluation of an automated haematology system (Technicon H.1). *Archives of Pathology and Laboratory Medicine*, **110**, 803–808.

28. Rümke CL (1960) Variability of results in differential cell counts on blood smears. *Triangle*, **4**, 154–157.

29. Simmons A & Elbert G (1975) Hemalog D and manual differential leukocyte counts. *American Journal of Clinical Pathology*, **64**, 512–517.

30. Talstad I (1981) Problems in microscopic and automatic cell differentiation of blood cell suspensions. *Scandinavian Journal of Clinical Haematology*, **26**, 398–406.

31. Wenz B, Ramirez MA & Burns ER (1987) The H*1 Hematology Analyzer. Its performance characteristics and value in the diagnosis of infectious disease. *Archives of Pathology and Laboratory Medicine*, **111**, 521–524.

5. Validating the blood count

Automated blood counts may be inaccurate and it is the responsibility of the laboratory staff performing a count or producing a report to detect inaccuracies whenever possible.

The validation of an automated blood count requires: (1) knowledge that an instrument is capable of measuring all parameters accurately and has been correctly calibrated, and that appropriate quality control procedures indicate normal functioning, and (2) assessment of each individual count as to the likelihood that it is correct.

A count should first be assessed as to whether results are likely. It is useful to check that the PCV (as a percentage) is about three times the Hb concentration, most easily done by verifying that the MCHC falls within or close to the reference limits. Since on most automated instruments the PCV/Hb ratio and the MCHC are derived from all three measured parameters, an abnormality can indicate an invalid result in any or all of these parameters. If results are abnormal then further assessment is necessary. This further assessment may include consideration of the diagnostic details provided to the laboratory in order to judge the likelihood that the result is valid, comparison with previous blood counts in the patient, comparison with a blood film and comparison of the data with cell size histograms or other visual representations produced by an automated counter. Laboratory results falling within reference limits may also be invalid; this may be detected by the same methods.

If the validation procedures raise the suspicion of inaccuracy then it may be necessary to inspect the sample and its labelling, repeat the analysis, examine a blood film (if this has not been done already) and check estimations by alternative methods.

Validating a laboratory result also includes confirming that all parameters required have been produced and that no parameter is beyond the linearity limits of the instrument.

Some of the causes of inaccuracy in automated FBCs are shown in Fig. 5.1 and subsequent figures. It should be noted that the relatively high frequency of reports of inaccuracy with Coulter counters reflects the fact that they have been widely used over a long period of time and have been studied in great detail.

VALIDATING THE WHITE CELL COUNT

Some of the causes of inaccurate WBCs are shown in Figs 5.2 and 5.3. WBCs which are inaccurate because of the presence of aggregated platelets or NRBC are relatively common in hospital practice whereas other causes of inaccurate WBC are uncommon.

WBCs which are beyond the linearity limits of an instrument may be flagged; those beyond the limits which can be printed may be shown by a count of 99.9 or by a code such as +++++ or HI. Instrument operators must be alert to the results which are beyond range and which require a dilution or the use of an alternative method. They should also consider whether a beyond-range WBC has interfered with other parameters.

A falsely high or low WBC is often only detected by examining a blood film and comparing the findings with the count. However in some circumstances noting the flags and examining the histogram produced by an automated counter will draw attention to an abnormality which may be associated with an erroneous result. The commonest such abnormality is platelet aggregation but other abnormalities which may be detected include malarial parasites (see Fig. 4.8b), NRBC (see Fig. 4.8c), non-lysed red cells (Fig. 5.4a), giant platelets and fibrin strands (Fig. 5.4b).

Fig.5.1 *Some causes of inaccurate automated blood counts.*

SOME CAUSES OF INACCURATE AUTOMATED BLOOD COUNTS	
Fault in specimen collection or storage	specimen diluted (e.g. intravenous infusion running, excess EDTA solution for volume of blood) specimen partly clotted specimen lysed aged blood haemoconcentration during phlebotomy (see page 2) blood from wrong patient, or sample and request form relate to different patients specimen contaminated with heparin
Faulty sampling	failure to prime instrument carryover from preceding very abnormal specimen poorly mixed specimen short specimen aspirator blocked by clot from previous specimen
Faulty calibration	
Instrument malfunction or reagent failure	
Inaccuracy inherent in methodology	underestimation of MCV and PCV and overestimation of MCHC in the presence of hypochromia by instruments using impedance technology and some instruments using light-scatter technology (see pages 23 and 25) inevitable carryover (very minor in current instruments)
Inaccuracy due to unusual characteristics of specimen	see following figures

SOME CAUSES OF FALSELY HIGH WHITE CELL COUNTS			
Cause of fault		**System on which error has been observed**	**Detection**	**Rectification**
non-lysis of red cells	in patients with uraemia or with various abnormal haemoglobins or with cord blood samples	Technicon Hemalog D and H 6000; occasionally with Technicon H.1 (in which case the basophil channel WBC is usually reported)	high WBC with reversed differential ('lymphocytes' > neutrophils); flagging on H.1	use alternative method
	with some neonatal red cells and some cases with target cells or sickle cells; some cases of multiple myeloma	Ortho instruments[29,51,57]	debris increased	
	in patients with cold agglutinins	Coulter instruments; Ortho instruments[47]	apparent macrocytosis and improbable red cell indices; flagging; abnormal histograms	warm specimen
NRBC present		all instruments	blood film; flagging and abnormal histogram on S Plus IV and related instruments; abnormal scattergram on Hemalog D and H 6000; scattergram and flagging on Technicon H.1	perform TNCC by alternative method; estimate NRBC percentage on blood film
thrombocytosis		Technicon Hemalog, Hemalog 8 and Hemalog D	blood film	haemocytometer count
numerous giant platelets		all instruments	blood film; S Plus series and Ortho histograms; scattergrams; and flagging on H.1	haemocytometer count

Fig.5.2 *Some causes of falsely high white cell counts.*

SOME CAUSES OF FALSELY HIGH WHITE CELL COUNTS			
Cause of fault	**System on which error has been observed**	**Detection**	**Rectification**
platelet aggregates	Coulter instruments;[44] Ortho instruments;[38] Technicon H.1[60]	blood film; histograms on Coulter S Plus series and Ortho instruments; flagging on H.1	haemocytometer count; rapid count before aggregation has occurred; count on heparinized sample
cryoglobulinaemia and cryofibrinogenaemia	Coulter instruments;[13,19] Toa-Sysmex instruments[7]	blood film; abnormal histogram and flagging	warm specimen
paraproteinaemia	Coulter instruments;[28] Ortho instruments[51]	blood film; abnormal histogram and flagging	haemocytometer count
fibrin strands	Coulter instruments[27]	blood film	haemocytometer count
hyperlipidaemia	Coulter instruments[32,33] Ortho instruments[30]	blood film; elevated MCHC	haemocytometer count
malarial parasites	Coulter instruments	blood film; abnormal histogram and flagging	haemocytometer count
unstable haemoglobin	Coulter instruments	blood film; abnormal histogram and flagging	haemocytometer count
heparin	Ortho instruments[38]	blood film	haemocytometer count
circulating mucin consequent on certain tumours	Ortho ELT-800[45]	blood film	haemocytometer count

SOME CAUSES OF FALSELY LOW WHITE CELL COUNTS			
Cause of fault	**System on which fault has been observed**	**Detection**	**Rectification**
WBC above linearity limits of instrument or above figure which can be printed	all instruments	blood film; flagging, count of 99.9, code, or no count produced	estimate WBC by alternative method or at greater dilution
cell lysis — disintegration of white cells in blood more than three days old	Coulter instruments (presumably other instruments also)	blood film; check date on specimen and request form; flagging	obtain fresh specimen
cell lysis — lysis associated with lymphocytosis	Hemalog and Hemalog 8	blood film	haemocytometer count
cell lysis — lysis associated with leukaemia, [42] uraemia[26] and immunosuppressive drugs[26]	earlier Coulter instruments	blood film	avoid reagents known to cause lysis of WBC
cell lysis — lysis associated with CLL	Ortho instruments [29,51,57]	blood film; histogram showing spilling of lymphocytes into debris area	haemocytometer count
cells clumped — WBC clumped due to antibody or other plasma constituent	Coulter instruments	blood film; abnormal histogram and flagging	haemocytometer count; blood taken into citrate
cells clumped — WBC clumped due to mucopolysaccharide produced by tumour	Hemalog[58]	blood film	accurate blood count may not be possible
cells clumped — WBC and platelets clumped	Coulter instruments[44]	blood film	haemocytometer count
potent cold agglutinin	Coulter instruments; Ortho instruments[16]	blood film; apparent macrocytosis and improbable red cell indices	warm specimen

Fig.5.3 *Some causes of falsely low white cell counts.*

Instruments vary as to the size threshold above which particles are counted as white cells and this determines whether some or all of any NRBC present are counted as white cells. The reagents used also have an influence since some instruments (for example the Coulter S Plus IV and related instruments) count the WBC following partial lysis which reduces the white cells to residues of considerably smaller size showing overlap with the residues of NRBC; the size of such residues depend on the specific reagents used. The Coulter S Plus IV includes

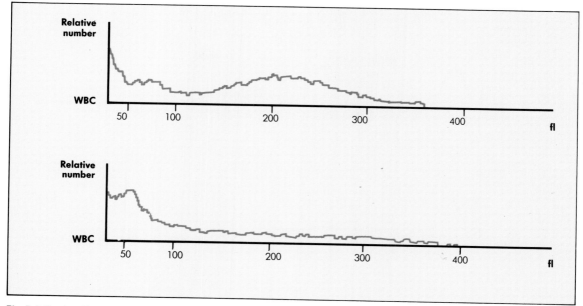

Fig.5.4 *Coulter Counter Model S Plus IV white cell histograms showing abnormalities which were associated with erroneously elevated white cell counts: (a) associated with a cold agglutinin: the automated WBC of 22.9 × 10⁹/l was backlit and had an R1 flag; following* warming to 37°C the WBC was 9.8 × 10⁹/l; (b) associated with fibrin strands; the automated WBC was 3.8 × 10⁹/l whereas the haemocytometer count was 0.4 × 10⁹/l; the automated WBC was backlit.

some but not all NRBC in the 'WBC'. To obtain a true white cell count with an instrument of this type it is necessary to first obtain an accurate total nucleated cell count (TNCC) using either a haemocytometer or a back-up primary instrument (such as a Coulter Counter of the B, F or Z series) on which the thresholds can be set low enough to count all the nucleated cells; the true WBC can then be obtained by counting on a blood film the percentage of the total nucleated cells which are red cells. With another automated counter based on electrical resistance of cells, the Sysmex CC-800/PDA-410 system, thresholds can be set manually so that it is possible to exclude at least some of the NRBC from the TNCC when the histogram indicates their presence.[14]

A factitious elevation of the WBC by platelet aggregates is a particular problem with capillary samples and with samples from neonates whether they are capillary or venous samples. In one study of the Ortho ELT-8, 2–3 percent of capillary samples had an elevated WBC and reduced platelet count for this reason.[28] Samples from patients who have EDTA-induced platelet aggregation

are similarly prone to pseudo-leucocytosis and pseudo-thrombocytopenia. Platelet aggregates are not always detected by the flagging system of the Coulter S Plus IV; large aggregates falling above the lower threshold for white cells will remain undetected. This has also been noted with the Ultra-Flo 100,[8] another impedance counter.

An abnormal histogram associated with factitious elevation of the WBC as the consequence of a cold agglutinin is shown in Fig.5.4a. In this circumstance the most likely mechanism of the factitious result is that agglutinated red cells are not adequately exposed to the lytic agent; paradoxically a cold agglutinin may also be associated with an erroneous WBC of zero (probably due to blocking of orifices). Fibrin strands causing a factitious elevation of the WBC may also be detected on the histogram (Fig.5.4b).

The factitious elevation of the WBC which may be consequent on non-lysis of RBC in the Technicon Hemalog D and H 6000 Counters may be detected by noting that 'lymphocytes' exceed neutrophils and also

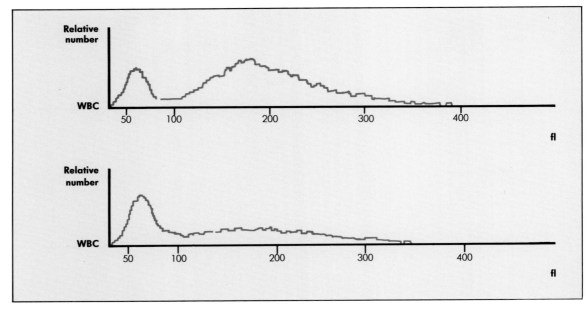

Fig.5.5 *Coulter Counter S Plus IV white cell histograms associated with an erroneously low white cell count due to white cell aggregation induced by an IgM cold antibody: (a) histogram produced when the specimen was kept at 37°C so that an accurate WBC of 9.1 × 10⁹/l and an accurate lymphocyte count of 17.9 percent were produced; (b) histogram produced when the specimen was left at room temperature allowing white cell aggregation to occur; white cell aggregates fell above the upper threshold of the white cell channel so that a falsely low WBC of 4.9 × 10⁹/l was recorded together with a falsely elevated lymphocyte count of 38.7 percent. This histogram was not flagged.*

by inspecting the instrument graphical output for a discrepancy between the WBC in the peroxidase channel and the WBC in the basophil channel, where normal red cell lysis occurs and the WBC is accurate. Failure of lysis in the peroxidase channel is common in the presence of haemoglobin C and occurs occasionally in a variety of other abnormalities (see page 110). This anomalous behaviour of the instrument may be seen as an advantage in that it may lead to the discovery of an abnormal haemoglobin but it is also an inconvenience since it requires a blood film for confirmation and a WBC by an alternative method. Non-lysis of red cells is less common with the Technicon H.1 counter; when it occurs the basophil channel WBC is reported, but is flagged to indicate the discrepancy between the two channels.

A falsely low WBC is uncommon unless blood has been subjected to prolonged storage at room temperature. Figure 5.5 shows an abnormal histogram associated with white cell clumping, a rare cause of a falsely low count.

VALIDATING THE HAEMOGLOBIN CONCENTRATION AND RED CELL PARAMETERS

Errors in haemoglobin concentration (Hb), RBC or MCV should be suspected if the calculated parameters, MCH and MCHC give improbably high or low results or if the PCV is not approximately three times the Hb concentration. On the H.1 the CHCM (see page 25) is useful in validating the MCHC and therefore the Hb. Apart from a factitious elevation of the Hb consequent on a high WBC, or factitious results due to cold agglutinins, errors in the Hb concentration and red cell parameters are uncommon.

INACCURACIES IN THE ESTIMATION OF THE HAEMOGLOBIN CONCENTRATION

Some causes of a falsely high estimation of the haemoglobin concentration are shown in Fig.5.6.

A falsely high Hb due to a grossly elevated WBC should be deliberately sought whenever the WBC

SOME CAUSES OF FALSELY HIGH ESTIMATIONS OF HAEMOGLOBIN CONCENTRATION			
Cause	**System in which fault has been observed**	**Detection**	**Rectification**
high WBC	Coulter instruments; Ortho instruments; Technicon instruments	should be checked for whenever WBC exceeds $100 \times 10^9/l$	manual estimation with centrifugation
hyperlipidaemia — endogenous[33] or due to parenteral nutrition with lipids[30,32]	Coulter instruments;[32,33] Ortho instruments;[30] Technicon instruments	improbable results; MCH and MCHC greatly elevated or MCH elevated and MCHC reduced; on H.1 flagging of discrepancy between MCHC and CHCM[60] (see page 25)	see text
turbidity due to non-lysed red cells in haemoglobinopathies	Coulter instruments	MCH and MCHC elevated	estimation in colorimeter after 1:1 dilution in distilled water
hyperbilirubinaemia	all instruments	MCH and MCHC slightly elevated	colorimeter estimation with plasma blank; the error is very minor and can usually be ignored
cryoglobulinaemia	Coulter instruments[53]	MCH and MCHC slightly elevated	warm specimen
paraproteinaemia or hyperglobulinaemia	Coulter instruments[28]	MCH and MCHC elevated	colorimeter estimation with addition of clearing agent (see page 13)
high levels of carboxyhaemoglobin	most instruments (minor effect only on Coulter S[8] and stated to have no effect on H.1[55])		inherent in cyanmethaemoglobin methodology

Fig.5.6 Some causes of falsely high estimates of haemoglobin concentration.

exceeds 100×10^9/l. On Coulter instruments some effect may be seen above a WBC of 60–70 $\times 10^9$/l; Ortho and Technicon instruments appear less sensitive to the effect of a high WBC on the Hb. Figure 5.7 is an example of erroneous results for the Hb and red cell indices consequent on a high WBC. When the Hb is falsely elevated the MCH and MCHC will show an equivalent error. The RBC will be falsely elevated by the inclusion of some or all of the white cells in the count. With instruments such as the Coulter S and the Ortho ELT-8 which have no upper threshold for red cell measurements all of the white cells will be counted and sized with the red cells. In the case of the Coulter S Plus IV and related instruments only white cells which fall below the 360 fl threshold will be included in these esti-

mates. In normal blood the ratio of red cells to white cells is approximately 200:1 so that no appreciable error is introduced into red cell indices by the presence of white cells. However in leukaemia with a high WBC the ratio may fall to 10:1. The inclusion of appreciable numbers of the larger white cells with red cells causes a false elevation of the MCV and RDW (Fig.5.7b). The errors in the RBC and MCV are compounded in the PCV. Reasonably accurate results can be obtained as follows.

The specimen is diluted to bring the count within linearity limits and obtain an accurate WBC. The haemoglobin is estimated on a colorimeter with the specimen being centrifuged to remove all white cell debris prior to reading the absorbance. A microhaematocrit

(a)	initial count	corrected results
WBC ($\times 10^9$/l)	+ + + + +	226
RBC ($\times 10^{12}$/l)	1.98	–
Hb (g/dl)	7.7	4.5
PCV	0.196	0.145
MCV (fl)	99.2	–
MCH (pg)	38.9	–
MCHC (g/dl)	39.2	31.7

Fig.5.7 *Erroneous Coulter Counter S Plus IV results consequent on a very high white cell count in acute myeloblastic leukaemia: (a) results produced by instrument compared with corrected results obtained by using the method described in the text; (b) blood count and red cell histogram of the blood sample as obtained from the patient in comparison with those of the sample when partly depleted of its buffy coat showing the effect of the excess white cells on red cell parameters; removing much of the buffy coat has returned parameters towards normal.*

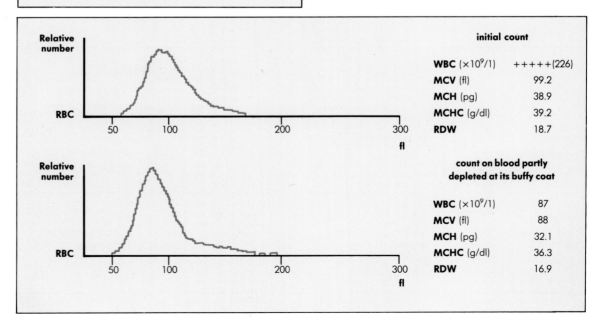

	initial count
WBC ($\times 10^9$/l)	+ + + + +(226)
MCV (fl)	99.2
MCH (pg)	38.9
MCHC (g/dl)	39.2
RDW	18.7

	count on blood partly depleted at its buffy coat
WBC ($\times 10^9$/l)	87
MCV (fl)	88
MCH (pg)	32.1
MCHC (g/dl)	36.3
RDW	16.9

estimation is performed. In the case of an instrument such as the Coulter S with no upper threshold in the red cell channel the RBC is corrected by subtraction of the WBC, and the MCV is calculated from the microhaematocrit and the corrected RBC. The MCH and MCHC can also be calculated. In the case of the S Plus IV it is not possible to determine what proportion of white cells fall below the 360 fl threshold, although in some cases it is clearly substantial. An alternative method which is applicable is to measure the MCV, MCH and MCHC on a blood sample from which the buffy coat has been removed. The RBC can then be calculated from the microhaematocrit and the MCV. The magnitude of the error introduced into the Hb and red cell parameters by a grossly increased white cell count is increased by the fact that anaemia and a low RBC usually coexist with a very high WBC.

Errors due to hyperlipidaemia may be suspected because of fuzzy cell outlines on the blood film (see Fig. 3.6), as well as from the highly abnormal indices (Fig. 5.8); the suspicion may be confirmed by centrifuging the specimen and observing the milky plasma. More accurate results may be obtained in various ways. A haemoglobin concentration can be estimated on a colorimeter with the absorbance of the plasma following addition of the appropriate reagent also being measured; the absorbance of the plasma blank multiplied by $(1 -$ microhaematocrit) is subtracted from the whole blood absorbance. The same technique can be applied on an automated instrument. Alternatively, plasma may be carefully removed and replaced with an equal volume of isotonic fluid prior to performing an automated count. The RBC before and after the replacement has been recommended to confirm that the replacement was done accurately; however hyperlipidaemia sometimes falsely elevates the RBC.[33] A third method can be used with an instrument which accepts a prediluted sample (for example, the Coulter S); the blood sample is mixed with diluent, centrifuged and the supernatant discarded; this is done twice prior to adding a lytic agent and estimating the haemoglobin concentration.

Inaccuracy due to partial failure of lysis of red cells is dealt with by making a more hypotonic lysate, and that due to interfering substances in the plasma by a colorimeter estimation with the use of a clearing agent (see page 13) or a plasma blank. False elevation of the Hb consequent on a paraprotein may be dependent on the interaction of the paraprotein with a specific lysing agent.[59]

(a)	initial count	corrected results
WBC ($\times 10^9/l$)	6.6	–
RBC ($\times 10^{12}/l$)	4.62	–
Hb (g/dl)	14.0	11.7*
PCV	0.364	0.35†
MCV (fl)	78.7	–
MCH (pg)	30.3	–
MCHC (g/dl)	38.5	33.4

(b)	initial count	count following one wash with isotonic diluent	count following two washes with isotonic diluent
WBC ($\times 10^9/l$)	28.4	27.8	26.3
RBC ($\times 10^{12}/l$)	3.37	3.24	2.98
Hb (g/dl)	13.7	10.3	8.3
PCV	0.289	0.278	0.256
MCV (fl)	85.9	85.9	86.0
MCH (pg)	40.7	31.8	27.9
MCHC (g/dl)	47.3	37.0	32.4

(c)	initial count	corrected results
RBC ($\times 10^{12}/l$)	5.36	5.35
Hb (g/dl)	21.5	15.7
PCV	0.435	0.436
MCV (fl)	82	82
MCH (pg)	39.2	28.6
MCHC (g/dl)	24.8	35.9

* following removal of plasma and replacement with isotonic diluent   † microhaematocrit

Fig.5.8 Erroneous results produced by hyperlipidaemia: (a) Coulter S Plus IV: attention is drawn to an error in the estimation of haemoglobin concentration by an improbable result for the MCHC; (b) Coulter S Plus IV: a moderately severe anaemia has been masked by hyperlipidaemia; attention is drawn to the likelihood of an erroneous result by the improbable results for the MCH and MCHC; (c) Coulter S: attention is drawn to a factitious result by the discrepancy between the Hb an the PCV and by the improbably low MCHC (due to a computational error);[32] with a lesser degree of abnormality the MCHC is elevated rather than lowered.

INACCURACIES IN THE RED CELL COUNT

Inaccuracies in the RBC (Fig. 5.9) may result from other particles (WBC or platelets) being counted as red cells, from RBC not being counted because they are below the size threshold or have been lysed, or from agglutination of RBC so that doublets or triplets are counted as single cells.

	SOME CAUSES OF INACCURATE RBC, MCV AND PCV ESTIMATIONS		
Fault	Cause	Instrument on which fault has been observed	Rectification
falsely high RBC	WBC very high	Coulter instruments; Technicon instruments	subtract true WBC from apparent RBC (Coulter S) or count RBC in haemocytometer
	numerous large platelets	Coulter instruments	haemocytometer count
	cryoglobulinaemia cryofibrinogenaemia	Coulter instruments[8]	warm specimen
	hyperlipidaemia (occasionally)	Coulter instruments[33]	use plasma replacement method
falsely low RBC	warm agglutinins	early models of Coulter Counter[5]	mix diluted specimen very thoroughly
	cold agglutinins	Coulter instruments; Ortho instruments; Technicon instruments	warm specimen
	EDTA-dependent pan-agglutination	Coulter instruments[39]	use heparinized sample
	in vitro red cell lysis	all instruments	Hb concentration is still valid and WBC may be accurate but other parameters are invalid
	extreme microcytosis (MCV < 50 fl) causing some cells to fall below the 36 fl lower threshold	Coulter instruments	perform RBC on primary instrument (Coulter B,Z and F series) with threshold set to include all microcytes
falsely high MCV	protein deposition in aperture	Coulter instruments	bleach aperture
	traces of bleach in instrument	Coulter instruments[64]	follow instructions for correct operation of instrument

Fig. 5.9 *Some causes of inaccurate RBC, MCV and PCV estimations.*

	SOME CAUSES OF INACCURATE RBC, MCV AND PCV ESTIMATIONS		
Fault	**Cause**	**Instrument on which fault has been observed**	**Rectification**
falsely high MCV (continued)	WBC very high	Coulter instruments; Ortho instruments [48]	remove buffy coat and repeat estimation
	warm and cold agglutinins and EDTA-dependent pan-agglutinin	see above	see above
	prolonged storage of blood	Coulter instruments	obtain fresh specimen
	hyperosmolar states	Coulter instruments (Coulter S Plus to a greater extent than Coulter S); [3,4,43] Ortho instruments [52]	predilute blood sample or estimate microhaematocrit and calculate MCV using automated RBC which will be valid
falsely low MVC	hypochromic red cells	Coulter instruments; Ortho instruments; Technicon H 6000	count RBC on a primary instrument (as above) and calculate the MCV from the RBC and the microhaematocrit
	increase in ambient temperature	Coulter instruments [64]	temperature control of laboratory is desirable
	hypo-osmolar states	Coulter instruments	predilute aliquot of sample or estimate MCV from microhaematocrit and automated RBC
falsely high PCV	factitious elevation of MCV (except when due to a cold agglutinin)	see above	see above
	factitious reduction of RBC	see above	see above
falsely low PCV	factitious reduction of MCV	see above	see above
	factitious reduction of RBC by extreme microcytosis or red cell lysis	see above	see above
	cold agglutinin	Coulter S Plus series; less often with Ortho instruments [47]	warm specimen

In vitro red cell lysis may have resulted from mishandling of a specimen (for example, accidental freezing), or from the presence of very pathological red cells as when then the erythrocyte membrane has been damaged by bacterial toxins in Clostridial infection. Since haemoglobin is correctly measured but red cell ghosts are not counted as cells, lysis will lead to a false elevation of the MCH and MCHC.

With early Coulter Counters red cell agglutination leading to a falsely low RBC was observed in warm autoimmune haemolytic anaemia,[5] but with the later automated counters the mixing of the diluted specimen within the instrument appears to be adequate to break up these agglutinates and produce an accurate count.[5] With all Coulter instruments, however, cold agglutinins produce a factitious lowering of the RBC and an elevation of the MCV (Fig.5.10a). The RBC is low both because doublets and triplets are counted as single cells,

and also, for the S Plus IV and related instruments, because clumps of cells greater than 360 fl in size are excluded entirely from the count. The size of doublets and triplets is underestimated. The combination of these factors means that although MCV is overestimated, PCV (MCV × RBC) is underestimated. The underestimation of the PCV means that there is a factitious elevation of the MCHC (Hb/PCV). The MCH is also elevated, as a consequence of the falsely low RBC. An erroneous result is usually suspected from the marked elevation of the MCHC (Fig.5.10a). Occasionally the red cell histogram of a Coulter S Plus IV may show an abnormality consequent on the presence of doublets or triplets but this is usually quite difficult to detect. As with hyperlipidaemic samples, a Coulter S counter may, when presented with blood containing a potent cold agglutinin, be unable to correctly compute the result and may produce a very low estimate of the

	count on specimen which had been at room temperature for several hours	count following rewarming specimen to 37°C
WBC (×10⁹/1)	6.2	6.7
RBC (×10¹²/1)	1.07	2.71
Hb (g/dl)	9.5	9.5
PCV	0.118	0.276
MCV (fl)	110	102
MCH (pg)	88.8	34.3
MCHC (g/dl)	80.5	33.7

	count on specimen which had been at room temperature for several hours	count following rewarming specimen to 37°C
WBC (×10⁹/1)	3.0	4.3
RBC (×10¹²/1)	0.40	3.31
Hb (g/dl)	12.4	12.4
PCV	0.154	0.352
MCV (fl)	385	106
MCH (pg)	99.9	37.5
MCHC (g/dl)	80.5	35.2

Fig.5.10 (a) *Erroneous results produced by a Coulter S Plus IV on a sample from a patient with a cold agglutinin. The patient had chronic cold haemagglutinin disease and had a mild macrocytosis due to reticulocytosis, superimposed on which was a factitious macrocytosis due to the cold agglutinin.*

(b) *Erroneous results produced by an Ortho ELT 1500 automated counter on a patient with a cold agglutinin.*

MCHC, half the figure which should have been calculated; with a lesser abnormality a falsely high MCHC is seen. Ortho instruments may also show a factitious elevation of the MCV in the presence of cold agglutinin (Fig. 5.10b). The MCHC may be elevated but this is not always so, and it is thus less readily apparent that the elevated MCV is factitious. The error in the PCV is also usually less than with the Coulter S Plus IV. The lesser effect on PCV and MCHC with Ortho instruments is attributable to there being no upper threshold in the red cell channel; large clumps are therefore not excluded although their size may be underestimated.[47] The lack of an upper threshold means that very high MCVs may be recorded (Fig. 5.10b). An elevated MCV is an indication to examine a blood film (see Fig. 3.7) so that all erroneous results due to cold agglutinins should be readily detected. The frequency of this phenomenon depends on the ambient temperature in the laboratory and the degree of chilling of the specimen which has occurred during transport. The detection of an erroneous elevation of the MCV on an automated counter often alerts laboratory staff to the presence of a cold agglutinin which may be of diagnostic significance.

INACCURACIES IN THE MCV
Falsely high MCVs due to a marked elevation of the white cell count or the presence of a cold agglutinin have been discussed above. Inaccuracy of lesser magnitude is introduced when there are appreciable numbers of large platelets falling above the threshold set for red cell detection and sizing. A falsely high MCV can also occur with faulty maintenance and operation of an instrument (Fig. 5.9).

When there is extreme microcytosis the exclusion from sizing of that proportion of the red cells which fall below the threshold could lead to an elevation of the measured MCV above the true value. This factor is generally more than counterbalanced by the fact that microcytic cells are usually also hypochromic and the size of hypochromic cells is underestimated by the majority of automated counters (see page 23). Only in the fragmentation syndromes where there may be numerous normochromic fragments is the net result of microcytosis likely to be an estimate of the MCV which is above the true value.

Various changes in plasma osmolarity also lead to artefacts in the measurement of the MCV. If a cell is in a hyperosmolar environment *in vivo* due, for example, to severe hypernatraemia or severe hyperglycaemia, then the cytoplasm of the cell will also be hyperosmolar.

When the blood is diluted within the automated counter in a medium of much lower osmolarity then the more rapid movement of water than of electrolytes, glucose or urea across the cell membrane will lead to acute swelling of the cell which will be detected in the measured MCV. Since the PCV is calculated from the MCV it will also be increased whereas the MCHC is correspondingly reduced. This phenomenon has been observed in hypernatraemic dehydration,[3] severe uraemia,[3] and in hyperglycaemia due to uncontrolled diabetes mellitus[52] or intravenous feeding with carbohydrate in high concentrations.[2] Not only may a factitious macrocytosis be produced, but true microcytosis may be masked. Spurious macrocytosis due to an osmotic effect is more important with the S Plus series of instruments than with the Coulter S as the interval between the dilution of the aliquot of blood and the sizing of the red cells is shorter with the former instrument.[43] The converse error of a falsely low MCV and PCV with elevation of the MCHC may be seen in patients with hyponatraemia[3] such as may be seen in chronic alcoholics and patients with inappropriate secretion of antidiuretic hormone. Hypo-osmolar states may lead to the masking of a true macrocytosis as well as to a factitious microcytosis. The prior dilution of a blood sample in a solution isotonic with normal blood allows equilibration of solutes across the red cell membrane so that the cellular swelling or shrinking on exposure to the diluent is no more or less than that of a normal cell and a more accurate estimation of MCV is produced.

The 'isotonic' diluents used in automated counters are in fact somewhat hypertonic, and diluents of somewhat different osmolarity are recommended for different instruments. This does not introduce any systematic inaccuracy into MCV measurements as long as instruments are standardized using PCV measurements of normal red cells. However when such a solution is being used to determine whether or not an erroneous result has occurred by the above mechanism a control sample should be pre-diluted and tested in parallel.

INACCURACIES IN THE PCV
Since in most automated instruments PCV is estimated from the RBC and the MCV inaccuracies in its estimation are consequent on inaccuracies in one or both of these parameters (Fig. 5.9). Older instruments which used alternative technology to estimate PCV had errors of other types (see page 18).

INACCURACIES IN THE MCH AND MCHC

Since the MCH and MCHC are computed from other parameters errors in their estimation are generally consequent on errors in one or more of the measured parameters (Fig.5.11). Since a true elevation of the MCHC is uncommon an elevation is an indication to consider the possibility of erroneous results.

Computational errors may lead to a very low MCHC on the Coulter S when the instrument is presented with a grossly abnormal sample as in hyperlipidaemia (Fig.5.8c) or when a potent cold agglutinin is present.

VALIDATING THE PLATELET COUNT

Automated and semi-automated haematology counters may count platelets in platelet-rich plasma or in whole blood, either in the presence of intact red cells or following red cell lysis. Some of the causes of inaccurate platelet counts are shown in Figs 5.12 and 5.13. Both falsely low counts and falsely normal counts in the presence of severe thrombocytopenia may have important consequences for patients and it is imperative that the laboratory detect such errors. A platelet count can only be considered validated when all unexpectedly low

Fig.5.11 Some causes of inaccurate estimations of the MCH and MCHC.

SOME CAUSES OF INACCURATE MCH AND MCHC ESTIMATIONS	
Fault	**Mechanisms**
MCH falsely high	factitious elevation of Hb concentration (see above)
	factitious reduction of RBC (see above)
	acute in vivo haemolysis with the presence of free plasma haemoglobin
	protein deposition in aperture of impedance counters[23]
MCH falsely low	in theory could occur with factitious elevation of RBC by giant platelets but does not occur with other causes of falsely elevated RBC since there is a simultaneous false elevation of the Hb
MCHC falsely high or true fall of MCHC masked	factitious elevation of Hb concentration
	acute in vivo haemolysis with free haemoglobin in plasma
	factitious reduction of PCV or the product of MCV and RBC (see above)
MCHC falsely low	computational error (see text)
	factitious elevation of MCV (with the exception of that due to cold agglutinins, unless a computational error also occurs) (see above)
	factitious elevation of RBC by giant platelets

SOME CAUSES OF FALSELY HIGH PLATELET COUNTS WITH AUTOMATED AND SEMI-AUTOMATED BLOOD CELL COUNTERS			
Methodology	Cause	Instrument on which fault may occur	Detection of fault
platelets counted in platelet-rich plasma	haemolysed sample; red cell fragments counted as platelets[6]	semi-automated impedance counters	observation of sample
	failure to correct for platelet-poor plasma trapped in red cells	early semi-automated impedance counters	will not occur if correct procedures are followed
platelets counted in whole blood in the presence of intact red cells	red cell fragments or microcytic red cells counted as platelets	impedance counters including Coulter S Plus series and other recent Coulter instruments, and also the Clay-Adams Ultra-Flo 100; Ortho ELT8 and ELT 1500; Technicon H 6000	blood film; flagging; abnormal histograms or scattergrams
	white cell fragments counted as platelets		
	red cell ghosts following in vitro lysis counted as platelets	H 6000[54]	
	haemoglobin H disease	Coulter and Ortho instruments[28]	blood film; histograms
	cryoglobulin[35]	Coulter instruments	blood film
	bacteria[15]	Ortho ELT-8	flagging
	RBC low	Coulter S Plus (prior to modification)[12]	
	RBC falsely low	UltraFlo 100	MCV raised
platelets counted in whole blood following lysis of red cells	white cells and NRBC counted with platelets		subtract white cells and NRBC from platelet count
	white cell fragments counted with platelets		blood film
	malarial parasites, Howell–Jolly bodies, Heinz bodies, Pappenheimer bodies, erythrocyte debris formed when red cells are aggregated by anti-bodies or agglutinating paraproteins[31]	Technicon Hemalog 8 and Autocounter	blood film
	abnormal plasma proteins generating particles counted as platelets[20]		blood film (rouleaux indicating presence of abnormal protein)
	low RBC[10]	Technicon Autocounter	

Fig.5.12 Some causes of falsely elevated platelet counts.

SOME CAUSES OF FALSELY LOW PLATELET COUNTS WITH AUTOMATED AND SEMI-AUTOMATED PLATELET COUNTING INSTRUMENTS			
Method	**Cause**	**Instrument**	**Detection**
all methodologies	partial clotting of specimen	all instruments	inspect sample
	platelet aggregation (including EDTA-induced aggregation)		blood film; flagging; abnormal histogram; HPX alarm
	platelet satellitism		blood film
platelets counted in platelet-rich plasma	loss of platelets during preparation (e.g. giant platelets)	semi-automated impedance counters	blood film; haemocytometer count
	contaminating red cells[6]		blood film
	high WBC (> $50 \times 10^9/1$)[6]		blood film and WBC
	failure to correct for coincidence	earlier semi-automated impedance counters without automatic coincidence correction	will not occur with correct laboratory procedures
platelets counted in whole blood in the presence of intact red cells	giant platelets	all commonly used instruments	blood film; flagging; abnormal histogram
	RBC high[10]	Coulter S Plus series	
platelets counted in whole blood following red cell lysis	RBC high	Technicon Autocounter[10]	

Fig.5.13 *Some causes of falsely low platelet counts.*

counts and all flagged counts have been verified on a blood film.

Falsely high platelet counts are consequent on particles other than platelets being counted with the platelets (Fig.5.12). Such particles may be present in a reagent (causing a high background count), may be present in the blood sample, or may be generated by an interaction between the blood sample and the reagents. The commonest particles to be falsely counted as platelets are microcytic red cells or red cell fragments.

When platelets are counted in the presence of intact red cells inaccuracies may be introduced by an overlapping in size between the red cell and platelet populations. This may be due either to giant platelets being counted with red cells or fragmented or microcytic red cells being counted with platelets. Most instruments in these circumstances will fail to produce a platelet count or will 'flag' the result (Fig.5.14). However sometimes inaccurate counts are produced and are unflagged (Fig.5.15). The degree of inaccuracy produced by giant platelets or microcytic red cells is determined by the threshold up to which particles are classified as platelets. The Technicon Hemalog 8 has no effective upper threshold so that all giant platelets will be counted (but so will be the white cells). Other instruments exclude particles above a certain size from the platelet count.

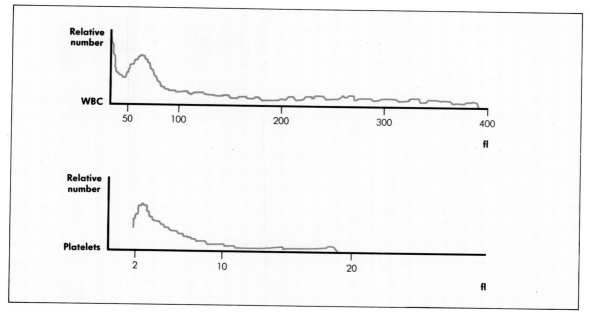

Fig.5.14 *White cell and platelet histograms from a Coulter S Plus IV counter showing an abnormality consequent on the presence of giant platelets in a patient with Bernard–Soulier syndrome. The platelet histogram was rejected for computation; the giant* platelets are apparent on the white cell histogram where they caused backlighting and an R1 flag. The count of particles between 2 and 20 fl was $30 \times 10^9/1$; the haemocytometer count was $35 \times 10^9/1$.

Before discussing inaccuracies with impedance counters consequent on the overlapping of red cell and platelet sizes it is necessary to consider how such instruments are calibrated. Originally there was no standard recommended procedure for platelet size calibration; this was carried out either by means of erythrocytes (from their MCVs) or by means of monodisperse polymer latex spheres of known diameter (and therefore of calculable volume). However the impedance counter responds differently to the two types of particle so that erythrocytes of 85 fl produce electrical pulses of similar height to those produced by latex spheres of about 65 fl. On current models of Coulter Counter such as the Coulter S Plus IV calibration of platelet size is by latex spheres and thresholds are set at 2 and 20 fl. After confirming a log-normal distribution of platelet size a curve is fitted which extrapolates to include particles between zero and 70 fl in the count; if criteria for fitting a curve are not met then the actual count of particles between 2 and 20 fl is available, but flagged. Other current Coulter instruments which also count platelets in whole blood, such as the S880 and the T660, classify as platelets only those particles between 2 and 20 fl, relative to latex calibration, and flag samples which lack the normal

trough below and above these thresholds. Earlier Coulter instruments which counted platelets in platelet-rich plasma such as the Thrombocounter and the Thrombocounter C were calibrated by means of red cells. Thresholds on early models were set at 3 and 30 fl[41] and on later models at 3 and 36 or 2.7 and 37 fl.[62] These thresholds are essentially the same as thresholds of 2 and 20 fl when latex spheres are used for calibrating. The setting of the upper threshold is less critical with instruments counting on platelet-rich plasma as contaminating red cells are not usually present. A further complication in platelet counting and sizing was introduced in 1983 when the size assigned to latex spheres used as calibrants in the UK was changed from 8.6 to 9.3 fl, bringing the calibration of UK instruments into line with those in the USA.

Impedance counters produced by other manufacturers classify as platelets particles between 2 or 3 fl and either 20, 30 or 40 fl. Some instruments will automatically set the upper threshold to a lower level if interference suggests that microcytic red cells are present; this avoids counting red cells as platelets although at the cost of excluding a small proportion of the platelets. One impedance counter, the Toa E-5000M, has moving lower and

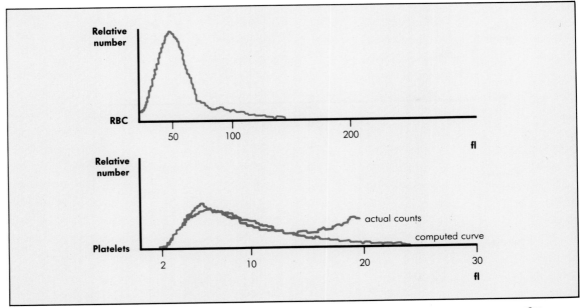

Fig.5.15 *Coulter S Plus IV platelet and red cell histograms associated with a factitiously high platelet count in a patient with severe microcytosis due to iron deficiency plus haemoglobin C trait. The automated MCV was 52 fl and the automated platelet count was 801×10⁹/l (unflagged). The blood showed the platelet count to be normal and the haemocytometer count was 456×10⁹/l.*

upper thresholds at 2–6 fl and 12–30 fl respectively which seek troughs in the histograms.

If no microcytic red cells are present then the logarithmic distribution of platelet size mean that the setting of the upper threshold is less critical than might be thought; unless platelet size is increased the proportion of the platelets which fall between 20 and 70 fl is small.

In whole blood counting methods fragments of white cells may be counted as platelets. Such factitious counts have been observed in acute myeloid leukaemia,[46] hairy cell leukaemia[49] and lymphoma;[50] it is theoretically possible that this could also occur with fragments of reactive neutrophils.[21]

When platelets are counted in whole blood following lysis of red cells any intracellular particles of similar size to the platelets are counted with them (see Fig.5.12). This will only be detected by comparison with a blood film. The presence of a paraprotein may also lead to a factitious elevation of the platelet count which may be due to an interaction of the paraprotein with red cells or to an abnormality in the plasma which does not require the presence of red cells to be manifest.[20]

When platelets are counted in platelet-rich plasma inaccuracy may be consequent on failure to correct for the platelet-free plasma which is trapped in the red cell column. The necessity for this correction was first demonstrated by Bull et al.[6] The need for it was subsequently questioned by Gottfried et al.[17] but the initial observations have been validated.[61,63]

One automated whole blood platelet counter using impedance technology to count platelets in whole blood (the Clay Adams Ultra-Flo 100) calculates the platelet count from the ratio of platelet-sized particles and red cell-sized particles. If the RBC (which has to be measured on another instrument and dialled into the platelet counter) is falsely low, for example because of the presence of a cold agglutinin, a falsely elevated platelet count will be produced.[18]

Falsely low platelet counts (see Fig.5.13) are more common than falsely high counts and the error is most often due to partial clotting of the specimen or platelet aggregation. Platelet counts which are unexpectedly low require the inspection of the specimen for small clots, and the examination of a blood film for platelet

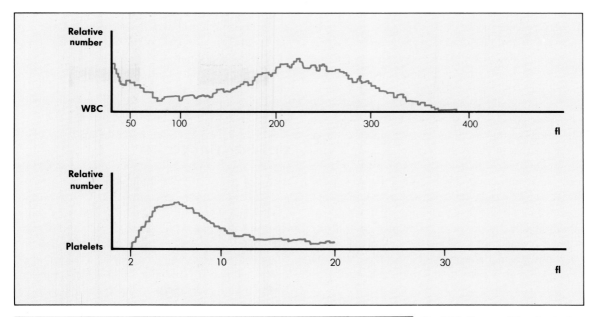

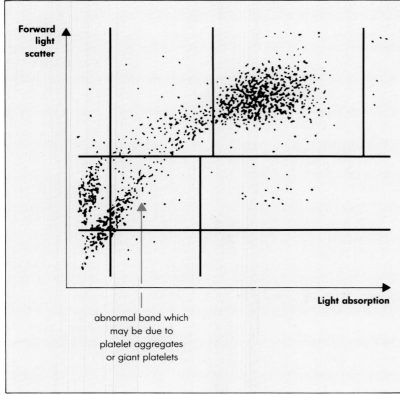

abnormal band which
may be due to
platelet aggregates
or giant platelets

Fig.5.16 *Abnormalities due to the presence of platelet aggregates: (a) Coulter S Plus IV white cell and platelet histograms showing respectively: (i) an abnormality below the 35fl white cell threshold due to the presence of platelet aggregates and (ii) an irregular histogram of smoothed data between 2 and 20 fl; as data do not conform to the expected distribution a logarithmic curve from 0–70 fl has not been fitted and a platelet count has not been computed; (b) Technicon H6000 peroxidase scattergram showing an abnormal pattern which may be due to either giant platelets or to platelet aggregates. Platelet aggregates may also cause an HPX alarm.*

aggregates or platelet satellitism. Although flagging, or an abnormal histogram or scattergram may alert the operator to the presence of platelet aggregates (Fig.5.16), these aids cannot always be relied on; sometimes a factitiously low platelet count is associated with the presence in the film of large masses of platelets despite a normal histogram and the absence of flagging. This is consequent on the platelet aggregates being large enough to fall into the size range of leucocytes. Platelet aggregation may be consequent on initiation of blood clotting and for this reason it is common in samples from neonates which are often difficult to obtain. It may also be an immunologically-mediated phenomenon. The platelet agglutinins responsible for pseudo-thrombocytopenia may be IgG or IgM antibodies active in the presence of EDTA. Such antibodies may be optimally active at a lower temperature $(0-4°C)$[37] and the aggregation may be time-dependent. In the presence of EDTA-dependent agglutinins an accurate count may be produced by using citrate or heparin as an anticoagulant. Platelet aggregation may also be due to an antibody acting independently of EDTA. Some such agglutinins are also cold agglutinins so that an accurate count may be produced on a fresh sample which has been kept warm.

It is particularly important for laboratory staff to be alert to factitiously low counts consequent on a platelet aggregation since this phenomenon has sometimes led to the misdiagnosis of a patient as suffering from idiopathic thrombocytopenia purpura and has even led to corticosteroid therapy and (in one case) splenectomy.[37]

When platelets are counted in platelet rich plasma a falsely low count may also be due to loss of giant platelets during the sedimentation or centrifugation process. Care in sampling from the platelet-rich plasma is also necessary since the platelet count on the top of the plasma column may be up to 12 percent lower than the platelet count from the middle of the column[25] and accidental aspiration of white cells (mainly a problem when the WBC is elevated) or of red cells will factitiously lower the platelet count.[6] This latter error is due to the presence of platelets being masked if they pass through the counting orifice simultaneously with the larger red cells or white cells. With semi-automated counters technical errors such as faulty setting of thresholds or failure to correct for coincidence will also falsely lower the count.

If a platelet count is very inaccurate then inspection of a blood film will be sufficient to reveal the inaccuracy. If the degree of error is less then it may be useful to estimate the platelet count by either (a) counting platelets in relation to red cells and calculating the platelet count from this ratio and the RBC or (b) counting the number of platelets per high power field. In one study based on the second method it was found that

subjects with a normal platelet count had 7–21 platelets per oil immersion field[1] while a second study found that the sum of platelets in ten oil immersion fields multiplied by two approximated to the platelet count.[34] These relationships will, of course, differ somewhat between different microscopes.

VALIDATING THE AUTOMATED DIFFERENTIAL COUNT

Automated differential counts should be regarded as a means of screening blood samples for an abnormality and, for the majority of instruments, as a means of producing a precise differential count when no major abnormality is present. A normal automated differential count does not totally exclude a significant abnormality; this can only be done by a careful visual examination of a blood film by a skilled observer. Nevertheless automated counts can compare favourably with a routine film examination and 100-cell differential count. The considerations which determine the extent to which a laboratory accepts an automated differential count as a replacement for examination of a blood film include the nature of the patient population, previous laboratory practice and an analysis of the balance between costs and benefits of any policy. Certain validation procedures are required before an automated count can be accepted as a valid result.

IMAGE RECOGNITION INSTRUMENTS
Image recognition instruments misclassify some normal cells but this is not frequent in well spread and stained films. Abnormal cells are usually classified as 'suspect', as are disintegrated cells and stain debris. All 'suspect' cells should be reviewed and identified. If they are few in number and are found to be normal cells their presence can generally be ignored since excluding them from the differential count does not introduce a great deal of inaccuracy. Any abnormal cells should be included in the differential count. Once suspect cells have been reviewed an image-recognition differential can be considered as validated.

FLOW-CYTOCHEMISTRY DIFFERENTIALS
Flow-cytochemistry differentials can be considered validated if there are no 'flags' and if the scattergram either is normal or conforms to what is expected in an

individual patient. An abnormal scattergram or the presence of a 'flag' is an indication to examine a blood film and perform a manual differential count. Some laboratories also consider that an abnormal haemoglobin concentration or platelet count is also an indication to examine a blood film to validate the automated differential count.

The Haemalog D and the H 6000 have generally been found accurate at flagging samples containing blast cells.[11,22,24,36] In the majority of cases the percentage of LUC (large unstained cells) is increased or other flags are present; in the minority of cases only an abnormal scattergram, pseudo-eosinophilia, or the presence of anaemia or thrombocytopenia draws attention to an abnormal sample.[24] Ross and Bardwell[40] found the Hemalog D to be more sensitive than the visual count to the presence of blasts, but the reverse was found by Cranendonk et al.[9] Early investigations of the H.1 counter suggest that the 'suspect blasts' flag is fairly sensitive to the presence of blasts.[60] Sensitivity can be altered by the user. The H.1, like the Hemalog D and the H 6000 may fail to flag the presence of NRBC.[60]

TWO AND THREE COMPONENT SCREENING DIFFERENTIAL COUNTS

The three part screening differential count of the Coulter Counter model S Plus IV and related instruments can be considered validated if there are no flags and if the differential count either is normal or shows only a quantitative abnormality which is consistent with the clinical situation. If flags occur or if an unexpected distributional abnormality is detected a blood film should be examined. Both false positive and false negative flags

occur with a screening differential. Among the abnormalities which may not be flagged are the presence of NRBC, blast cells, lymphoma cells and a elevated eosinophil count. In order to reduce the number of false negatives most laboratories also include an abnormal haemoglobin concentration or platelet count as an indication to examine a blood film. Others consider a blood film should be examined on all new patients, even if the blood count and screening differential count are normal. Yet others consider that an ideal compromise is to examine a blood film on all samples processed, in order to detect morphological abnormalities and abnormal cells present in low frequency, but to make use of the automated granulocyte and lymphocyte counts since their precision is much superior to that of a conventional 100-cell differential count. The automated differential count should be rejected even if unflagged in patients with chronic lymphocytic leukaemia, circulating lymphoma cells, eosinophilia or abnormal cell populations. Similar principles are applicable to the use of other two or three component differential counts based on impedance measurements.

Three component differential counts produced by Ortho instruments using light-scatter methodology can be considered validated if the histograms appear normal and no flags are present. Such instruments may on occasion fail to flag or reject samples containing blast cells, NRBC, hairy cells or Sézary cells.[29,56] The lymphocyte count may be falsely elevated by the presence of NRBC or by non-lysis of red cells but such results are usually flagged. Instruments with a faster throughput (such as the ELT 1500) reject the majority of samples from patients with chronic lymphocytic leukaemia but slower instruments (such as the ELT 8) do not.

References

1. Abbey AP & Belliveau RR (1978) Enumeration of platelets. *American Journal of Clinical Pathology,* **69,** 55–56.
2. Allen SC, Balfour IC & Wise CC (1980) The red cell osmometer. A useful inaccuracy in measurement of mean corpuscular volume. *Journal of Clinical Pathology,* **33,** 430–433.
3. Beautyman W & Bills T (1974) Osmotic error in the measurement of red cell volume. *Lancet,* **ii,** 905–906 (letter).
4. Beautyman W & Bills T (1983) Interference of serum tonicity with the measurement of red cell mean corpuscular volume. *Acta Haematologica,* **70,** 140–141.

5. Brittin GM, Brecher G, Johnson C & Stuart J (1969) Spurious macrocytosis of antibody-coated red cells. *American Journal of Clinical Pathology,* **52,** 237–241.
6. Bull BS, Schneiderman MA & Brecher G (1965) Platelet counts with the Coulter Counter. *American Journal of Clinical Pathology,* **44,** 678–688.
7. Clarke A, Garvey B & Lewis SM (1986) *An evaluation of the Sysmex TOA E5000 analyser.* Department of Health and Social Security.
8. Cornbleet J (1983) Spurious results from automated hematology cell counters. *Laboratory Medicine,* **14,** 509–514.

9. Cranendonk E, Abeling NGGM, Bakker A, de Jong ME & van Gennip AH (1984) Evaluation of the use of the Hemalog D in acute lymphoblastic leukaemia and disseminated non-Hodgkin's lymphoma in childhood. *Acta Haematologica*, **71**, 18–24.

10. Dalton WT, Bollinger P & Drewinko B (1980) A side-by-side evaluation of four platelet-counting instruments. *American Journal of Clinical Pathology*, **74**, 119–134.

11. d'Onofrio D & Mango G (1984) Automated cytochemistry in acute leukaemias. A new approach to the FAB classification based on cell distribution pattern. *Acta Haematologica*, **72**, 221–230.

12. Drewinko B, Bollinger P, Rountree M, Johnston D, Corrigan G, Dalton WT & Trulillo JM (1982) Eight-parameter automated haematology analyzers: comparison of two flow cytometric systems. *American Journal of Clinical Pathology*, **78**, 738–747.

13. Emori HW, Bluestone R & Goldberg LS (1973) Pseudo-leukocytosis associated with cryoglobulinemia. *American Journal of Clinical Pathology*, **60**, 202–204.

14. Gauvin GP, Fox SM, Chin NT & Penoyer K (1987) Evaluation of the Sysmex CC-800/PDA-410 system with trimodal histogram for white cell differential analysis. *Laboratory Medicine*, **18**, 373–381.

15. Gloster ES, Strauss RA, Jiminez JF, Neuberg RW, Berry DH & Turner EJ (1985) Spurious elevated platelet counts associated with bacteremia. *American Journal of Haematology*, **18**, 329–332.

16. Gloster ES & Strauss RA (1985) More on spurious red cell parameters. *American Journal of Clinical Pathology*, **84**, 775–776 (letter).

17. Gottfried EL, Wehman J & Wall B (1976) Electronic platelet counts with the Coulter Counter. *American Journal of Clinical Pathology*, **66**, 506–511.

18. Guthrie DL & Priest CJ (1980) The Ultra-Flo 100 platelet counter: a new approach to platelet counting. *Clinical and Laboratory Haematology*, **2**, 231–242.

19. Haeney MR (1976) Erroneous values for the total white cell count and ESR in patients with cryoglobulinaemia. *Journal of Clinical Pathology*, **29**, 894–897.

20. Hall PC & Ibbotson RM (1974) The influence of paraproteinaemia on the Technicon automated platelet counter. *Journal of Clinical Pathology*, **27**, 583–584.

21. Hanker JJ & Giammara BL (1983) Neutrophil pseudoplatelets: their discrimination by myeloperoxidase determination. *Science*, **220**, 415–417.

22. Hinchcliffe RF, Lilleyman JS, Burrows NF & Swan HT (1981) Use of the Hemalog D automated leucocyte differential counter in the diagnosis and therapy of leukaemia. *Acta Haematologica*, **65**, 79–84.

23. Koepke JA & Protextor TJ (1980) Quality assurance for multichannel hematology instruments. *American Journal of Clinical Pathology*, **75**, 28–33.

24. Lai AP, Martin PJ, Richards JDM, Goldstone AH & Cawley JC (1986) Automated leucocyte differential counts in acute leukaemia: a comparison of the Hemalog D, H 6000 and Coulter S Plus IV. *Clinical and Laboratory Haematology*, **8**, 33–41.

25. Lewis SM, Skelly JV & Cousins S (1981) Automated platelet counting – a reevaluation of the sedimentation method. *Clinical and Laboratory Haematology*, **3**, 215–222.

26. Luke RG, Koepke JA & Siegal RR (1971) The effects of immunosuppresive drugs and uremia on automated leukocyte counts. *American Journal of Clinical Pathology*, **56**, 503–507.

27. Maeda K & Pohlad R (1980) Pseudoleukocytosis due to fibrin strands. *American Journal of Clinical Pathology*, **74**, 497 (Abstract).

28. Mayer K, Chin B, Magnes J, Thaler HT, Lotspeich C & Baisley A (1980) Automated platelet counters. A comparative evaluation of latest instrumentation. *American Journal of Clinical Pathology*, **74**, 135–150.

29. Midyett RA (1985) Let the buyer beware, let the user be aware. *Laboratory Medicine*, **16**, 564 (letter).

30. Moore R, Mahnovski V, Pinkney DS & Lipsey A (1984) Correction for the effects of lipemia in Ortho ELT-8 results. *Laboratory Medicine*, **15**, 476–477.

31. Morton BD, Orringer EP, La Hart LA & Stass SA (1980) Pappenheimer bodies. An additional cause for a spurious platelet count. *American Journal of Clinical Pathology*, **74**, 310–311.

32. Nicholls PD (1977) The erroneous haemoglobin–hyperlipidaemia relationship. *Journal of Clinical Pathology*, **30**, 638–640.

33. Nonsanchuk JS, Roark MF & Wanser C (1974) Anemia masked by triglyceridemia. *America Journal of Clinical Pathology*, **62**, 838–839.

34. Nosanchuk JS, Chang J & Bennett JM (1978) The analytic basis for the use of platelet estimates from peripheral blood smears. *American Journal of Clinical Pathology*, **69**, 383–387.

35. Patel KJ, Hughes CG & Parapia LA (1987) Pseudoleucocytosis and pseudothrombocytosis due to cryoglobulinaemia. *Journal of Clinical Pathology*, **40**, 120–121 (letter).

36. Patterson KG, Cawley JC, Goldstone AH, Richards JDM & Janossy D (1980) A comparison of automated cytochemical analysis and conventional methods in the classification of acute leukaemia. *Clinical and Laboratory Haematology*, **2**, 281–291.

37. Pegels JG, Bruynes ECE, Engelfreit CP & von dem Bornw AEGKr (1982) Pseudothrombocytopenia: an immunological study on platelet antibodies dependent on ethylene diamine tetraacetate. *Blood*, **59**, 157–161.

38. Rabinovitch A (1984) Anticoagulants, platelets and instrument problems. *American Journal of Clinical Pathology*, **82**, 132.

39. Reid ME, Bottenfield LK, Toy PT, Ellison SS & Hart CA (1985) Agglutination of an EDTA blood sample caused by an EDTA-dependent panagglutinin. *American Journal of Clinical Pathology*, **83**, 534–535.

40. Ross DW & Bardwell A (1980) Automated cytochemistry and the white cell differential in leukaemia. *Blood Cells*, **6**, 455–470.

41. Rowan RM, Fraser C, Gray JH & McDonald GA (1977) Evaluation of a semiautomated platelet counting system. *Journal of Clinical Pathology*, **30**, 361–366.

42. Sanders C (1966) Fragility of leucocytes in chronic lymphatic leukaemia. *Journal of Clinical Pathology*, **19**, 526 (letter).

43 Savage RA & Hoffman GC (1983) Clinical significance of osmotic matrix errors producing spurious macrocytosis. *American Journal of Clinical Pathology*, **80,** 861–865.

44 Savage RA (1984) Pseudoleukocytosis due to EDTA-induced platelet clumping. *American Journal of Clinical Pathology*, **81,** 317–322.

45 Schaub CR & Farhi DC (1987) Circulating mucin in Wilms' tumor: a cause of artificial elevation of leukocyte counts (Abstr). *American Journal of Clinical Pathology*, **87,** 413.

46 Shulman G & Yapit MK (1980) Whole blood platelet counts with an impedance-type particle counter. *American Journal of Clinical Pathology*, **73,** 104–106.

47 Solanki DL & Blackburn BC (1985) Spurious red cell parameters due to serum cold agglutinins: observations on the Ortho ELT-8 Cell Counter. *American Journal of Clinical Pathology*, **83,** 218–222.

48 Solanki DL (1985) More on spurious red blood cell parameters. *American Journal of Clinical Pathology*, **84,** 776 (letter).

49 Stass SA, Holloway ML, Slease RB & Schumacher HR (1977) Spurious platelet counts in hairy cell leukemia. *American Journal of Clinical Pathology*, **68,** 530–531.

50 Stass SA, Holloway ML, Peterson V, Creegan WJ, Gallivan M & Schumacher HR (1979) Cytoplasmic fragments causing spurious platelet counts in the leukemic phase of poorly differentiated lymphocytic lymphoma. *American Journal of Clinical Pathology*, **71,** 125–128.

51 Strange CA, Mackie MJ, Marnell JH & McEvoy P (1985) An assessment of the Ortho ELT-800 WBC and three-part WBC screen. *Clinical and Laboratory Haematology*, **7,** 151–156.

52 Strauchen JA, Alston W, Anderson J, Gustafson Z & Fajardo LF (1981) Inaccuracy in automated measurement of hematocrit and corpuscular indices in the presence of severe hyperglycaemia. *Blood*, **57,** 1065–1067.

53 Taft EG, Grossman J, Abraham GN, Leddy JP & Lichtman MA (1973) Pseudoleukocytosis due to cryoprotein crystals. *American Journal of Clinical Pathology*, **60,** 669–671.

54 Technicon Instruments Corporation (1981) *Technicon™ Product Labelling Technicon™ H 6000 system.* Tarrytown, New York: Technicon Instruments Corporation.

55 Technicon Instruments Corporation (1986) *Technicon H.1™ System. (H∗1™) Operators' Guide.* International Division Edition. Tarrytown, New York: Technicon Instruments Corporation.

56 Tisdall PA (1985) Evaluation of a laser-based three-part leukocyte differential analyzer in detection of clinical abnormalities. *Laboratory Medicine*, **16,** 228–233.

57 Tisdall PA (1985) Let the buyer beware, let the user be aware. *Laboratory Medicine*, **16,** 564 (letter).

58 Waddell CC & Shapiro DM (1977) Spuriously low automated blood counts in mucin-producing adenocarcinoma. *American Journal of Clinical Pathology*, **67,** 115–116 (letter).

59 Wallis JP & Ford JM (1987) Incorrect haemoglobin estimation on the Coulter Counter S Plus IV in some patients with IgM paraproteinaemia. *Clinical and Laboratory Haematology*, **9,** 95–96 (letter).

60 Watson TS & Davis RA (1987) Evaluation of the Technicon H.1 Haematology System. *Laboratory Medicine*, **18,** 316–322.

61 Weisbrot IM (1977) Electronic platelet counts. *American Journal of Clinical Pathology*, **67,** 313 (letter).

62 Wertz RK & Koepke JA (1977) A critical analysis of platelet counting methods. *American Journal of Clinical Pathology*, **68,** 195–201.

63 Willson G & Bain BJ (1983) Unpublished observations.

64 Young M & Lawrence ACK (1975) The influence of extraneous factors on Coulter S measurements of the mean corpuscular volume *Journal of Clinical Pathology*, **28,** 12–15.

6. Normal ranges

The interpretation of any laboratory test result requires assessment of whether or not the result is normal. In this context the word normal implies that the test result is that expected in a healthy subject. Ideally the test result would be compared with the result in that particular individual when in a state of optimal health. Since that information is rarely available recourse must be had to comparison with the results of healthy subjects as biologically similar to the subject as possible. Test results have conventionally been compared with normal ranges, such ranges often deriving from text books and being of obscure origin. More recently the concept of reference values has been introduced from clinical chemistry[46] into haematology. Relevant concepts are as follows.

A reference individual is one selected using defined criteria. The reference individual derives from a population which includes all individuals who meet these criteria. A reference sample is a number of reference individuals chosen to represent the reference population. Reference values are test results derived from reference individuals and can be analysed and statistically described: they will have a certain distribution; they will fall within certain limits. The usual method of describing a collection of reference values is in terms of the reference limits which exclude 2.5 percent of the values at either end of the observed range; that is, a reference interval representing the central 95 percent of the observed values is produced. Such a reference interval derived from the sample individuals will be representative of the reference interval of the population from which the sample is derived; the closeness of fit of the two intervals can be represented by the confidence limits of each of the reference limits. Closeness of fit is determined by the size of the sample and by whether the reference individuals have been chosen from the reference population in a way which is free of bias. Reference individuals can be derived from the reference population by random sampling, or can be carefully selected to reflect the mix of age, sex, social class and other variables in the reference population. Reference intervals are commonly described as reference ranges, but this term is not one which has been recommended.

A reference individual is not necessarily healthy, but if a state of good health is included as a criterion for selection then it will be seen that a reference interval may be very similar to a traditional normal range, although more carefully defined.

If reference intervals are to be derived for use by laboratories as normal ranges for the assessment of test results on patients then they should be derived from a population which is in good health but is otherwise similar to the patient population. Allowance must be made for the biological factors which influence test results. Defining criteria must therefore include age, sex and ethnic origin. Pregnant women would normally be excluded unless deriving a reference interval for the assessment of test results during pregnancy. Reference intervals are often derived from test results obtained in carefully controlled conditions with fasting and rested subjects who have abstained from alcohol, cigarettes and drugs, and whose blood samples are collected at a set time of day. Such conditions are not commonly met by patient populations and if reference intervals derived in this manner are used for assessing patients then the known effects of exercise, alcohol and cigarette smoking on laboratory tests must be considered. The site of blood sampling and other variables in the technique of obtaining a blood specimen will also influence the reference values and therefore the reference intervals (Fig.6.1).

In this chapter I have used the term 'normal range' rather than 'reference interval'. The reason for this is that the great majority of ranges for haematological variables which have been published up till now have not been based on samples collected in the carefully controlled circumstances laid down for reference samples. The careful sampling of a reference population is a difficult and expensive procedure which is often beyond the resources of an individual laboratory. The terms 'reference interval' or 'reference range' should not be loosely applied to data collected in other ways.

Normal ranges can be derived not only from a sample of a reference population but also from subjects attending health screening clinics or having annual medical examinations. Blood donors and hospital staff are also often used but are not ideal since their age distribution may not be representative of the community and, in the case of blood donors, some haematological parameters may have been affected by previous blood donations.

Particular problems occur when attempting to derive normal ranges for use in the elderly because of the high prevalence of known and occult disease. It is desirable, if possible, to separate the effects of the increasing prevalence of disease from the effect of the ageing process itself. Similarly it may be difficult in an underdeveloped country to select an adequate population sample which is not adversely affected by malnutrition and subclinical disease. In such circumstances it may be necessary to derive normal ranges from 'elite' individuals (such as the army, police force, nursing staff and medical staff); such individuals will not be typical of the communities from which they are drawn, but their test results will more closely approximate to those which would be expected in an optimal state of health. Problems also occur in communities with a high prevalence of genetic

EFFECT OF METHOD OF OBTAINING BLOOD SPECIMEN ON HAEMATOLOGICAL PARAMETERS

Site of obtaining blood specimen
During the first week of life the Hb, PCV and RBC are approximately 15 percent higher in heel-prick capillary specimens than in venous specimens;[54] in older infants, children and adults no consistent differences have been reported between finger-prick and venous specimens but ear-lobe capillary specimens have Hb, PCV and RBC values 6–17 percent higher than finger-prick or venous specimens.[5,25] In neonates heel-prick specimens have WBC, neutrophil and lymphocyte counts about 20 percent higher than arterial or venous samples.[24] Platelet counts are sometimes lower on capillary samples; counts are most likely to approximate to those of venous blood if there is a free flow of blood and if early drops, excluding the first, are used for the count.

Position of arm
PCV,[33] Hb, and RBC are 2–3 percent higher if the arm is hanging down than if it is at the level of the atrium of the heart.

Use of tourniquet
Hb, PCV and RBC are increased by 2–3 percent by prolonged application of a tourniquet (see page 2).

Nature of anticoagulant
The dilution caused by using a liquid anticoagulant causes a slight reduction of cell counts, Hb and PCV.

Fig. 6.1 *Some effects of the method of obtaining the blood specimen on haematological parameters.*

abnormalities. In deriving normal ranges for red cell parameters it is necessary to exclude subjects with β-thalassaemia trait in communities where this disorder is common, and in Black populations where there is a high prevalence of both haemoglobinopathies and thalassaemia it is preferable that these conditions should be specifically excluded. In deriving reference ranges for red cell parameters in children it is desirable to exclude sub-clinical iron deficiency.

Once a set of test results are available they must be dealt with by a statistical technique which is appropriate for the distribution of the data. If data have a Gaussian distribution then a mean and standard deviation (SD) can be estimated and the mean ± 1.96 SD will represent the central 95 percent of the data; the commonly used mean ± 2 SD represents 95.4 percent of the data. The Hb concentration and other red cell parameters can usually be treated as if they have a Gaussian distribution, although even they are not strictly Gaussian.[40] Other haematological data have a skewed distribution with a tail of higher values; this is so for the total WBC and for absolute counts of the various types of leucocytes. If data with this type of distribution are treated inappropriately as if they were Gaussian then the estimates of both the upper and lower limits are too low, and the lower limit is often a negative value. The appropriate management may be a logarithmic transformation of the data, or a more complex transformation may be necessary.[79] If a Gaussian distribution cannot be produced by transformation of the data then a non-parametric analysis must be carried out, that is, one which makes no assumptions about the distribution of the data. The advantage of using transformation to a Gaussian distribution is that a smaller sample is adequate, of the order of 36 samples as opposed to the 120 samples which is the smallest adequate sample for non-parametric analysis.[3] The normal ranges given in this chapter are restricted to those which appear to have been derived in a manner appropriate to the distribution of the data.

Use of the central 95 percent range is arbitrary but gives a reasonable balance between missing a clinically significant abnormality and misclassifying a normal subject as abnormal. However, comparison of a patient's observed value with the laboratory's normal range should be done with the constant awareness that for each test 5 percent of values of healthy subjects will be expected to fall outside the normal range. Conversely an individual may, as a result of a pathological process, have an alteration of the measured parameter away from his own normal value while still remaining within the normal range.

If a laboratory does not derive its own normal ranges but adopts those of others it is necessary to be certain not only that the type of population is similar and the appropriate statistical techniques have been employed but also that the blood sampling techniques and laboratory methods, including methods of calibrating instruments, are identical.

DEMOGRAPHIC VARIABLES AFFECTING HAEMATOLOGICAL PARAMETERS

Sex

Hb, PCV, and RBC are higher in men than in women.

Women in the reproductive age range have a higher WBC than men[6,40] whereas in post-menopausal women the WBC is lower than in men.[29,40]

The platelet count is higher in women than in men.[10,13,71]

Age

Normal values of neonates, infants and children differ widely from those of adults (see Figs 6.8–6.11).

MCV rises gradually during adult life.[21,40,44,65]

Hb rises in women and falls in men between the fifth and seventh decades.[21,29]

Lymphocyte counts fall in old age.

Ethnic origin

The WBC and neutrophil count are lower in Blacks than in Caucasians[43,76] (see Figs 6.4 & 6.6), and are also low in Yemenite Jews.[77] WBCs and differential counts of Indian and Oriental subjects are essentially the same as those of Caucasians of European origin.[12] Eosinophil counts do not vary between healthy subjects of different ethnic groups.[12]

In some studies[14,35,39] but not others[71] Blacks have been found to have lower platelet counts than Caucasians.

Hb, PCV, RBC, MCV and MCH are lower in Blacks than in Caucasians[56] (see Figs 6.5 & 6.7).

Geographic location

Hb, PCV and RBC are higher at higher altitude; in one study the response to moderate altitude was a rise in RBC alone with the MCV being lower whereas at a greater altitude Hb and PCV also rose.[66]

Fig. 6.2 *Some demographic variables affecting haematological parameters.*

EXTRANEOUS INFLUENCES AND BIOLOGICAL VARIABLES AFFECTING HAEMATOLOGICAL PARAMETERS

Diurnal variation
WBC and neutrophil counts are higher in the afternoon than in the morning.[6,36] The eosinophil count is lowest at 10am to midday, and up to twice as high between midnight and 4am.

The platelet count is higher in the afternoon and evening.[70]

The Hb and the PCV are higher in the morning than in the evening.[80]

Pregnancy
The WBC, neutrophil count and monocyte count rise; left shift occurs; lymphocyte, eosinophil and basophil counts fall.[34]

Hb, PCV and RBC fall: MCV rises, on average about 6 fl.

Erythrocyte sedimentation rate rises.

Neutrophil alkaline phosphatase score rises.

The platelet count has been observed to fall during pregnancy[19] but if subjects with pregnancy-related hypertension are excluded no fall is observed.[38]

Labour
There is a further marked rise of the WBC and the neutrophil count together with a steep fall of the eosinophil count and a slight further fall of the lymphocyte count during labour.

Postpartum
WBC and neutrophil counts remain markedly elevated for some days post partum then fall gradually over 4–6 weeks.

Hb, PCV and RBC fall with the lowest level at 3–4 days post partum.

Menstruation
WBC, neutrophil count, and monocyte count fall steeply during menstruation;[7] a reciprocal change is seen in the eosinophil count; the basophil count falls mid-cycle.

Menopause
The WBC and the neutrophil count fall post-menopausally.[2]

The Hb concentration rises.[21,29]

Exercise
WBC and absolute counts of all leucocyte types rise with exercise.

The Hb, PCV and RBC rise.

Bed rest
The Hb, PCV and RBC fall by 5–8 percent after as little as half an hour of bed rest.[81]

Cigarette smoking
WBC, neutrophil, monocyte and lymphocyte counts are higher in smokers[23,44] as are Hb, PCV, MCV and MCH.[23,44]

The ESR is higher in smokers.[45]

Alcohol ingestion
The MCV and MCH rise as a chronic effect of alcohol ingestion; heavy alcohol intake may cause anaemia, leucopenia and thrombocytopenia.

Fig. 6.3 *Some extraneous influences and biological variables affecting haematological parameters.*

Normal ranges in haematology are influenced by a number of biological variables and extraneous influences (Figs 6.2 and 6.3).

Number of subjects		Age (years)		WBC (× 10⁹/l)		Neutrophils (× 10⁹/l)		Lymphocytes (× 10⁹/l)		Monocytes (× 10⁹/l)	
Male	Female	M	F	M	F	M	F	M	F	M	F
198	71	19–30		4.6–11.0	4.5–11.7	1.9–7.3	1.9–8.2	1.3–5.2		0.0–0.87	
642	–	–		4.1–12.1	–	1.8–8.1	–	1.3–4.8	–	0.0–0.85	–
204	22	16–44		4.6 – 10.1		2.0–6.8		1.5–4.0		0.2–0.95	
85	76	54–65		4.0–9.6	3.4–8.2	2.1–6.6	1.8–5.5	1.0–3.8	0.8–3.5	0.06–0.66	0.06–0.7
292	215	15–>70		4.1–10.9		2.3–7.7		0.8–3.1		0.12–0.80	
100	100	18–60		3.5–9.5	4.1–10.9	1.6–6.0	2.0–7.3	1.2–3.5		0.22–0.84	
50	100	18–65		3.6–10.4	4.0–11.6	1.5–7.1	1.7–7.5	1.05–3.55		0.2–0.95	
100	100	18–65		–	4.0–11.6	**Granulocytes** 1.8–7.5	2.1–8.9	1.15–3.25		**Mononuclear cells** 0.16–0.91	0.20–0.8?
86	104	24–56	23–55	4.1–10.9	4.0–10.4	**Granulocytes** 2.1–8.7		1.3–2.9		**Mononuclear cells** 0.2–0.8	
140	159	20–80		4.5–10.3		**Neutrophils** 1.8–6.9		1.2–3.6		**Monocytes** 0.05–0.94	
						2.1–6.8		1.3–3.4 plus LUCᵃ 0.02–0.12		0.05–0.77	
52	50	18–60		4.1–8.4	4.5–11.0	2.0–5.6	2.2–7.7	1.3–3.1 plus LUCᵃ 0.04–0.18		0.19–0.99	

ᵃLUC = large unstained cells; in healthy subjects these are likely to be mainly lymphocytes.   ᵇSubjects with hayfever excluded.

Fig. 6.4 *95 percent ranges for white cell counts in Caucasians.*

NORMAL RANGES FOR ADULTS

Normal ranges for white cell counts and red cell parameters for adult Caucasian subjects are shown in Figs 6.4 and 6.5 and those applicable to adult Black subjects in Figs 6.6 and 6.7. The lower haemoglobin concentration, RBC, PVC and MCV which are observed in Blacks in comparison with Caucasians are not explicable on the basis of a different frequency of iron deficiency. The differences persist when subjects with a haemoglobinopathy or β-thalassaemia trait are excluded but it is very likely that the explanation lies in the high frequency of α-thalassaemia trait (25–30 percent) in Black subjects. The lower WBCs which are observed in Blacks in

Eosinophils (× 10⁹/l)		Basophils (× 10⁹/l)		Methods	Cells counted	Reference
M	F	M	F			
0.0–0.6		0.0–0.19		haemocytometer WBC; manual diff.	200	59; recalculated 6
0.0–0.47	–	0.0–0.27	–	haemocytometer WBC; manual diff.	100	16
0.03–0.86		0.0–0.16		Coulter A or F WBC; manual diff.	200	58
–		–		Coulter B WBC; manual diff.	200	31
0.0–0.49		0.0–0.16		Coulter counter (model unspecified)	200	84
0.02–0.59[b]		0.0–0.13		Coulter S WBC; manual diff.	500	6
0.02–0.9[c]	0.02–0.66[c]	–		Coulter S Plus IV WBC; manual diff.	500	11
–		–		Coulter S Plus IV WBC; automated diff.	≈ 20 000	
–		–		Coulter S Plus IV WBC; automated diff.	≈ 20 000	62
0.0–0.94[c]		0.0–0.16		Coulter S WBC; manual diff.	200	20
0.05–0.73[c]		0.01–0.1		Coulter S WBC; Hemalog D diff.	10 000	
0.03–0.37		0.01–0.11		Hemalog D	10 000	8

[c]Subjects with hayfever not excluded.

comparison with Caucasians may be partly explicable by diet and other extraneous influences, but a true biological difference appears to exist. No difference is observed at birth[22] but a difference appears before the age of one year.[68] Higher eosinophil counts which have been described in Blacks and Indians in the past do not represent a biological difference from Caucasians; such high counts are explicable on the basis of sub-clinical disease, particularly the presence of parasites.

Number of subjects		Age (years)	Country	RBC ($\times 10^{12}$/l)		Haemoglobin concentration (g/dl)		PCV (l/l)	
Male	Female			M	F	M	F	M	F
950[a]	–	17–29	USA	4.31–5.96	–	13.1–16.7	–	0.41–0.51	–
100	100	18–60	UK	4.28–5.49	3.86–4.94	13.1–16.5	12.0–14.7	0.38–0.49	0.36–0.4
183	218	25–34[b]	Canada	4.32–5.74	3.82–5.12	13.4–17.2	11.3–15.2	0.40–0.50	0.35–0.4
4000		21–70	Australia	4.28–5.73	3.83–5.17	12.9–16.9	11.5–15.1	0.37–0.49	0.33–0.4
194	189	20–60	Italy	4.37–5.77	3.87–5.15	13.4–16.8	11.8–15.2	0.39–0.50	0.34–0.4
75	128	17–40	Mexico	4.40–5.90	3.89–5.40	13.7–18.3	11.9–16.3	0.43–0.56	0.38–0.5
74[d]	91[d]			4.96–6.30	4.32–5.58	15.3–19.9	13.1–17.5	0.47–0.59	0.41–0.5
895	991	25–34[b]	USA	4.5–5.4	3.8–5.0	13.8–17.0	11.7–15.2	0.40–0.485	0.35–0.4
51	50	18–60	Australia	4.4–5.7	4.0–5.1	13.1–16.6	11.8–15.0	0.38–0.50	0.34–0.4
				4.4–5.6	3.97–5.11	13.1–16.5	11.8–15.0	0.37–0.49	0.34–0.4
100	100	18–65	UK	4.38–5.71	3.9–4.99	13.4–16.7	11.9–14.7	0.40–0.51[f]	0.36–0.4
86	104	23–56	USA	4.44–5.51	3.89–5.03	12.9–16.6	11.6–14.9	0.386–0.48	0.345–0.4

[a] 92 percent Caucasian, 7 percent Black, 1 percent Oriental.

[b] For ranges for other age bands see original publications.

[c] Iron deficiency and β-thalassaemia trait excluded.

[d] These subjects were living at an altitude of 2670 metres.

Fig. 6.5 *95 percent ranges for red cell parameters in Caucasians.*

MCV (fl)		MCH (pg)		MCHC (g/dl)		Methods	Reference
M	F	M	F	M	F		
81–96	–	26.1–31.5	–	30.4–34.8	–	Hb by haemoglobinometer; RBC by Coulter A; microhaematocrit	41
82–97.1		27.7–32.9		32.1–35.5		Coulter S	6
81–98	80–97	27.4–33.5	26.7–32.7	32.9–35.3	32.1–35	Coulter S	47
77–93	77.3–93.1	26.6–32.8	31.9–37.7	31.9–37.7	32.5–36.5	Coulter S	64
80–96	79–97	27.0–32.7	26.7–33.3	31.7–36.4	32.2–36.2	Coulter S^c	69
87–105	85–103	–		31.7–31.8	30.7–33.5	Coulter S^e	66
86–103	87–103	–		31.8–34.6	31.2–34		
82–98	82–99	27.5–33	27.5–33.5	32.7–36.3	31.9–35.8	Hb by haemoglobinometer; RBC by Coulter ZB1; microhaematocrit	56
80–94		26.5–31.7		31.6–35.5		Hemalog 8	9
80–92		25.0–30.0		31.6–34.5		Coulter S	
82.5–99^f		27.0–32.8		31.7–34.2^f		Coulter S Plus IV	11
.2–95.1	81.6–98.3	27.4–33	27.4–33	33.3–35.2	33.1–34.4	Coulter S Plus IV	62

^{e} Iron deficiency excluded; sampling after overnight fasting.

^{f} 3 percent plasma trapping correction.

Number of subjects		Age (years)	Ethnic origin	WBC (× 10⁹/l)		Neutrophils (× 10⁹/l)		Lymphocytes (× 10⁹/l)	
Male	Female			M	F	M	F	M	F
65	—	16–49	USA Blacks	3.6–10.2	—	1.3–7.4	—	1.45–3.75	—
122	137	18–59	Lesotho	2.5–8.4	2.9–9.1	0.96–6.4		1.0–3.0	0.8–3.3
—	158	16–45	African and West Indian in UK	—	3.1–8.7[a]	—	1.1–6.1[a]	—	1.0–3.6[a]
35	—	18–53	African and West Indian in UK	3.1–10.1[b]	—	1.1–6.2[b]	—	1.3–3.6[b]	—

[a]Subjects rested and fasted; 30 percent African, 70 percent West Indian.

Fig. 6.6 *95 percent ranges for white cell count in Blacks.*

Number of subjects		Age	Ethnic origin	RBC (× 10¹²/l)		Haemoglobin concentration (g/dl)		PCV (l/l)	
Male	Female			M	F	M	F	M	F
122	137	18–59	Lesotho[a]	4.49–5.9	3.85–5.25	13.7–17.8	11.7–16.0	0.41–0.52	0.35–0.4
136	141	25–34	USA Blacks[b]	4.1–5.6	3.6–4.9	12.4–15.9	10.8–14.3	0.38–0.48	0.33–0.4
715	994	21–30	USA Blacks[c]	4.14–5.89	3.67–5.26	12.8–17.2	11.2–15.5	0.38–0.53	0.33–0.4

[a]Biochemical abnormalities and deficiency of iron, vitamin B₁₂ and folic acid excluded.

[b]For other age bands see original publication; this group is directly comparable with the Caucasian subjects in Fig. 6.5.

Fig. 6.7 *95 percent ranges for red cell parameters in Blacks.*

Monocytes (× 10⁹/l)		Eosinophils (× 10⁹/l)		Basophils (× 10⁹/l)		Method	Cells counted	Reference
M	F	M	F	M	F			
0.21–1.05	—	0.03–0.72	—	0–0.16	—	Coulter A or F; manual differential	200	58
0.08–0.6		0–0.28			—	Sysmex electronic counters (CC 110 and CC 120)	200	28
—	0.14–0.77ᵃ	—	0.01–0.82ᵃ	—	0–0.08ᵃ	Coulter S; manual differential	500	12
0.21–0.87ᵇ	—	0.01–0.79ᵇ	—	0–0.14ᵇ	—	Coulter S Plus IV; manual differential	500	15

ᵇSubjects ambulatory and not fasted; 57 percent African, 43 percent West Indian.

MCV (fl)		MCH (pg)		MCHC (g/dl)		Methods	Reference
M	F	M	F	M	F		
81–99		27.2–33.6		32.1–35.5		microhaematocrit; Sysmex electronic counters (CC110 and CC120)	28
79–100	80–100	26.0–32.5	26.0–34.0	31.6–35.3	30.9–35.1	haemoglobinometer; microhaematocrit; Coulter ZBI	56
76–103	74–103	24.9–34.9	24.4–35.1	30.4–38.1	29.9–38.0	JTB 700 electronic counter	21

ᶜFor other age bands see original publication; these are 94 percent ranges rather than 95 percent.

Age	Category	Number	Ethnic origin	Total nucleated cell count ($\times 10^9$/l)	WBC ($\times 10^9$/l)	Neutrophils ($\times 10^9$/l)
cord blood	full term, healthy	106	Caucasian	—	6.0–22.0	4.5–12.0
96 hours	full term, healthy	53	presumably Caucasian	—	—	1.3–6.9
≃ ½ hour	29–44 weeks gestation, basically healthy	434[b]	Caucasian and Black[c]	—	—	~1.9–~5.8
12–14 hours						~7.8–~14.5
72 hours						~1.7–~7.0
5–28 days						~1.8–~5.4
cord blood	full term, unselected	100	Caucasian	5.7–25.1	5.4–23.3	1.7–19.0
		50	Indian	5.3–22.5	4.8–21.2	1.3–16.5
		50	Black	4.9–24.2	4.5–22.7	1.5–15.6
8 days	healthy	52	Caucasian	—	9.0–18.4	2.1–8.0

[a]Observed range, not 95 percent range, for NRBC.   [b]904 counts on 434 babies between birth and 28 days.

Fig. 6.8 95 percent ranges for white cell counts in neonates of various ethnic origins

NORMAL RANGES FOR NEONATES

Some normal ranges for red cell parameters in neonates are shown in Figs 6.8 and 6.9. Ranges applicable to the fetus from 8 weeks of gestation onwards are also available. [53,63]

The haemoglobin concentration, PCV and RBC of the neonate are considerably influenced by the time of umbilical cord clamping since inflow from the placenta increases the blood volume of the neonate by up to 50–60 percent during the first few minutes after birth. The rate of transfer of placental blood to the neonate is increased if ergometrine is administered to the mother to stimulate uterine contraction and is decreased if the baby is held above the level of the mother. During the first few hours of life the plasma volume decreases so that the Hb, PCV and RBC rise appreciably, particularly when late cord clamping has been practiced. WBC and neutrophil counts rise after birth to a peak level at about 12 hours and thereafter fall sharply; the lymphocyte count falls in the first few days of life. [83]

Haematological parameters in the neonate are influenced by certain maternal factors. Maternal fever, prolonged oxytocin administration and rapid or stressful delivery increase the neonate neutrophil count. [49]

Lymphocytes (×10⁹/l)	Monocytes (×10⁹/l)	Eosinophils (×10⁹/l)	NRBC (×10⁹/l)	Methods	Reference
1.0–6.0	0.2–1.6	0.0–0.8	0.0–5.4[a]	haemocytometer; 200-cell differential	50
2.2–7.1	0.2–1.8	0.2–1.9	—	capillary sample; Coulter electronic counter; 200-cell differential	83
—	—	—	—	capillary sample; Coulter S; 100-cell differential	49
1.5–11.1	0.11–3.69	0.05–2.03	0.03–4.8		
0.7–8.0	0.1–3.91	0.03–1.93	0.04–5.6	Coulter S; 500-cell differential	22
1.5–8.6	0.12–3.38	0.03–1.75	0.06–4.6		
3.1–8.4 plus 0.2–0.97 LUC[d]	0.03–0.98	0.16–0.94	0.03–0.11	capillary sample; Hemac 630L WBC; Hemalog D differential	27

[c]No effect of ethnic group on neutrophil count was observed.   [d]LUC=large unstained cells which are mainly large lymphocytes.

Maternal smoking causes a small increase in the neonatal Hb, PCV and MCV and a more substantial decrease in the neutrophil count which persists at least for the first days after birth.[42]

In the neonate, crying increases the WBC and violent crying also causes a left shift of the neutrophils.[24]

Premature babies have lower WBC, neutrophil and lymphocyte counts and higher counts of immature myeloid cells than term babies.[26,83] The reticulocyte count and the MCV are higher.[85] In the premature baby eosinophil counts commonly become elevated at 2–3 weeks of age.[37]

NORMAL RANGES IN INFANTS AND CHILDREN

Some normal ranges applicable to infants and children are shown in Figs 6.10 and 6.11. The iron stores of the neonate are adequate to sustain erythropoiesis for 3 to 5 months depending on whether the infant was full term or premature, and on whether the cord was clamped early or late. Thereafter iron deficiency is common. In deriving normal ranges for red cell parameters it is desirable to exclude infants with iron deficiency, even if apparently healthy, since one of the purposes of having such ranges is to facilitate the diagnosis of deficiency

Age	Period of gestation	Category		Number	Ethnic origin	RBC ($\times 10^{12}$/l)	Haemoglobin concentration (g/dl)
Cord blood	full term	healthy; early cord clamping		221		3.5–6.7	13.7–20.1
Birth–12 hours	full term	healthy			Caucasian (Capetown)	–	
			early	17			15.6–24.0
			late	31			16.3–24.0
13–24 hours		cord clamping	early	46			14.3–22.1
			late	39			16.1–23.6
72–96 hours			early	18			14.2–21.8
			late	19			16.2–23.3
1 day	full term	healthy; early cord clamping		19	Caucasion	3.77–6.51	15.0–23.6
1–2 weeks				32		3.23–6.37	12.8–21.8
3–4 weeks				17		2.82–5.18	10.1–18.3
1 day	24–25 weeks	within 2 SD of weight for gestation; early cord clamping		7	Caucasian	3.81–5.49	16.5–22.3
1 day	28–29 weeks			7		3.15–6.09	15.8–22.8
1 day	32–33 weeks			23		3.51–6.49	14.6–22.4
1 day	36–37 weeks			20		3.94–6.60	15.9–22.5
cord blood	full term	healthy		61	Indian	4.38–5.76	12.9–16.6
1 day				29		4.80–6.02	15.0–22.0
1 day	full term	healthy; haemoglobinopathy and β-thalassaemia trait excluded; α-thalassaemia trait not excluded		191	Black (Jamaica)	4.61–7.55	15.7–27.5
1 week				99		4.02–6.88	13.4–22.4
4 weeks				79		3.12–5.94	9.5–18.1
1 day	full term	healthy; early cord clamping; haemoglobinopathies and thalassaemia not excluded		304	Black (Nigeria)	2.69–5.31	11.6–19.6
2 weeks				233		2.35–4.55	9.4–16.8
4 weeks				117		2.07–3.95	7.5–13.6
1 week	27–36 weeks (mean 33.8)			51		2.88–5.12	11.3–18.8
2 weeks				36		2.25–4.45	8.5–15.7
4 weeks				26		1.69–3.77	6.5–13.5

aFor other periods of gestation see the original publication.

Fig. 6.9 95 percent ranges for red cell parameters in Black, Indian and Caucasian neonates.

PCV (l/l)	MCV (fl)	MCH (pg)	MCHC (g/dl)	Methods		Reference
0.47–0.59	90–118	30.5–36.5	30.9–36.5 (observed range)	haemoglobinometer (oxyhaemoglobin); Wintrobe haematocrit; haemocytometer RBC		50
–	–	–	–	capillary blood; haemoglobinometer (oxyhaemoglobin)		48
0.46–0.75	101–137	37.5 (mean)	27.9–35.3	capillary blood; haemoglobinometer; microhaematocrit; electronic counter		51
0.38–0.70	75–149	39.9 (mean)	26.4–37.8			
0.32–0.54	90–120	35.5 (mean)	30.4–36.6			
0.55–0.71	–	41.7 (mean)	30.8 (mean)	capillary blood; haemoglobinometer; microhaematocrit; electronic counter		85[a]
0.46–0.74	104–157	41.8 (mean)	32.2 (mean)			
0.44–0.76	92–154	37.0 (mean)	30.8 (mean)			
0.50–0.78	96–145	36.4 (mean)	30.0 (mean)			
0.45–0.58	88–116	25.2–38.8	26.0–36.6	cord blood	methods not specified	4
0.48–0.62	–	–	–	venous blood		
	90–118	28.4–42.6	29.4–39.2	capillary blood; haemoglobinometer; microhaematocrit; Coulter ZBI6		75
–	88–116	28.1–37.9	29.5–36.5			
	83–107	25.9–35.3	29.9–36.1			
0.32–0.58	113 (mean)	38.9 (mean)	34.6 (mean)	venous blood; haemoglobinometer; microhaematocrit; haemocytometer		73
0.31–0.47	113 (mean)	37.9 (mean)	33.5 (mean)			
0.24–0.41	108 (mean)	35.1 (mean)	33.2 (mean)			
0.34–0.57	113 (mean)	37.7 (mean)	33.3 (mean)			
0.27–0.47	110 (mean)	36.0 (mean)	32.6 (mean)			
0.18–0.41	107 (mean)	36.6 (mean)	34.2 (mean)			

Age	Number	Ethnic origin	WBC (×10⁹/l)	Neutrophils (×10⁹/l)	Lymphocytes (×10⁹/l)
4–7 years	43 male, 43 female	Caucasian (USA)	6.3–16.2	1.6–9.0	2.2–9.8
8–14 years	83 male, 72 female		4.9–13.7	1.4–7.5	1.9–7.6
9 days–1 year	47		7.3–16.6		3.4–9.4
1 year	67		5.6–17.0	1.5–6.9	2.5–8.6
2	82				2.2–7.7
3	55				1.7–5.5
4	56		4.9–12.9	1.8–7.7	
5	71				
6	81		4.4–10.6		1.6–4.3
7	85	Caucasian (Holland)			
8	77			1.5–5.9	
9	86				
10	78				
11	87		3.9–9.9		1.4–3.8
12	56				
13	87				
14	53			1.4–5.6	
15 & 16	96			1.7–5.7	

ªRecalculated to make allowances for skewed distribution of white cell counts.

Fig. 6.10 *95 percent ranges for white cell counts in Caucasian infants and children.*

Monocytes ($\times 10^9$/l)	Eosinophils ($\times 10^9$/l)	Basophils ($\times 10^9$/l)	Large unstained cells ($\times 10^9$/l)	Methods	Reference
0.06–1.0	0.0–1.4	0.0–0.26	—	venous blood haemocytometer; 200-cell manual differential	60[a]
0.06–0.8	0.0–0.75	0.0–0.2	—		61[a]
0.21–1.64		0.02–0.17	0.09–0.61		
	0.06–0.62		0.13–0.72		
		0.02–0.12	0.11–0.68		
	0.04–1.19		0.09–0.48		
			0.09–0.38		
	0.09–1.04	0.03–0.12	0.08–0.32		
				capillary blood; Ortho Hemac 630L Counter total WBC; Hemalog D automated differential count (approx. 10 000 cells)	27
0.15–1.28	0.08–1.01				
		0.02–0.12			
			0.07–0.26		
	0.04–0.76				
		0.02–0.1			

Age	Status		Number	Ethnic origin	RBC ($\times 10^{12}$/l)	Haemoglobin concentration (g/dl)
7–8 weeks	full term; early cord clamping		17	Caucasian	2.62–4.18	8.9–13.2
11–12 weeks			13		3.11–4.29	9.5–13.1
8 weeks	see Fig. 6.9	full term	80	Black (Nigeria)	2.46–3.64	7.5–11.3
12 weeks			71		—	7.4–11.8
8 weeks		premature	18		1.92–4.08	6.9–11.2
12 weeks			15		—	7.7–11.0
2 months	see Fig. 6.9 (iron deficiency not excluded)		42	Black (Jamaica)	3.18–4.78	9.1–13.5
3 months			25		3.52–5.20	9.4–13.4
6 months			73		3.90–5.62	9.0–13.0
1 year			73		3.84–5.48	7.6–12.6
2 years			68		3.85–5.53	7.8–13.2
3 years			60		3.51–5.47	8.6–13.4
4 years			35		3.64–5.24	9.6–13.6
5 years			16		3.67–5.13	9.3–14.3
1 month	full term; delayed cord clamping; iron deficiency excluded		240	Caucasian (Finland)	3.3–5.3	10.8–17.0
2 months			241		3.1–4.3	9.4–13.0
4 months			52		3.5–5.1	10.3–14.1
6 months			52		3.9–5.5	11.1–14.1
1 year			56		4.1–5.3	11.3–14.1
4–5 years	iron deficiency not excluded		143	Black (USA)	3.8–5.0	10.2–13.4
7–8 years			151		4.0–5.2	10.3–14.7

[a]For a wider range of ages see reference.   [b]For ranges at higher altitude see reference.

Fig. 6.11 95 percent ranges for red cell parameters in infants and children.

PCV (l/l)	MCV (fl)	MCH (pg)	MCHC (g/dl)	Methods	Reference
0.26–0.40	75–125	32.3 (mean)	28.6–38.8	see Fig. 6.9	51
0.27–0.39	73–103	30.5 (mean)	30.5–39.1		
0.23–0.34	94 (mean)	30.8 (mean)	32.7 (mean)	see Fig. 6.9	73[a]
0.24–0.35	—	—	32.4 (mean)		
0.20–0.32	91 (mean)	30.2 (mean)	31.8 (mean)		
0.20–0.32	—	—	32.8 (mean)		
	77–101	24.3–32.6	29.5–36.0	see Fig. 6.9; capillary blood up to 1 year of age, venous blood thereafter	75[a]
	71–95	22.6–29.6	29.8–36.0		
	62–86	19.1–27.7	28.6–35.2		
	58–86	16.2–27.5	26.4–35.0		
	58–90	16.4–28.6	27.6–35.8		
	64–92	18.7–30.5	28.9–36.7		
	70–94	21.1–31.3	29.8–37.6		
	69–97	21.3–32.3	30.5–37.5		
0.33–0.55	91–112	29–36	28.1–35.5		
0.28–0.42	84–106	27–33.8	28.3–35.3		
0.32–0.44	76–97	25–32.2	28.8–36.6	Coulter S; venous blood	67
0.31–0.41	68–85	24–29.6	32.7–37.3		
0.33–0.41	71–84	24–29.6	32.1–36.5		
0.31–0.40	70–89.5	23.0–30.2	30.6–36.2	Coulter S; capillary blood	72
0.32–0.42	72–89	23.4–30.6	30.8–35.2		

[a]These figures are 94 rather than 95 percent ranges.

(continued next page)

Age	Status	Number		Ethnic origin	RBC (×10¹²/l)	Haemoglobin concentration (g/dl)	
		M	F			M	F
3 months	full term; iron deficiency excluded	404		97 percent Caucasian (Bristol, UK)	—	9.3–13.8	
6 months		152				9.9–13.9	
12 months		107				9.8–13.7	
18 months		81				9.7–15.1	
2 years		86				9.6–14.8	
7 years	healthy; allowance made for effect of iron deficiency	25	29	Caucasian (Norway)	—	10.9–14.2	10.7–14.2
8 years		28	22			11.6–14.4	11.4–14.
9 years		27	23			11.3–13.7	11.2–14.
10 years		84	80			11.5–14.7	11.9–14.6
11 years		19	25			11.9–15.2	11.9–15.0
12 years		33	37			11.8–15.4	12.0–15.2
13 years		34	37			11.5–15.2	11.7–15.0
15 years		80	83			12.6–16.8	11.9–16.4
16 years		90	83			12.9–17.1	11.8–16.0
17 years		67	91			13.1–17.4	12.0–15.7
18 years		121	108			13.8–17.1	11.5–16.3
1–4 years	healthy; altitude 750m; deficiency of iron, folate and vitamin B_{12} excluded	34		Central America & Panama	3.69–5.28	10.7–15.0	
5–8 years		74			3.47–5.37	10.3–15.0	
9–12 years		54			3.67–5.47	11.3–15.2	
6 months–1 year	healthy; iron\deficiency largely excluded	9946 for Hb; 2314 for MCV		Caucasian (USA & Finland)		11.0–14.1	
2–5 years						11.0–14.5	
5–9 years						11.5–14.6	
9–12 years						12.0–15.1	
12–14 years						12.5–15.8	12.0–15.3
14–18 years						13.0–17.0	12.0–15.4

[a]For a wider range of ages see reference.   [b]For ranges at higher altitude see reference.

Fig. 6.11   *95 percent ranges for red cell parameters in infants and children (continued)*

PCV (l/l)		MCV (fl)		MCH (pg)	MCHC (g/dl)		Methods	Reference
M	F	M	F		M	F		
—		—		—			haemoglobinometer; capillary blood	18°
0.35–0.43	0.33–0.44				29.5–35.1	28.5–36.3		
0.39–0.45	0.36–0.44				31.1–35.0	28.6–36.4		
0.32–0.42	0.33–0.46				30.2–37.0	27.9–35.7		
0.33–0.46	0.38–0.45				29.3–37.7	29.6–37.2		
0.36–0.42	0.35–0.45				29.0–37.6	31.1–35.9	haemoglobinometer; microhaematocrit; capillary blood	55
0.36–0.45	0.35–0.47	—	—		30.3–36.5	29.4–37.0		
0.37–0.46	0.35–0.46				27.8–37.2	29.7–36.2		
0.37–0.50	0.37–0.50				29.7–38.5	29.4–40.2		
0.37–0.44	0.37–0.50				30.2–38.4	29.5–38.0		
0.38–0.53	0.38–0.52				30.1–37.7	29.8–37.8		
0.38–0.52	0.39–0.52				30.4–38.2	29.5–37.3		
0.31–0.45		72–100		23.9–34.1	31.4–36.5		haemoglobinometer; microhaematocrit; Coulter B; venous blood	82[b]
0.31–0.44		71–99		24.7–33.3	31.1–36.9			
0.34–0.44		73–99		24.1–33.9	31.2–36.7			
		70–84						
		73–86						
		75–88					Coulter S· venous blood	32[c]
		76–91						
		77–91	76–92					
		78–92	77–92.5					

These figures are 94 rather than 95 percent ranges.

states. Iron deficiency may be excluded by requiring a normal serum ferritin level or transferrin saturation or by administering iron supplements to the infants.

NORMAL RANGES IN PREGNANCY

The haematological changes in normal pregnancy are listed in Fig.6.3 and discussed in Chapter 3. Some ranges applicable to pregnant women are shown in Fig.6.12.

The fall of haemoglobin concentration, PCV and RBC which occurs in pregnancy is consequent on a greater expansion of plasma volume than of total red cell mass. Lowest levels are seen at about 30 weeks. The haemoglobin concentration is usually above 10 g/dl unless there is iron deficiency or some other complicating factor.

NORMAL RANGES FOR PLATELET COUNTS

Some normal ranges for platelet counts at different ages are shown in Fig.6.13. Inaccuracies in platelet counting are common and this is the probable cause of the considerable discrepancies between published ranges.

A recent study found children to have higher platelet counts than adults (Fig.6.13),[57] although in an earlier investigation babies and older children had similar mean counts to adults.[74] Neonates including healthy premature infants have similar mean counts to adults though with a greater spread;[1] it has been suggested that a platelet count of less than 100×10^9/l in a neonate should be regarded as abnormal.[1]

SOME 95% RANGES FOR HAEMATOLOGICAL PARAMETERS DURING PREGNANCY		
Period of gestation (weeks)	Number	Haemoglobin concentration (g/dl)
7–14	26	12.8–13.6
15–22	43	11.4–13.8
23–30	25	10.9–13.8
31–38	86	11.1–13.6
WBC		5.9–13.7×10^9/l**
Neutrophils plus metamyelocytes		3.7–10.8×10^9/l**
Lymphocytes		1.0–3.1×10^9/l*
Monocytes		0.3–1.1×10^9/l**
Eosinophils		0.02–0.33×10^9/l
Basophils		0.0–0.90×10^9/l

** $P < 0.001$
* $P < 0.05$ } Significance of difference from values in non-pregnant women.[6]

Fig. 6.12 *95 percent ranges for haemoglobin concentration and white cell counts during pregnancy:*
(a) *haemoglobin concentration;*[30]

(b) *leucocyte counts in 50 unselected women in the third trimester.*[34]

Number of subjects		Age		Ethnic origin		95 percent range (× 10⁹/l)		Method	Reference
Male	Female					M	F		
50	–	'young'		Caucasian		140–440	–	phase-contrast microscopy	17
45	35	18–29		Caucasian		127–351	165–359	light microscopy[a]	78
						140–340			
1011		not stated		not stated		170–430		Coulter S plus	38
180		not stated		not stated		145–375		phase-contrast microscopy	52
51	50	18–60		Caucasian		162–346		Hemalog 8	9
59	69	18–55		Caucasian		143–379	156–417	Coulter Thrombofuge & Thrombocounter C	10
148	225	18–65	17–63	Caucasian		168–411	188–445	Coulter S Plus III & IV	14
86	104	23–56		not stated		184–370	196–451	Coulter S Plus IV	62
46[b]	–	18–45		Black (Nigeria)		95–278	–	phase-contrast microscopy	35
31[c]	–	24–45				114–322			
200	–	18–30		Black (Zambia)		36–258	–	Coulter FN	39
12	13	median age 29		Black	African	128–365	166–377	Coulter S Plus III or IV	14
10	63	median age 26			West Indian	210–351	160–411		
1417		1–12 months		not stated		300–750[d]		Coulter S Plus IV (795); Ortho ELT 8(622)	57
		1–3 years				250–600[d]			
		3–7 years				250–550[d]			
		7–12 years				200–450[d]			

Adults	Children

[a]Capillary blood.
[b]Mainly peasant farmers; sex not stated but probably male.
[c]'Elite' subjects; sex not stated but probably male.
[d]90 percent ranges.

Fig. 6.13 95 percent ranges for platelet counts in Blacks and Caucasians at all ages.

References

1. Aballi AJ, Puapondh Y & Desposito F (1968) Platelet counts in thriving premature infants. *Pediatrics*, **42**, 684–689.
2. Allen RN & Alexander MK (1968) A sex difference in the leucocyte count. *Journal of Clinical Pathology*, **21**, 691–694.
3. Amador E (1975) Health and normality. *Journal of the American Medical Association*, **232**, 953–955.
4. Aneja S, Manchanda R, Patwari A, Sagreiya K & Bhargava SK (1979) Normal hematological values in newborns. *Indian Pediatrics*, **16**, 781–786.
5. Avoy DR, Canuel ML, Otton BM & Mileski EB (1977) Hemoglobin screening in prospective blood donors: a comparison of methods. *Transfusion*, **17**, 261–264.
6. Bain BJ & England JM (1975) Normal haematological values: sex difference in the neutrophil count. *British Medical Journal*, **i**, 306–309.
7. Bain BJ & England JM (1975) Variations in leucocyte count during menstrual cycle. *British Medical Journal*, **ii**, 473–475.
8. Bain BJ, Neill PJ, Scott D, Scott TJ & Innis MD (1980) Automated differential leucocyte counters: an evaluation of the Hemalog D and a comparison with the Hematrak. I. Principles of Operation; reproducibility and accuracy on normal blood samples. *Pathology*, **12**, 83–100.
9. Bain BJ (1980) Unpublished observations on the Hemalog 8 and Hemalog D, including a comparison with the Coulter S.
10. Bain BJ (1980) A sex difference in the bleeding time. *Thrombosis and Haemostasis*, **43**, 131–132.
11. Bain BJ (1984) Unpublished observations on the S Plus III and S Plus IV.
12. Bain BJ, Seed M & Godsland I (1985) Normal values for peripheral blood white cell counts in women of four different ethnic origins. *Journal of Clinical Pathology*, **37**, 188–193.
13. Bain BJ (1985) Platelet count and platelet size in males and females. *Scandinavian Journal of Haematology*, **35**, 77–79.
14. Bain BJ & Seed M (1986) Platelet count and platelet size in healthy Africans and West Indians. *Clinical and Laboratory Haematology*, **8**, 43–48.
15. Bain BJ (1987) Unpublished observations on WBC in Black men.
16. Blackburn CRB (1947) The normal leucocyte count. *Medical Journal of Australia*, **i**, 525–528.
17. Brecher G & Cronkite EP (1950) Morphology and enumeration of human blood platelets. *Journal of Applied Physiology*, **3**, 365–377.
18. Burman D (1972) Haemoglobin levels in normal infants aged 3 to 24 months, and the effect of iron. *Archives of Diseases in Childhood*, **47**, 261–271.
19. Cairns JW, Mahon A, Waters DAW & Chanarin I (1977) Platelet levels in pregnancy. *Journal of Clinical Pathology*, **30**, 392 (letter).
20. Cairns JW, Healy MJR, Vitek P & Waters DAW (1977) Evaluation of the Hemalog D differential leucocyte counter. *Journal of Clinical Pathology*, **30**, 997–1004.
21. Castro OL, Haddy TB, Rana SR, Worrell KD & Scott RB (1985) Electronically determined red blood cell values in a large number of healthy black adults. *American Journal of Epidemiology*, **121**, 930–936.
22. Chan PCY, Hayes L & Bain BJ (1985) A comparison of white cell counts of cord blood from babies of different ethnic origins. *Annals of Tropical Paediatrics*, **5**, 153–155.
23. Chan-Yeung M, Ferreira P, Frohlich J, Schulzer M & Tan F (1981) The effects of age, smoking and alcohol on routine laboratory tests. *American Journal of Clinical Pathology*, **75**, 320–326.
24. Christensen RD & Rothstein G (1978) Pitfalls in the interpretation of leucocyte counts of newborn infants. *American Journal of Clinical Pathology*, **72**, 608–611.
25. Coburn TJ, Miller WV & Parrill WD (1977) Unacceptable variability of hemoglobin estimation on samples obtained by ear punctures. *Transfusion*, **17**, 265–268.
26. Coulombel L, Dehan M, Tchernia G, Hill C & Vial M (1979) The number of polymorphonuclear leukocytes in relation to gestational age in the newborn. *Acta Paediatrica Scandinavica*, **68**, 709–711.
27. Cranendonk E, van Gennip AH, Abeling NGGM & Behrendt H (1985) Reference values for automated cytochemical differential count of leukocytes in children 0–16 years old: comparison with manually obtained counts from Wright-stained smears. *Journal of Clinical Chemistry and Clinical Biochemistry*, **23**, 663–667.
28. Cross JP & Heyns ADUP (1983) Haematological reference values for the Basotho. *South African Medical Journal*, **63**, 480–483.
29. Cruickshank JM (1970) Some variations in the normal haemoglobin concentration. *British Journal of Haematology*, **18**, 523–529.
30. Cruickshank JM (1970) The effect of parity on the leucocyte count in pregnant and non-pregnant women. *British Journal of Haematology*, **18**, 531–540.
31. Cruickshank JM & Alexander MK (1970) The effect of age, sex, parity, haemoglobin level, and oral contraceptive preparations on the normal leucocyte count. *British Journal of Haematology*, **18**, 541–550.
32. Dallman PR & Siimes MA (1979) Percentile curves for hemoglobin and red cell volume in infancy and childhood. *Journal of Pediatrics*, **94**, 26–31.
33. Eisenberg S (1963) Effect of posture and the position of venous sampling site on the hematocrit and serum protein concentration. *Journal of Laboratory and Clinical Medicine*, **61**, 755–760.
34. England JM & Bain BJ (1976) Annotation: Total and differential leucocyte count. *British Journal of Haematology*, **33**, 1–7.
35. Essien EM, Usanga EA & Ayeni O (1973) The normal platelet count and platelet factor 3 availability in some Nigerian population groups. *Scandinavian Journal of Haematology*, **10**, 378–383.
36. Garrey WE & Bryan WR (1935) Variations in the white blood cell counts. *Physiological Review*, **15**, 597–638.

37. Gibson EL, Vaucher Y & Corrigan JJ (1979) Eosinophilia in premature infants: relationship to weight gain. *Journal of Pediatrics*, **95**, 99–101.

38. Giles C (1981) The platelet count and mean platelet volume. *British Journal of Haematology*, **48**, 31–37.

39. Gill GV, England A & Marshal C (1979) Low platelet counts in Zambians. *Transactions of the Royal Society of Tropical Medicine and Hygiene*, **73**, 111–112.

40. Giorno R, Clifford JH, Beverly S & Rossing RG (1980) Hematology reference values. Analysis by different statistical technics and variations with age and sex. *American Journal of Clinical Pathology*, **74**, 765–770.

41. Greendyke RM, Meriwether WA, Thomas ET, Flintjer JD & Bayliss MW (1962) A suggested revision of normal values for hemoglobin, hematocrit, and erythrocyte count in healthy adult men. *American Journal of Clinical Pathology*, **37**, 429–436.

42. Harrison KL (1979) The effect of maternal smoking on neonatal leucocytes. *Australian and New Zealand Journal of Obstetrics and Gynaecology*, **19**, 166–168.

43. Hawgood BC (1969) Leucocyte levels in East Africa. *East African Medical Journal*, **46**, 680–682.

44. Helman N & Rubenstein LS (1975) The effect of age, sex and smoking on erythrocytes and leukocytes. *American Journal of Clinical Pathology*, **63**, 33–44.

45. Howell RW (1970) Smoking habits and laboratory tests. *Lancet*, **ii**, 152 (letter).

46. International Federation of Clinical Chemistry, Expert panel on the Theory of Reference Values (1978) Provisional Recommendations on the theory of reference values. *Clinica Chimica Acta*, **26**, 383–391.

47. Kelly A & Munan L (1977) Haematological profile of natural populations: red cell parameters. *British Journal of Haematology*, **35**, 153–160.

48. Lazkowsky P (1960) Effects of early and late clamping of umbilical cord on infant's haemoglobin level. *British Medical Journal*, **ii**, 1777–1782.

49. Manroe BL, Weinberg AG, Rosenfeld CR & Browne R (1979) The neonatal blood count in health and disease. I Reference values for neutrophilic cells. *Journal of Pediatrics*, **95**, 89–98.

50. Marks J, Gairdner D & Roscoe JD (1955) Blood formation in infancy. Part III. Cord Blood. *Archives of Diseases in Childhood*, **30**, 117–120.

51. Matoth Y, Zaizov R & Varsano I (1971) Postnatal changes in some red cell parameters. *Acta Paediatrica Scandinavica*, **60**, 317–323.

52. Miale JB (1982) *Laboratory Medicine Hematology*, Sixth Edition. St Louis: CV Mosby.

53. Millar DS, Davis LR, Rodeck CH, Nicolaides KH & Mibashan RS (1985) Normal blood cell values in the early mid-trimester fetus. *Prenatal Diagnosis*, **5**, 367–373.

54. Moe PJ (1981) Nordic attempts to standardize skin-blood specimen collection in infants and children: the newborn baby, a preliminary report. In *Reference Values in Laboratory Medicine*. Edited by R Gräsbeck & W Alström. Chichester: John Wiley & Sons.

55. Natvig H, Vellar OD & Andersen J (1967) Studies on hemoglobin values in Norway. VII. Hemoglobin, hematocrit and MCHC values among boys and girls aged 7–20 years in elementary and grammar schools. *Acta Medica Scandinavica*, **182**, 183–191.

56. (NCHS) National Centre for Health Statistics, Health and Nutrition Examination Survey (HANES II) 1976–1980, derived from Koepke, JA. *Laboratory Hematology, Volume 2*. New York: Churchill Livingstone.

57. Novak RW, Tschantz JA & Krill CE (1987) Normal platelet and mean platelet volumes in pediatric patients. *Laboratory Medicine*, **18**, 613–614.

58. Orfanakis NG, Ostlund RE, Bishop CR & Athens JW (1970) Normal blood leukocyte concentration values. *American Journal of Clinical Pathology*, **53**, 647–651.

59. Osgood EE, Brownlee IE, Osgood MW, Ellis DM & Cohen W (1939) Total, differential and absolute leukocyte counts and sedimentation rates determined for persons nineteen years of age and over. *Archives of Internal Medicine*, **64**, 105–120.

60. Osgood EE, Baker RL, Brownlee IE, Osgood MW, Ellis DM & Cohen W (1939) Total, differential and absolute leukocyte counts and sedimentation rates of healthy children four to seven years of age. *American Journal of Diseases of Children*, **58**, 61–70.

61. Osgood EE, Baker RL, Brownlee IE, Osgood MW, Ellis DM & Cohen W (1939) Total, differential and absolute leukocyte counts and sedimentation rates of healthy children. Standards for children eight to fourteen years of age. *American Journal of Diseases of Children*, **58**, 282–294.

62. Payne BA & Pierre RV (1986) Using the three-part differential. Part 1. Investigating the possibilities. *Laboratory Medicine*, **17**, 459–462.

63. Playfair JHL, Wolfendale MR & Kay HEM (1963) The leucocytes of peripheral blood in the human foetus. *British Journal of Haematology*, **9**, 336–344.

64. Pun ASL, Holliday J & Biggs JC (1979) A survey of haematological values including serum ferritin in two Sydney populations. *Australian and New Zealand Journal of Medicine*, **9**, 615 (Abstract).

65. Pun ASL, Holliday J, Simons LA, Biggs JC & Jones AS (1982) A survey of haematological values in Sydney. *Pathology*, **14**, 149–151.

66. Ruíz-Argüelles GJ, Sánchez-Medal L, Loría A, Piedras J & Córdova MS (1980) Red cell indices in normal adults residing at altitudes from sea level to 2670 meters. *American Journal of Hematology*, **8**, 265–271.

67. Saarinen UM & Siimes MD (1978) Developmental changes in red blood cell counts and indices in infants after exclusion of iron deficiency by laboratory criteria and continuous iron supplementation. *Journal of Pediatrics*, **92**, 412–416.

68. Sadowitz PD & Oski FA (1983) Differences in polymorphonuclear cell counts between healthy white and black infants: response to meningitis. *Pediatrics*, **72**, 405–407.

69. Salvati AM, Camagna A, Samoggia P & Tentori L (1979) Reference values in Haematology. A survey in Italy: report from Latium. *Haematologica*, **64,** 296–308.

70. Saunders A (1980) Predictive value and efficiency of haematology data: discussion. *Blood Cells*, **6,** 185–197.

71. Saxena S, Cramer AD, Weiner JM & Carmel R (1987) Platelet counts in three racial groups. *American Journal of Clinical Pathology*, **88,** 106–109.

72. Schmaier AH, Maurer HM, Johnston CL, Scott RB & Stewart LM (1974) Electronically determined red cell indices in a predominantly urban population of children 4–8 years of age. *Journal of Pediatrics*, **84,** 559–561.

73. Scott-Emuakpor AB, Okolo AA, Omene JA & Ukpe SI (1985) The limits of physiological anemia in the African neonate. *Acta Haematologica*, **74,** 99–103.

74. Sell EJ & Corrigan JJ (1973) Platelet counts, fibrinogen concentrations, and Factor V and Factor VII levels in healthy infants according to gestational age. *Journal of Pediatrics*, **82,** 1028–1032.

75. Serjeant GR, Grandison Y, Mason K, Serjeant B, Sewell A & Vaidya S (1980) Haematological indices in normal negro children: a Jamaican cohort from birth to five years. *Clinical and Laboratory Haematology*, **2,** 169–178.

76. Shaper AG & Lewis P (1971) Genetic neutropenia in people of African origin. *Lancet*, **ii,** 1021–1023.

77. Shoenfeld Y, Weinberger A, Avishar R, Zamir R, Gazit E, Joshua H & Pinkhas J (1978) Familial leukopenia among Yemenite jews. *Israel Journal of Medical Science*, **14,** 1271–1274.

78. Sloan AW (1951) The normal platelet count in man. *Journal of Clinical Pathology*, **4,** 37–46.

79. Solberg EK (1981) Statistical treatment of collected reference values and determination of reference limits. In *Reference Values in Laboratory Medicine*. Edited by R Gräsbeck & W Alström. Chichester: John Wiley & Sons.

80. Stengle JM & Schade AL (1957) Diurnal–nocturnal variations of certain blood constituents in normal human subjects: plasma iron, siderophilin, bilirubin, copper, total serum protein and albumin, haemoglobin and haematocrit. *British Journal of Haematology*, **3,** 117–124.

81. Tombridge TL (1968) Effect of posture on hematology results. *American Journal of Clinical Pathology*, **49,** 491–493.

82. Viteri FE, de Tuna V & Gúzman MA (1972) Normal haematological values in the Central American population. *British Journal of Haematology*, **23,** 189–204.

83. Xanthou M (1970) Leucocyte blood picture in full term and premature babies during neonatal period. *Archives of Diseases in Childhood*, **45,** 242–249.

84. Zacharski LR, Elveback LR & Linman JW (1971) Leukocyte counts in healthy adults. *American Journal of Clinical Pathology*, **56,** 148–150.

85. Zaizov R & Matoth Y (1976) Red cell values on the first postnatal day during the last sixteen weeks of gestation. *American Journal of Haematology*, **1,** 275–278.

7. Important supplementary tests

This chapter deals with some cytochemical techniques which can be usefully applied to peripheral blood cells. Recommended methods are shown in Fig. 7.1.

SOME RECOMMENDED METHODS FOR CYTOCHEMICAL STAINS	
Procedure	**Recommended method**
reticulocyte count	new methylene blue[9] with 15 minutes incubation
haemoglobin H preparation	brilliant cresyl blue with 2 hours incubation[9]
detection of haemoglobin F-containing cells	acid elution[9]
Heinz body preparation	rhodanile blue with 2 minutes incubation[9] or methyl violet
Perls' reaction for iron	potassium ferrocyanide[9]
neutrophil alkaline phosphatase stain	naphthol AS-MX phosphate + fast blue RR*[1]
myeloperoxidase stain	p-phenylenediamine + catechol + H_2O_2*[14]
sudan black B stain	sudan black B*[9]
naphthol AS-D chloroacetate esterase (chloroacetate esterase) stain	naphthol AS-D chloroacetate + hexazotized new fuchsin[33] or fast blue BB[15] or corinth V*
α naphthyl acetate esterase (ANAE) stain OR naphthol AS-D acetate esterase (NASDA) stain	α naphthyl acetate + hexazotized pararosaniline[33] or fast blue RR* naphthol AS-D acetate + fast blue BB[9]
periodic acid-Schiff (PAS) stain	periodic acid + Schiff's reagent[9]
acid phosphatase stain and tartrate-resistant acid phosphatase	naphthol AS-BI phosphate + fast garnet GBC, with and without tartaric acid[17]

* Reagents suitable for these methods can be purchased from Sigma Diagnostics, Sigma Chemical Company, St Louis, Missouri or Sigma Diagnostics, Poole, Dorset BH17 7NH.

Fig. 7.1 *Some recommended methods for cytochemical stains.*

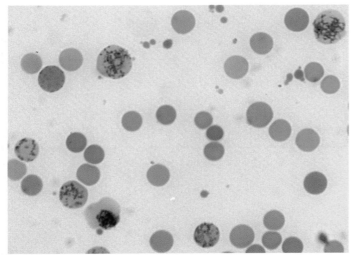

Fig. 7.2 *Reticulocytes stained with new methylene blue:*
(a) *a group I reticulocyte with a dense clump of reticulum*[1], *several group II reticulocytes with a wreath or network of reticulum*[2] *and several group III reticulocytes with a disintegrated wreath of reticulum*[3];

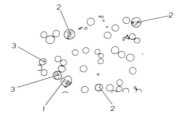

(b) *group II*[1], *III*[2] *and IV*[3] *reticulocytes. The group IV reticulocyte has two granules of reticulum. There is also a cell with a single dot of reticulum*[4]. *By some criteria th would also be classified as a reticulocyte;*

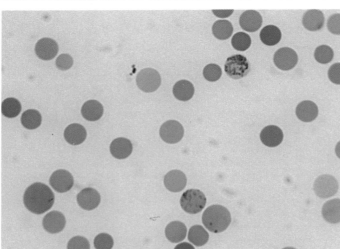

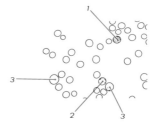

(c) *three reticulocytes*[1] *and a Howell–Jolly body*[2].

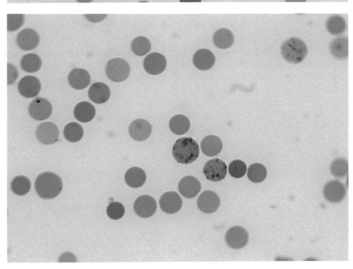

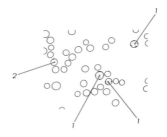

RETICULOCYTES AND THE RETICULOCYTE COUNT

Reticulocytes are young red cells, newly released from the bone marrow, which still contain ribosomal RNA. On exposure of the unfixed cells to certain dyes such as brilliant cresyl blue or new methylene blue the ribosomes are precipitated and stained by the dye, to appear as a reticular network; as the cells are still living when exposed to the dye this may be referred to as supravital staining. With new methylene blue, red cells stain a pale greenish-blue while the reticulum stains bluish-purple.

The amount of reticulum in a reticulocyte varies from a large clump in the most immature cells (Group I reticulocytes) to a few granules in the most mature forms (Group IV reticulocytes) (Fig. 7.2). The difficulty in determining whether one or two dots of appropriately stained material represent RNA has led to various definitions of a reticulocyte being proposed. The minimum requirement varies from a single dot, through two or three dots to a minimum network. Because the majority of reticulocytes in the peripheral blood are Group IV the precise definition of a reticulocyte will

have an appreciable effect on the reticulocyte count. The USA National Committee for Clinical Laboratory Standards classifies as a reticulocyte 'any non-nucleated red cell containing two or more particles of blue stained material corresponding to ribosomal RNA'.[20]

The RNA which, with vital dyes, is responsible for forming the recticulum, gives rise, on a Romanowsky-stained film, to diffuse cytoplasmic basophilia. Not all reticulocytes contain enough RNA to cause polychromasia on a Romanowsky-stained blood film, but whether polychromatic cells correspond only to the least mature reticulocytes (equivalent to Group I reticulocytes)[25] or to all but the most mature reticulocytes (Group I, II and III reticulocytes)[8] is not certain.

In a reticulocyte preparation Heinz bodies, Howell–Jolly bodies and Pappenheimer bodies are also stained (Fig. 7.3). Heinz bodies and Howell–Jolly bodies can be recognized by their characteristic size, shape and position in the cell. Pappenheimer bodies tend to stain a slightly darker blue than the reticulum but they can sometimes be difficult to distinguish from late reticulocytes with only a few granules of reticulo-filamentous material. If necessary, a reticulocyte preparation can be

THE CHARACTERISTIC APPEARANCE OF VARIOUS RED CELL INCLUSIONS ON A NEW METHYLENE BLUE RETICULOCYTE PREPARATION		
Inclusion	**Nature**	**Morphology**
reticulum	ribosomal RNA	reticulo-filamentous material or scanty small granules
Pappenheimer bodies	iron-containing inclusions	one or more granules towards the periphery of the cell; may stain a deeper blue than reticulum
Heinz bodies	denatured haemoglobin	larger than Pappenheimer bodies, irregular in shape, usually attached to the cell membrane and may protrude through it; pale blue
Howell–Jolly bodies	DNA	larger than Pappenheimer bodies, regular in shape, distant from the cell membrane; pale blue
haemoglobin H inclusions	denatured haemoglobin H	usually do not form with short incubation periods; if present they are multiple and spherical giving a 'golf-ball' appearance; pale greenish-blue

Fig. 7.3 The characteristic appearance of various red cell inclusions in a new methylene blue reticulocyte preparation.

counterstained by a Perls' stain (see below), to identify Pappenheimer bodies, or by a Romanowsky stain, to identify Howell–Jolly bodies. Because of the relatively short incubation period haemoglobin H inclusions are not usually apparent in a reticulocyte preparation. However, if present, their characteristic 'golf-ball' appearance (see below) allows their identification. When a reticulocyte preparation is fixed in methanol and counterstained with a Romanowsky stain the vital dye (for example, the new methylene blue) is washed out during the methanol fixation; the reticulum is then stained by the basic component of the Romanowsky stain.[22]

Reticulocytes are usually counted as a percentage of red blood cells. The reticulocytes among at least 1000 red cells should be counted. The use of an eyepiece containing a Miller ocular micrometer disc (Fig. 7.4) facilitates counting; reticulocytes are counted in the large squares and total red cells in the small squares, which are one ninth of the size of the large squares. If 20 fields are counted the reticulocyte count is equal to:

$$\frac{\text{reticulocytes in 20 large squares} \times 100}{\text{erythrocytes in 20 small squares} \times 9} \%$$

When 20 fields are counted then the reticulocytes among approximately 2000 red cells are counted. This gives superior precision to counting the reticulocytes among 1000 red cells without use of an ocular insert.[4] Consecutive rather than random fields should be counted since there is otherwise a tendency to subconsciously select fields with more reticulocytes.[4] Reticulocytes can be counted on blood films prepared by centifugation or by wedge-spreading; they may be more evenly distributed on a film prepared by centrifugation and it has been suggested that precision may therefore be improved.[29]

Reticulocyte counts have traditionally been expressed as a percentage. If the red cell count is available an absolute reticulocyte count, which gives a more accurate impression of bone marrow output, can be calculated. As an alternative a result which is more meaningful than a percentage can be produced by correcting for the degree of anaemia as follows:

$$\frac{\text{reticulocyte}}{\text{index}} = \frac{\text{reticulocyte percentage} \times \text{observed PCV}}{\text{normal PCV}}$$

for example, reticulocyte index $= \frac{1.2 \times 0.29}{0.45} = 0.77$

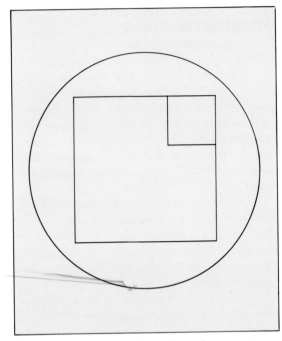

Fig. 7.4 The appearance of a Miller ocular micrometer for use in counting reticulocytes.

This example shows that a reticulocyte percentage which is apparently normal can be demonstrated to be low if allowance is made for the presence of anaemia. This procedure and the use of an absolute reticulocyte count give similar information. A more complex correction[16] can be made which allows for the fact that in anaemic subjects, under the influence of increased levels of erythropoietin, reticulocytes are released prematurely from the bone marrow and spend longer in the blood before becoming mature red cells. The reticulocyte index and the absolute reticulocyte count both give a somewhat false impression of the marrow output of cells in this circumstance. The reticulocyte production index[16] is calculated by dividing the reticulocyte index by the average maturation time of a reticulocyte in the peripheral blood at any degree of anaemia.

Although the absolute reticulocyte count or one of the reticulocyte indices is to be preferred as an indicator of bone marrow output the reticulocyte percentage has the advantage that it gives an indication of red cell life span. If a patient with a stable haemolytic anaemia has a reticulocyte count of 10 percent it is apparent that 1 cell in 10 is less than 1 to 3 days old.

The reticulocyte count is stable with storage of EDTA-anticoagulated blood for up to 24 hours at room temperature.[11]

SOME 95 PERCENT RANGES FOR THE RETICULOCYTE COUNT

Number of subjects	Age in years	Range	Method	Reference
78	20–40	0.8–2.5 percent (mean 1.65) for 48 males; 0.8–4.1 percent (mean 2.45) for 30 females	new methylene blue with Perls' reaction counterstain; cells with a single granule classified as reticulocytes	10
32	not stated	0.4–2.0 percent (mean 1.2) on a wedge-spread film; 0.8–2.4 percent (mean 1.6) on a spun film	new methylene blue; Wright counterstain for spun film	8*
not stated	not stated	$18–158 \times 10^9/l$; (mean $88 \times 10^9/l$)	new methylene blue	21

* 95 percent range calculated from mean and SD assuming a Gaussian distribution.

Fig. 7.5 *Some 95 percent ranges for the reticulocyte count.*

Automated reticulocyte counting is possible either with traditional staining methods and an image recognition instrument, or by flow cytometry following exposure to a dye, such as acridine orange or thioflavin-T, which fluoresces following combination with RNA.[29] Flow cytometry methods are likely to lead to an increase of precision because of the greater number of cells which can be counted and because detection of group IV reticulocytes is more consistent; if reticulocytes with only a single granule of RNA are detectable then it would be expected that counts would be higher than with current techniques.

Some normal ranges for reticulocyte counts are shown in Fig. 7.5 and some causes of high and low reticulocyte counts in Fig. 7.6. When the reticulocyte count is expressed as a percentage it is higher in women than in men[10] (Fig. 7.5). There is no certainty as to what should be regarded as a normal absolute reticulocyte count. It has been suggested that the count should be below $84 \times 10^9/l$[23] or below $40 \times 10^9/l$[7] whereas others have found average counts of $88 \times 10^9/l$[21] and approximately $60 \times 10^9/l$[2] respectively. The reticulocyte count is higher in the neonatal period than later in life. At birth the count is 2–6 percent; there is a rise during the first three days to levels of 3–9 percent followed by a fall around day 8–10 to levels similar to those of the adult.[13,22]

SOME CAUSES OF INCREASED AND DECREASED PERCENTAGES OF RETICULOCYTES

Some causes of an increased percentage of reticulocytes

neonatal period
pregnancy
ascent to altitude
response to haemorrhage or haemolysis
shock or hypoxia
replacement of iron, vitamin B_{12} or folic acid in a deficient patient
recovery from bone marrow failure or suppression
bone marrow infiltration
idiopathic myelofibrosis

Some causes of a decreased reticulocyte percentage (and absolute count)

suppression of erythropoiesis, e.g. by infection or inflammation
pure red cell aplasia
aplastic anaemia
ineffective erythropoiesis, e.g. thalassaemia major
severe iron deficiency
megaloblastic anaemia

Fig. 7.6 *Some causes of increased and decreased percentages of reticulocytes.*

HEINZ BODIES

Heinz bodies are red cell inclusions composed of denatured haemoglobin. They can be seen as refractile bodies in dry unstained films viewed with the condenser wound down. They can be stained by a variety of vital dyes including methyl violet, cresyl violet, new methylene blue, brilliant cresyl blue, brilliant green and rhodanile blue. Their characteristic size and shape (see Figs 7.3 and 7.7) aid in their identification. Heinz bodies are not seen in normal subjects since they are removed from the cell by the spleen, a process known as 'pitting'. Small numbers are seen in the blood of splenectomized subjects. Larger numbers are found following exposure to oxidant drugs or chemicals, particularly in subjects who are deficient in glucose-6-phosphate dehydrogenase or who have been splenectomized, and in patients with an unstable haemoglobin who have been splenectomized. Patients with an unstable haemoglobin who have not been splenectomized may not show Heinz bodies, but some may form after prolonged *in vitro* incubation.

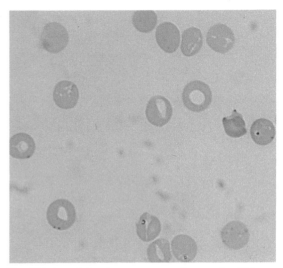

Fig. 7.7 *A methyl violet preparation showing five Heinz bodies. The blood sample was from a patient who had been exposed to dapsone, an oxidant drug.*

HAEMOGLOBIN H DETECTION

Haemoglobin H (a haemoglobin with no α chains but with a β chain tetramer) is denatured and stained by the same vital dyes which stain reticulocytes. The characteristic small regular 'golf-ball' inclusions (Fig. 7.8a) take longer to appear than the reticulum of a reticulocyte. An incubation period of 2 hours is recommended. It is important that either new methylene blue or brilliant cresyl blue is used in a haemoglobin H preparation in order to demonstrate the characteristic inclusions. Methylene blue (which is sometimes sold by manufacturers wrongly identified as new methylene blue) does not give the typical appearance.[12,32] Patients with haemoglobin H who have not been splenectomized show the characteristic 'golf-ball' appearance; patients who have been splenectomized have, in addition, preformed inclusions of haemoglobin H which are similar to Heinz bodies (Fig. 7.8b). Cells containing haemoglobin H are readily detected in patients with haemoglobin H disease, in whom they may comprise the majority of the cells. In patients with α-thalassaemia trait their frequency is of the order of one per thousand cells (when two of four α genes are missing) or less (when one of four α genes is missing); even when a prolonged search is made, they are not always detectable. Haemoglobin H inclusions are not found in the red cells of haematologically normal subjects; apparently similar inclusions may be seen, however, in very occasional cells in normal subjects so that a control blood should always be incubated in parallel with a haemoglobin H preparation.

DETECTION OF HAEMOGLOBIN F-CONTAINING CELLS

Haemoglobin F-containing cells are identified cytochemically by their resistance to haemoglobin elution in acid conditions (Fig. 7.9); the procedure is commonly called a Kleihauer test from its originator, although Kleihauer's method is often modified. This test is useful for the detection of fetal cells in the maternal circulation, and also for the detection of autologous cells containing appreciable concentrations of haemoglobin F such as may be seen in hereditary persistence of fetal haemoglobin (HPFH) and δβ-thalassaemia, and in some patients with β-thalassaemia trait, sickle cell disease, dyshaemopoietic states and various other conditions. The distribution of haemoglobin F in adult cells may be homogeneous (in some types of HPFH) or heterogeneous (in other types of HPFH and in other conditions). Both a positive and a negative control should be tested in parallel with the sample under investigation. A positive control can be prepared by mixing together adult and fetal red cells.

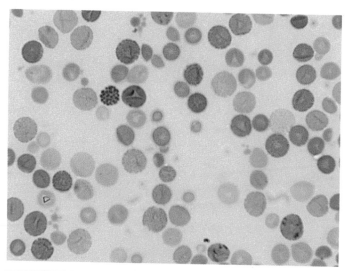

Fig. 7.8 *Haemoglobin H preparations showing:*
(a) *haemoglobin H-containing cells[1] and reticulocytes[2] in the blood of a patient with haemoglobin H disease;*

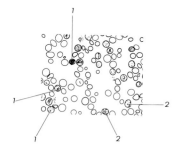

(b) *haemoglobin H-containing cells[1], reticulocytes[2] and Heinz bodies[3] in the blood of a patient with haemoglobin H disease who had had a splenectomy.*

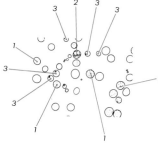

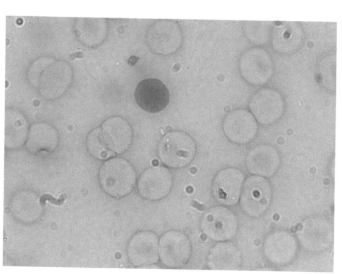

Fig. 7.9 *Acid elution technique for Haemoglobin F- containing cells; the blood sample was taken from a post-partum woman who had suffered a feto-maternal haemorrhage. A single stained fetal erythrocyte is seen against a background of maternal red cell ghosts.*

PERLS' REACTION FOR IRON

Perls' stain is based on a reaction between acid ferrocyanide and the ferric ion (Fe^{+++}) of haemosiderin to form ferric ferrocyanide which has an intense blue colour (prussian blue). Ferritin, which is soluble, does not give a positive reaction. Perls' stain is most often performed on the bone marrow but it can be used to stain peripheral blood cells in order to detect siderocytes and sideroblasts.

On a Romanowksy-stained blood film, haemosiderin appears as small blue granules which are designated Pappenheimer bodies (see page 80). When their nature has been confirmed by a positive Perls' reaction they are referred to as siderotic granules and the cells containing them are designated siderocytes (Fig. 7.10a). Siderocytes are rarely detectable in the peripheral blood of normal subjects; siderotic granules are present in reticulocytes newly released from the bone marrow but disappear during maturation of the reticulocyte in the spleen, probably because the haemosiderin is utilized for further haemoglobin sythesis. When haematologically normal subjects are splenectomized small numbers of siderocytes are seen in the blood. When red cells containing abnormally large or numerous siderotic granules are released from the bone marrow, as in sideroblastic anaemia and in thalassaemia major, many of the abnormal inclusions are 'pitted' by the spleen. Some remain detectable in the peripheral blood, in both reticulocytes and mature red cells. If a patient with a defect of iron incorporation has been splenectomized or is hyposplenic for any other reason very numerous siderocytes are seen.

A sideroblast is a nucleated red blood cell which contains siderotic granules. Sideroblasts are normally present in the bone marrow but, since nucleated red cells do not normally circulate, it is unusual to see peripheral blood sideroblasts. When they do appear they may be morphologically normal, containing only one or a few fine granules, or abnormal, with the granules being increased in number and/or in size. Abnormal sideroblasts include ring sideroblasts, in which a ring of siderotic granules are present close to the nucleus (Fig. 7.10b). Whenever nucleated red blood cells are present in the peripheral blood they can be stained by Perls' reaction to allow any siderotic granules present to be studied. Abnormal sideroblasts may be detected in the blood in sideroblastic anaemias (Fig. 7.10b), megaloblastic anemias and thalassaemias. They are seen in larger numbers when anaemia is severe or when the spleen is absent or hypofunctional. Sideroblastic anaemia is usually diagnosed by bone marrow aspiration but strong support for the diagnosis is obtained if ring sideroblasts are detected in the blood, if necessary in a buffy coat preparation in which any nucleated red cells are concentrated.

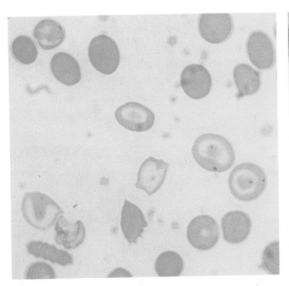 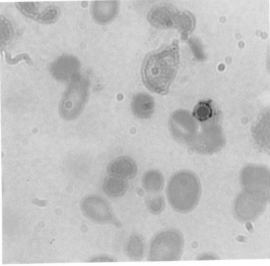

Fig. 7.10 (a) *siderocytes in the blood of a patient with thalassaemia major;*   **(b)** *a ring sideroblast in the blood of a patient with sideroblastic anaemia.*

CYTOCHEMICAL STAINS USED IN THE DIAGNOSIS AND CLASSIFICATION OF LEUKAEMIAS

Cytochemical stains used in the diagnosis and classification of leukaemias can be applied to both the bone marrow and the peripheral blood. Studies of peripheral blood cells are essential when bone marrow aspiration is difficult or impossible. In other circumstances studies of blood and of bone marrow are complementary. Cytochemical staining for neutrophil alkaline phosphatase is usually performed only on peripheral blood.

NEUTROPHIL ALKALINE PHOSPHATASE

Mature neutrophils, but not eosinophils, have alkaline phosphatase activity in specific cytoplasmic organelles[27] which have been designated phosphosomes. Neutrophil alkaline phosphatase (NAP) has also been designated leukocyte alkaline phosphatase (LAP) but the former designation is the more accurate since it is the neutrophils which are assessed. A number of cytochemical stains can be used for demonstrating NAP activity. One suitable stain[1] depends on the following reaction:

naphthol AS-MX phosphate

↓ alkaline phosphatase

arylnaphthol amide + phosphate

↓

diazonium salt → insoluble precipitate of
(fast blue RR)   blue dye

Following a cytochemical reaction such as this the strength of the NAP activity can be graded as shown in Figs 7.11 and 7.12 to give an NAP score which will fall between 0 and 400. The normal range is dependent on the substrate used. As there is an element of subjectivity in the scoring, laboratories should establish their own normal ranges. With the above method the normal range is of the order of 30–180. The NAP score is preferably determined on blood films made from native blood or heparinized blood. The cytochemical staining reaction is best carried out within 8 hours of obtaining the blood, but if this is not possible the films can be fixed

Score of cell	volume of cytoplasm occupied by precipitated dye (percent)	size of granules	intensity of staining	cytoplasmic background
0	none	–	none	colourless
1	50	small	faint to moderate	colourless to very pale blue
2	50–80	small	moderate to strong	colourless to pale blue
3	80–100	medium to large	strong	colourless to blue
4	100	medium and large	very strong	not visible

SCORING NEUTROPHIL ALKALINE PHOSPHATASE ACTIVITY (AFTER KAPLOW[18]) ONE HUNDRED NEUTROPHILS ARE INDIVIDUALLY SCORED AS FOLLOWS:

Following the scoring of individual neutrophils the scores are summed to produce the final NAP score. This is most easily done by multiplying each score by the number of cells having that score and adding the results together.

Fig. 7.11 *Scoring neutrophil alkaline phosphatase activity.*

and stored, in the dark, at room temperature. EDTA-anticoagulated blood is not ideal as enzyme activity is inhibited; if it is used the films should be made within 10–20 minutes of obtaining the blood, but even then there is some loss of activity. A low, normal and high control should be stained together with the test sample.

A low control can be obtained from a patient with chronic granulocytic leukaemia, or can be prepared by immersing an appropriately fixed film of normal blood in boiling water for 1 minute. A high control can be obtained from a patient with infection or from a pregnant or post-partum woman or a woman taking oral

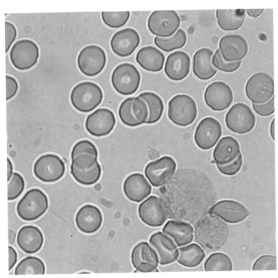

Fig. 7.12 *Cells stained for neutrophil alkaline phosphatase activity (method of Ackerman[1]) showing typical cells graded 0 to 4;* **(a)** *neutrophil with a score of zero plus a lymphocyte which is also negative;*

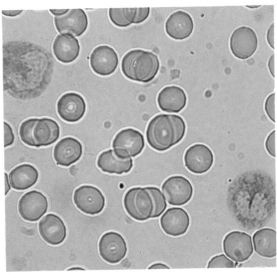

(b) *two band cells with a score of 1;*

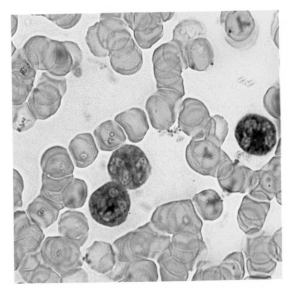

(c) *two neutrophils with a score of 2 and one with a score of 3;*

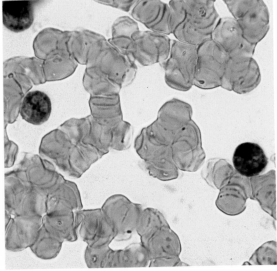

(d) *one neutrophil with a score of 2 and another with a score of 4.*

contraceptives. Positive and negative control films which have been appropriately fixed and wrapped in parafilm can be stored at −70°C for at least a year.

Some causes of high and low NAP scores are shown in Fig. 7.13. Neonates have very high NAP scores, usually exceeding 200; a fall to levels more typical of childhood occurs between 5 and 10 months of age.[24] Premature and low birth weight babies have lower scores than full term babies. Children have higher NAP scores than adults with a gradual fall to adult levels occurring before puberty.[26] Women in the reproductive age range have higher NAP scores than men with the

SOME CAUSES OF HIGH AND LOW NAP SCORES[15,19]	
High NAP	**Low NAP**
cord blood and neonate	chronic granulocytic leukaemia
mid-cycle in menstruating females	paroxysmal nocturnal haemoglobinuria
oral contraceptive intake	some cases of infectious mononucleosis and other viral infections
pregnancy and post-partum	
bacterial infection	inherited hypophosphatasia (NAP absent)
inflammation	
surgery and trauma	lactoferrin deficiency[5]
tissue infarction	some cases of acute myeloid leukaemia, particularly acute myeloblastic leukaemia with differentiation
leukaemoid reactions	
corticosteroids and ACTH administration	
acute stress	
some cases of acute myeloid leukaemia, particularly acute monoblastic leukaemia	some cases of idiopathic myelofibrosis
	some cases of aplastic anaemia
most cases of idiopathic myelofibrosis	most cases of sideroblastic anaemia
most cases of aplastic anaemia	
most cases of polycythaemia rubra vera	
some cases of myelodysplastic syndrome	
acute lymphoblastic leukaemia	
hairy cell leukaemia	
some cases of chronic lymphocytic leukaemia	
multiple myeloma	
Hodgkin's disease	
Down's syndrome	
cirrhosis of the liver (particularly when decompensated)	

Fig. 7.13 *Some causes of high and low neutrophil alkaline phosphatase scores.[15,19]*

score varying during the menstrual cycle (Fig. 7.14). After the menopause NAP scores of women approach those of men[26,30] (Fig. 7.15).

The NAP score is low in 95 percent of patients with Ph' positive chronic granulocytic leukaemia. The test is useful in distinguishing between CGL and other chronic myeloproliferative disorders which usually have a normal or elevated NAP score, and between CGL and reactive neutrophilias since the latter almost invariably have a high NAP score. Patients with CGL may have a

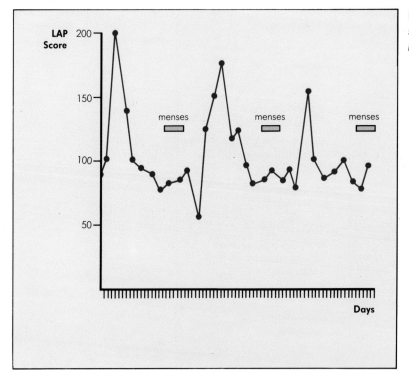

Fig. 7.14 *Changes in the NAP score during the menstrual cycle. in a healthy woman*

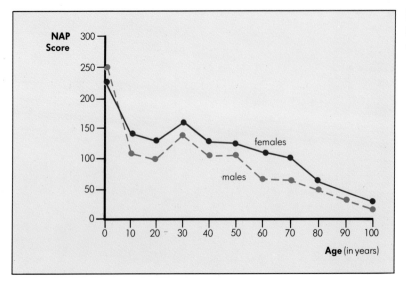

Fig. 7.15 *Changes of the NAP score with age in men and women derived from reference 30.*

normal or elevated NAP during pregnancy, postoperatively (particularly following splenectomy), during bacterial infection, when rendered hypoplastic by therapy, and following the onset of transformation.

The NAP score is also of use in distinguishing between polycythaemia rubra vera, which usually has an elevated score, and secondary polycythaemia, in which the NAP is usually normal.

The NAP has been recommended for distinguishing between hydatidiform mole (high NAP) and choriocarcinoma (normal NAP) and for the diagnosis of ectopic pregnancy (high score).[19]

MYELOPEROXIDASE

Peroxidases are enzymes which catalyse the oxidation of substrates by hydrogen peroxide. The granules of neutrophils and eosinophils contain a peroxidase which is designated leucocyte peroxidase or myeloperoxidase. The demonstration of myeloperoxidase activity is useful in establishing and confirming the diagnosis of acute myeloblastic leukaemia since lymphoblasts are uniformly negative. The French–American–British (FAB)´ classification[3] (see page 208) requires more than 3 percent of bone marrow blasts to show peroxidase activity for an acute leukaemia to be classified as myeloid.

Myeloperoxidase was initially demonstrated with benzidine or one of its derivatives as a substrate. A suitable non-carcinogenic substitute is used in the method of Hanker:[14]

$$\text{p-phenylene diamine} + \text{catechol} + H_2O_2$$
$$\downarrow \text{peroxidase}$$
$$\text{brownish-black insoluble reaction product}$$

Myeloperoxidase is demonstrable in the granules of neutrophils and their precursors (Fig. 7.16), eosinophils and their precursors and the precursors of basophils. In neutrophils and in eosinophils both the primary granules and the specific granules contain peroxidase; neutrophil peroxidase and eosinophil peroxidase enzymes differ from one another, for example in their pH optima and in their sensitivity to inhibition by cyanide. Auer rods are peroxidase-positive. Monocytes and their precursors are either negative or have a much weaker reaction so that peroxidase activity is of use in the further classification of the acute myeloid leukaemias (see page 214). An inherited partial deficiency of neutrophil peroxidase is quite common, and several cases of inherited deficiency of eosinophil peroxidase have also been described.

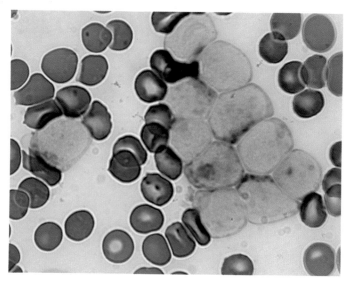

Fig. 7.16 *Leukaemic blast cells stained by the Hanker technique[14] for myeloperoxidase, showing a brownish-black deposit in the cytoplasm. The patient had AML (FAB class M2).*

SUDAN BLACK B

Sudan black B (Fig. 7.17) has an affinity for leukocyte granules. In general the intensity of a positive staining reaction parallels myeloperoxidase activity and a positive reaction in more than 3 percent of bone marrow blasts is accepted in the FAB classification for designating an acute leukaemia as as myeloid. Sudan black B positivity is slightly more sensitive than the demonstration of myeloperoxidase activity for the detection of myeloblasts. Sudan black B stains the granules of neutrophils (both the azurophilic and the specific granules), the specific granules of eosinophils and to a variable extent the specific granules of basophils. The staining of eosinophil granules may be peripheral with the central core remaining unstained. Auer rods are stained. Monoblasts are either negative or show scattered fine positively-staining granules; the staining of monocytes varies from a few fine dots to a particulate dusting of the cytoplasm. In hereditary myeloperoxidase deficiency neutrophils and monocytes are sudan black B negative and in hereditary deficiency of eosinophil peroxidase, eosinophils are similarly negative with sudan black B. Lymphoblasts can have occasional fine positive dots which may represent staining of mitochondria.[15] Very rarely a stronger reaction is seen in the lymphoblasts of acute lymphoblastic leukaemia[31] or in lymphoma of T or B cell origin.[28]

NAPHTHOL AS-D CHLOROACETATE ESTERASE

Naphthol AS-D chloroacetate esterase ('chloroacetate esterase', CAE) activity is found in neutrophils and their precursors (Fig. 7.18). Auer rods are positive. Normal eosinophils and basophils are negative but the eosinophils of eosinophilic leukaemia may be positive.[9] Monocytes are usually negative, but may have a weak positivity. Chloroacetate esterase is generally less sensitive than either myeloperoxidase or sudan black B in the detection of myeloblasts, although some cases have been noted to be positive for chloroacetate esterase despite being negative for peroxidase.[15,33]

'NON-SPECIFIC' ESTERASES

Esterase activity is common in haemopoietic cells. Nine isoenzymes have been demonstrated of which four are found in neutrophils, and are responsible for the naphthol AS-D chloroacetate activity. Five are found in monocytes and a variety of other cells and the esterase activity of these cells has been designated 'non-specific' esterase.[6,15] Different isoenzymes ae preferentially detected by different substrates and at different pHs. The most specific cytochemical reaction to detect the esterase activity of monocytes is α naphthyl acetate esterase activity (Fig. 7.19) at acid pH (ANAE); α naphthyl butyrate esterase (ANBE) activity is very similar. With

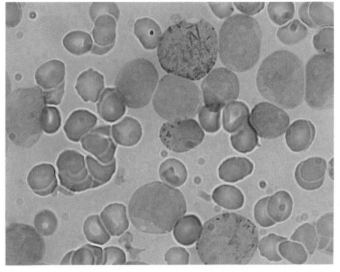

Fig. 7.17 *Leukaemic blast cells stained with sudan black B. One large blast cell contains both granules and Auer rods. Several other blast cells contain granules. This patient with AML (FAB class M1) had very few granules and very rare Auer rods visible on a Romanowksy stain.*

ANAE, strongly positive reactions are given by monocytes and their precursors, and by megakaryocytes and platelets; plasma cells give a weaker reaction. Monocyte and megakaryocyte non-specific esterase activity can also be detected as naphthol AS-D acetate esterase activity (NASDA esterase) or the very similar naphthol AS acetate esterase (NASA esterase). NASDA esterase is weakly positive in neutrophils and their precursors. It is therefore less suitable than ANAE for differentiating between the monocyte lineage and the neutrophil lineage; the specificity of the reaction can be improved by doing the test with and without fluoride since the monocyte and megakaryocyte enzymes are inhibited by fluoride whereas the neutrophil enzyme is fluoride-resistant. The ANAE activity of monocytes and megakaryocytes is also fluoride sensitive, but ANAE allows a clearer distinction between neutrophils and monocytes and the addition of fluoride is not necessary. Non-specific esterase activity is often demonstrable in normal T lymphocytes and also in acute and chronic leukaemias of T cell origin. With ANAE a characteristic focal or dot positivity is often demonstrable in T-acute lymphoblastic leukaemia and in T-prolymphocytic leukaemia; ANAE is superior to NASDA esterase in this regard.[9] The abnormal erythroblasts of erythroleukaemia or megaloblastic anaemia may also have non-specific esterase activity. NASDA esterase is recommended for identification of the monocyte lineage in the FAB classification of acute myeloid leukaemias.[3]

A combined cytochemical reaction for α naphthyl acetate esterase and chloroacetate esterase[33] allows both reactions to be studied on the one blood film.

PERIODIC ACID-SCHIFF

The periodic acid-Schiff (PAS) reaction stains a variety of carbohydrates including the glycogen which is often found in haemopoietic cells. The main clinical application of this stain is in the differential diagnosis of the acute leukaemias. Lymphoblasts of acute lymphoblastic leukaemia (ALL) are PAS-positive in the great majority of cases, with positivity often being in the form of coarse granules or large blocks (Fig. 7.20). A negative PAS reaction is commoner in T-ALL than in common ALL. Myeloblasts and monoblasts may be PAS-negative or may have a faint diffuse or fine granular positivity; coarse positive granules are sometimes seen in monoblasts. Block positivity is rare in acute myeloid leukaemia but it has been observed in monoblasts, megakaryoblasts and erythroblasts.

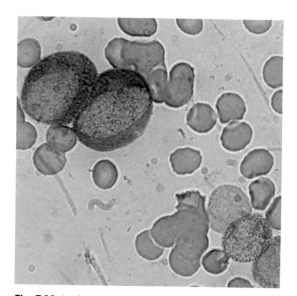

Fig. 7.18 *Leukaemic blast cells stained for chloroacetate esterase activity, using Corinth V as the dye. The patient had AML (FAB class M2).*

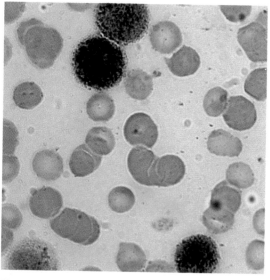

Fig. 7.19 *Leukaemic blast cells stained for α naphthyl acetate esterase activity using fast blue RR as the dye. The patient had AML (FAB class M5).*

Many other haemopoietic cells are PAS-positive but the reaction is rarely of diagnostic importance. Platelets, megakaryocytes and the more mature megakaryoblasts are positive. Mature neutrophils have fine granules packing the cytoplasm whereas eosinophils and basophils have a positive cytoplasmic reaction with PAS-negative granules. Monocytes have fine scattered granules. Normal erythroblasts are PAS-negative. Strong, diffuse or block PAS-positivity may be seen in erythroleukaemia; quite strong reactions, either diffuse or granular, may also be seen in thalassaemia major and severe iron deficiency and weaker reactions in sideroblastic anaemia, severe haemolytic anaemia and a number of other disorders of erythropoiesis. Most normal lymphocytes are PAS-negative; lymphocytes containing PAS-positive granules become more frequent in reactive conditions such as infectious mononucleosis and other virus infections and in lymphoproliferative disorders such as chronic lymphocytic leukaemia and non-Hodgkin's lymphoma. A circlet of PAS-positive granules surrounding the nucleus may be found in Sézary cells. A PAS stain can be performed on a blood film which has previously been stained by a Romanowksy stain. The PAS stain finds a limited application in the diagnosis of erythroleukaemia and megakaryoblastic leukaemia.

ACID PHOSPHATASE

Acid phosphatase activity is demonstrated by a variety of haemopoietic cells. Its two main applications are in the diagnosis of hairy cell leukaemia and the diagnosis of leukaemias of T lineage (Fig. 7.21).

A number of isoenzymes of acid phosphatase are found in haemopoietic cells. That of hairy cells is characteristically tartrate-resistant whereas that of other cells is sensitive to inhibition by tartrate. The demonstration of tartrate-resistant acid phosphatase activity (TRAP) is thus important in the diagnosis of hairy cell leukaemia; it is present in the great majority of cases. TRAP activity is rare in conditions other than hairy cell leukaemia but it has been reported in occasional cases of infectious mononucleosis, chronic lymphocytic leukaemia, prolymphocytic leukaemia, non-Hodgkin's lymphoma and the Sézary syndrome.

Acid phosphatase activity is usually stronger in acute and chronic leukaemias of T lineage than in those of B lineage where it is often negative. The focal nature of acid phosphatase activity is of use in the diagnosis of T acute lymphoblastic leukaemia.

Acid phosphatase activity is also demonstrable in granulocytes and their precursors, in the monocyte lineage, and in platelets, megakaryocytes and the more mature megakaryoblasts. Auer rods are positive.

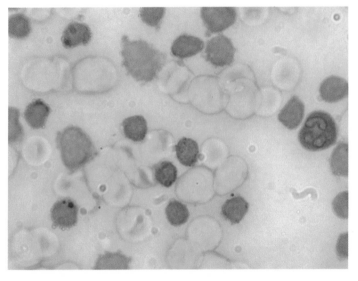

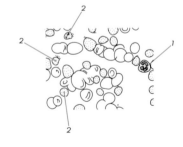

Fig. 7.20 *Periodic acid-Schiff stain of the blood of a patient with acute lymphoblastic leukaemia (FAB class L1) showing a neutrophil with positive cytoplasmic granules[1] and several blast cells with block positivity[2].*

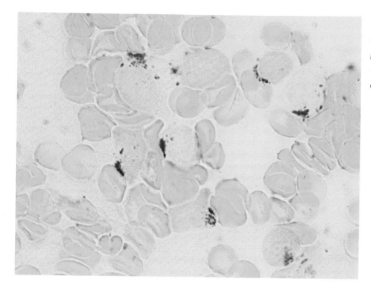

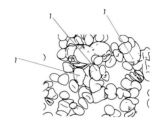

Fig. 7.21 *Acid phosphatase stain by the method of Janckila [17] on the blood of a patient with acute lymphoblastic leukaemia (FAB class L2). Several blasts show focal activity*[1]

References

1. Ackerman GA (1962) Substituted naphthol AS phosphate derivatives for the localization of leukocyte alkaline phosphatase activity. *Laboratory Investigation*, **11**, 563–567.
2. Atwater J & Erslev AJ (1983) In *Haematology*. Edited by WJ Williams, E Beutler, AJ Erslev & MA Lichtman. New York: McGraw Hill Book Company.
3. Bennett JM, Catovsky D, Daniel MT, Flandrin G, Galton DAG, Gralnick HR & Sultan C (1976) Proposals for the classification of acute leukaemias. *British Journal of Haematology*, **33**, 451–458.
4. Brecher G & Schneiderman MR (1950) A time-saving device for the counting of reticulocytes. *American Journal of Clinical Pathology*, **20**, 1079–1083.
5. Breton-Gorius J, Mason DY, Buriot D, Vilde J-L & Griscelli C (1980) Lactoferrin deficiency as a consequence of a lack of specific granules in neutrophils from a patient with recurrent infections. *American Journal of Clinical Pathology*, **99**, 413–419.
6. Catovsky D (1980) Leucocyte enzymes in leukaemia. In *Topical Reviews in Haematology, Volume 1*. Edited by S Roath. Bristol: John Wright and Sons Ltd.
7. Cline MJ & Berlin NI (1963) The reticulocyte count as an indicator of the rate of erythropoiesis. *American Journal of Clinical Pathology*, **39**, 121–128.
8. Crouch JY & Kaplow LS (1985) Relationship of reticulocyte age to polychromasia, shift cells, and shift reticulocytes. *Archives of Pathology and Laboratory Medicine*, **109**, 325–329.
9. Dacie JV & Lewis SM (1984) *Practical Haematology*, sixth edition. Edinburgh: Churchill Livingstone.
10. Deiss A & Kurth D (1970) Circulating reticulocytes in normal adults as determined by the New Methylene Blue method. *American Journal of Clinical Pathology*, **53**, 481–484.
11. Fannon M, Thomas R & Sawyer L (1982) Effect of staining and storage times on reticulocyte counts. *Laboratory Medicine*, **13**, 431–433.
12. Gadson D, Hughes M, Dean A & Wickramasinghe SN (1986) Morphology of redox-dye-treated Hb H-containing red cells: confusion caused by wrongly identified dyes. *Clinical and Laboratory Haematology*, **8**, 365–366.
13. Gairdner D, Marks J & Roscoe JD (1952) Blood formation in infancy. Part II. Normal erythropoiesis. *Archives of Diseases of Childhood*, **27**, 214–221.
14. Hanker JS, Yates PE, Metz CB & Rustioni A (1977) A new specific, sensitive and non-carcinogenic reagent for the demonstration of horseradish peroxidase. *Histochemical Journal*, **9**, 789–792.

15. Hayhoe FGJ & Quaglino D (1980) *Haematological Cytochemistry*. Edinburgh: Churchill Livingstone.

16. Hillman RS & Finch CA (1969) The misused reticulocyte. *British Journal of Haematology*, **17**, 313–315.

17. Janckila A, Li C-Y, Lam K-W & Yam LT (1978) The cytochemistry of the tartrate-resistant acid phosphatase — technical considerations. *American Journal of Clinical Pathology*, **70**, 45–55.

18. Kaplow LS (1963) Cytochemistry of leukocyte alkaline phosphatase. *American Journal of Clinical Pathology*, **39**, 439–449.

19. Kaplow LS (1968) Leukocyte alkaline phosphatase cytochemistry: applications and methods. *Annals of the New York Academy of Sciences*, **155**, 911–947.

20. Koepke JF & Koepke JA (1986) Reticulocytes. *Clinical and Laboratory Haematology*, **8**, 169–179.

21. Lee GR (1981) In *Clinical Haematology*, eighth edition. Edited by MM Wintrobe, GR Lee, DR Boggs, TC Bithell, J Foerster, JW Athens & JN Lukens. Philadelphia: Lea & Febiger.

22. Lowenstein ML (1959) The mammalian reticulocyte. *International Review of Cytology*, **9**, 135–174.

23. Myhre E (1961) Reticulocyte count. *Nordisk Medicin*, **65**, 37, quoted by Dacie JV & Lewis SM (*op cit*).

24. O'Kell RT (1968) Leukocyte alkaline phosphatase activity in the infant. *Annals of the New York Academy of Sciences*, **155**, 980–982.

25. Perrotta AL & Finch CA (1972) The polychromatophilic erythrocyte. *American Journal of Clinical Pathology*, **57**, 471–477.

26. Rosner F, Lee SL, Schultz FS & Gorfien PC (1968) The regulation of leukocyte alkaline phosphatase. *Annals of the New York Academy of Sciences*, **155**, 902–910.

27. Rustin GJS, Wilson PD & Peters TJ (1979) Studies on the subcellular localization of human neutrophil alkaline phosphatase. *Journal of Cell Science*, **36**, 401–412.

28. Savage RA, Fishleder J & Tubbs RR (1983) Confirming myeloid differentiation. *American Journal of Clinical Pathology*, **80**, 412 (letter).

29. Savage RA, Skoog DP & Rabinovitch A (1985) Analytic inaccuracy and imprecision in reticulocyte counting: a preliminary report from the College of American Pathologists Reticulocyte Project. *Blood Cells*, **11**, 97–112.

30. Stavridis J, Creatsas G, Lolis D, Traga G, Antonopoulos M & Kaskarelis D (1981) Relationships between leucocyte alkaline phosphatase and nitroblue tetrazolium reduction activities in the peripheral blood polymorphonuclear leucocytes in normal individuals. *British Journal of Haematology*, **47**, 157–159.

31. Stein P, Peiper S, Butler D, Melvin S, Williams D & Stass S (1983) Granular acute lymphoblastic leukaemia. *American Journal of Clinical Pathology*, **79**, 426–430.

32. Wickramasinghe SN, Hughes M, Fucharoen S & Wasi P (1985) The morphology of redox-dye-treated Hb H-containing red cells: difference between cells treated with brilliant cresyl blue, methylene blue and new methylene blue. *Clinical and Laboratory Haematology*, **7**, 353–358.

33. Yam LT, Li CY & Crosby WH (1971) Cytochemical identification of monocytes and granulocytes. *American Journal of Clinical Pathology*, **55**, 283–290.

8. Interpretation – white cells

There are three main reasons for the haematology laboratory to produce a blood count and examine a blood film.

Firstly, a specific diagnosis may be made with certainty or near certainty. Such is the case in many patients with leukaemia.

Secondly, a blood count and film may suggest a diagnosis or give supporting evidence for a diagnosis already under consideration. This is so, for example, when the detection of neutrophil leucocytosis in a patient with symptoms of myocardial ischaemia gives support for a diagnosis of myocardial infarction rather than merely angina, or when the finding of numerous spherocytes suggests that the patient might have hereditary spherocytosis or warm autoimmune haemolytic anaemia.

Thirdly, the blood count and film may allow disease severity to be gauged or the effects of treatment to be monitored. This is the case when the response to therapy of an infective or inflammatory condition is being judged, or when the effects of cytotoxic chemotherapy are being followed.

When interpreting a blood film and count it is necessary to bear in mind the provisional diagnosis and the likely reason the test has been requested in order to be certain to note all relevant abnormalities and fulfil the intended purpose of the test.

This chapter and the following one deal with the differential diagnosis of common quantitative and qualitative haematological abnormalities and discuss the characteristic findings of various disease states.

When assessing haematological parameters the age, sex and ethnic origin of the subject (see chapters 2 and 6) should be considered. In assessing the blood count it must also be remembered that if comparison is made with 95 percent reference intervals or 95 percent normal ranges then, by definition, 5 percent of healthy subjects will fall outside these limits. Furthermore, as the number of parameters measured increases, an increasing number of healthy subjects will have at least one parameter falling outside the reference limits — if seven independent parameters are measured 30 percent of healthy subjects will have at least one 'abnormal' result.

NEUTROPHIL LEUCOCYTOSIS (NEUTROPHILIA)

Neutrophil leucocytosis or neutrophilia is the elevation of the absolute neutrophil count above that which would be expected in a healthy subject of the same age, sex, race and physiological status.

Some of the causes of a neutrophil leucocytosis are shown in Fig. 8.1.

In assessing an apparent neutrophilia it is necessary to consider whether the elevated count is physiological or pathological. Since healthy neonates have higher neutrophil counts than subjects of any other age they should be regarded as having neutrophilia only if their neutrophil counts exceed what is expected at that age.

Likewise a left shift is a physiological feature in a neonate. Similarly women have higher neutrophil counts than men with the count varying with the menstrual cycle. During pregnancy a marked rise in the neutrophil count occurs and this is further accentuated during labour and in the post-partum period. It is difficult to distinguish between the effects of normal pregnancy and a pathological condition on the basis of the blood

---

SOME CAUSES OF NEUTROPHIL LEUCOCYTOSIS

infections
many acute and chronic bacterial infections, including miliary tuberculosis[120]
some rickettsial infections — typhus (some cases), Rocky Mountain Spotted Fever
some viral infections — chickenpox, herpes simplex infection, rabies, polio, St Louis encephalitis,[99] eastern equine encephalitis[99]
some fungal infections — actinomycosis, coccidiodomycosis, North American blastomycosis
some parasitic infestations — liver fluke, hepatic amoebiasis, filariasis,[174] some *Pneumocystis carinii* infections[174]

tissue damage
trauma, burns, surgery (particularly splenectomy), acute hepatic necrosis, acute pancreatitis

tissue infarction
myocardial infarction, pulmonary embolism causing pulmonary infarction, sickle cell crisis, atheroembolic disease[33]

acute inflammation or severe chronic inflammation
gout, rheumatic fever, rheumatoid arthritis, ulcerative colitis, polyarteritis nodosa, familial mediterranean fever, scleroderma,[67] familial cold urticaria[162]

metabolic and endocrine
diabetic ketoacidosis, acute renal failure, Cushing's syndrome, thyrotoxic crisis

malignant disease
(particularly but not only when there is extensive disease or tumour necrosis) carcinoma, sarcoma, melanoma, Hodgkin's disease[136]

post-neutropenia rebound
following dialysis neutropenia, recovery from agranulocytosis and cytoxic chemotherapy, treatment of megaloblastic anaemia

myeloproliferative and leukaemic disorders
chronic granulocytic leukaemia, chronic myelomonocytic leukaemia, neutrophilic leukaemia, acute myeloid leukaemia (uncommonly), other rare leukaemias, primary proliferative polycythaemia (polycythaemia rubra vera), essential thrombocythaemia, myelofibrosis (early in the disease process)

drugs
adrenaline, corticosteroids, lithium

acute haemorrhage

cigarette smoking

poisoning by various chemicals and drugs

hypersensitivity reactions including those due to drugs

hereditary neutrophilia[81]

inherited deficiency of CR3 complement receptors[109]

vigorous exercise

acute pain, epileptic convulsions, electric shock, paroxysmal tachycardia

eclampsia and pre-eclampsia (toxaemia of pregnancy)

acute anoxia

Fig.8.1 *Some causes of a neutrophil leucocytosis.*

film appearances alone, since pregnancy causes a number of haematological changes which are otherwise usually indicative of disease. Not only is there neutrophilia but also a left shift (including myelocytes (see Fig. 3.56) and even occasionally promyelocytes), 'toxic' granulation, Döhle bodies, a fall in the haemoglobin concentration, increased rouleaux formation and elevation of the ESR. A knowledge that the patient is pregnant is necessary to avoid misinterpretation.

The commonest and most important cause of neutrophilia is increased bone marrow output of neutrophils due to infection, inflammation or tissue damage (including surgery). In these circumstances neutrophilia may be associated with a left shift, toxic granulation and Döhle bodies (Fig. 8.2 and see also Figs 3.13, 3.21, 3.25 and 3.32a). Eosinopenia and lymphopenia may coexist. Associated alterations in those serum proteins known as acute phase reactants (for example, α_2 macroglobulin and fibrinogen) may cause increased rouleaux formation and an elevation of the ESR. Many of this group of conditions also cause a reactive thrombocytosis, but thrombocytopenia may also occur as a consequence of defective bone marrow function or peripheral consumption of platelets.

Neutrophilia can also be due to an alteration of neutrophil distribution rather than to increased bone marrow output. Exercise can cause neutrophilia by mobilizing cells previously marginated along the walls of blood vessels. Vigorous exercise can double the neutrophil count with the absolute numbers of the other granulocytes — and of monocytes and lymphocytes — also being considerably elevated. If the exercise is both severe and prolonged a left shift may occur, indicating that there is increased bone marrow output of immature granulocytes rather than merely redistribution. Patients do not usually undergo vigorous exercise before having a blood specimen taken but adrenaline administration and epileptiform convulsions mobilize neutrophils in a similar way, and even severe pain may have an effect on the neutrophil count.

Corticosteroids elevate the neutrophil count by altering kinetics. The input of neutrophils from the bone marrow is increased and the egress to the tissues is decreased but the neutrophil marginal turnover rate does not alter. A rise of the white cell count starts within a few hours of intravenous administration or within a day of oral administration. White cell counts as high as $20 \times 10^9/l$ occur, the elevation being predominantly due to neutrophilia with some increase also in the absolute monocyte count, and with a fall in the absolute eosinophil and lymphocyte counts.

Since both corticosteroids and some of the conditions for which they are commonly prescribed predispose to infection the differentiation between neutrophilia due to corticosteroids and neutrophilia due to infection can be important. It can also be necessary to consider whether neutrophilia in a patient who has suffered an epileptiform convulsion is due to the convulsion or is

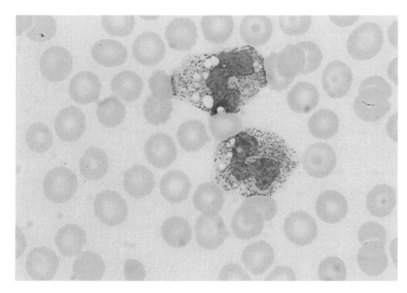

Fig.8.2 *Neutrophil morphology in a patient with reactive neutrophilia; there is vacuolation and marked toxic granulation.*

indicative of underlying infection, such as meningitis. When an elevated neutrophil count is due to corticosteroid administration or an alteration of neutrophil distribution there is no associated toxic granulation or formation of Döhle bodies and except for very vigorous exercise there is no left shift. Observation of the lack of these features together with a knowledge of the clinical circumstances avoid misinterpretation.

A blood count is often performed in the hope of establishing whether or not a patient has an infection. As we have seen, neutrophilia, toxic granulation and Döhle bodies are not specific for infection although when the changes are marked they are certainly strongly suggestive. Neutrophil vacuolation (see Fig. 3.21) is a more specific finding, very commonly indicating septicaemia, although this finding also is not totally specific.[99] The

SOME FEATURES WHICH MAY AID IN THE DIFFERENTIATION BETWEEN REACTIVE NEUTROPHILIA AND CHRONIC GRANULOCYTIC LEUKAEMIA		
feature	reactive neutrophilia	chronic granulocytic leukaemia
WBC	rarely > 60×10^9/l	usually 20–500×10^9/l or higher
left shift	may be moderate or marked; if slight in relation to neutrophilia supports reactive neutrophilia	proportional to WBC; may be marked
white cell morphology	toxic granulation, neutrophil vacuolation and Döhle bodies may be present	toxic changes not present
absolute eosinophil count	usually reduced	usually elevated; eosinophil myelocytes may be present
absolute basophil count	usually reduced	almost invariably elevated; basophil myelocytes may be present
absolute monocyte count	may be elevated	usually moderately elevated
erythropoiesis	anaemia may be present; usually normocytic and normochromic but if hypochromic and microcytic supports a reactive neutrophilia; rouleaux may be present	anaemia may be present; normocytic and normochromic
platelet count	thrombocytosis or thrombocytopenia may occur; if there is a reactive thrombocytosis the platelets are usually small	the platelet count is usually normal or high; giant platelets may be present; platelets are large, even in the presence of thrombocytosis; megakaryocytes may be present
neutrophil alkaline phosphatase	usually elevated	almost always reduced

Fig.8.3 *Some features which may aid in the differentiation between reactive neutrophilia and chronic granulocytic leukaemia.*

vacuolation may be associated with partial neutrophil degranulation so that there are reduced numbers of granules which are 'toxic' in appearance. The observation of bacteria within neutrophils in a blood film made without delay (see Fig. 3.27) allows a specific diagnosis of bacteraemia, but this is a rare finding. It has been observed mainly but not exclusively in hyposplenic patients, some of whom have also had a defect of antibody production, and is associated with a very poor prognosis. Extracellular organisms may also be seen. Microorganisms which have been detected on routine examination of a peripheral blood film include pneumococci, meningococci (Fig. 3.27), staphylococci, streptococci, *Clostridium perfringens*, *Pasteurella pestis*, *Bacteroides* species, the DF-2 organism, *Borrelia recurrentis*, *Candida* and *Histoplasma*. If blood is being examined specifically for bacteria then a buffy coat film is recommended. The nature of the organism can be further elucidated by a Gram stain or a silver stain for histoplasma.

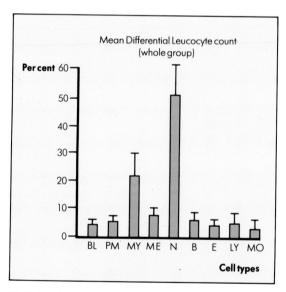

Fig.8.4 *A diagrammatic representation of the typical differential count in chronic granulocytic leukaemia based on 1500 cell differential counts in 50 patients with Ph'-positive CGL. BL=blasts, PM=promyelocytes, MY=myelocytes, ME=metamyelocytes, N=neutrophils, B=basophils, E=eosinophils, LY=lymphocytes, MO=monocytes. Standard deviation is indicated by the lines surmounting the shaded bars.*

In examining a blood film characterized by neutrophilia a specific diagnosis is rarely made. Most often the haematological findings suggest the possibility of infection, inflammation or tissue damage, or are used to assess the severity of a known pathological process, or to monitor the progress of the disease or the response to treatment. Rarely a specific diagnosis of leukaemia or of a bacterial infection can be made.

CHRONIC GRANULOCYTIC LEUKAEMIA (CGL)

Chronic granulocytic leukaemia (CGL) is a neoplastic proliferation of myeloid precursors, characterized by maturation of progenitors into granulocytes of all types. Chronic myeloid leukaemia (CML) is an alternative designation; the term chronic granulocytic leukaemia may be preferred since it emphasizes the maturation which occurs and sets this condition apart from various other types of chronic leukaemia of myeloid lineage. CGL is rare in childhood but occurs throughout adult life. Common clinical features are anaemia and splenomegaly.

The distinction between CGL and a reactive neutrophilia is usually straightforward. The WBC is usually higher in CGL, commonly in excess of 100×10^9/l and occasionally in the region of $500–700 \times 10^9$/l. A reactive neutrophilia may occasionally reach extreme levels (for example, $40–60 \times 10^9$/l, or even higher) but in such cases the cause of the neutrophilia is usually readily apparent. Some of the other features which help to make the distinction between CGL and a reactive neutrophilia are shown in Fig. 8.3. In CGL the differential count (Fig. 8.4) and the blood film (Fig. 8.5 and see also Fig. 3.57) are highly characteristic with neutrophils and myelocytes being the two dominant cell types, promyelocytes being less numerous than myelocytes, and myeloblasts in turn being less numerous than promyelocytes.[153] The almost invariable occurrence of basophilia and the common occurrence of eosinophilia are important diagnostic features. There are often some eosinophils in which there are occasional granules with basophilic staining characteristics (see Fig. 3.39) and, in addition, abnormal cells which appear to be eosinophil–basophil hybrids.[169] In CGL the absolute monocyte count is increased but not in proportion to the increase in the granulocyte series. A low platelet count favours reactive neutrophilia but a normal or high platelet count is unhelpful in making the distinction between the two conditions. Consideration of the relationship between

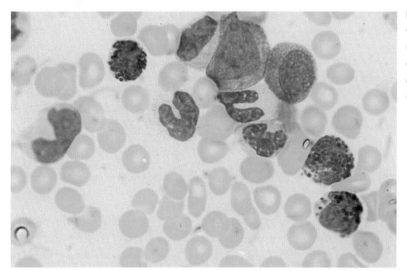

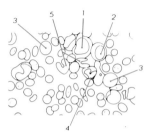

Fig.8.5 *Blood film of a patient with Ph'–positive CGL showing* **(a)** *a promyelocyte[1], an eosinophil myelocyte[2], three basophils[3] and a number of neutrophils[4] and band forms[5];*

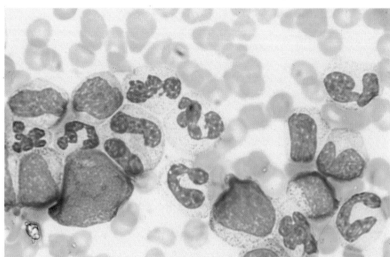

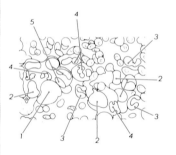

(b) *a promyelocyte[1], several myelocytes[2], neutrophil band forms[3] and neutrophils[4]; there is one binucleate neutrophil[5] — an unusual feature;*

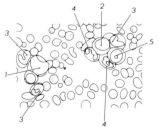

(c) *a promyelocyte[1], myelocyte[2], band forms[3] and neutrophils[4]; there is one neutrophil with a ring nucleus[5] — these forms are uncommon.*

the platelet count and platelet size may be useful (Fig. 8.3). Circulating megakaryocytes and megakaryocyte fragments are much commoner in CGL than in reactive neutrophilia, and a small number of NRBC are usually present. A minority of patients have extensive bone marrow fibrosis at presentation and the red cell features of myelofibrosis (see page 220) are superimposed on the usual features of CGL.

In CGL, in contrast to other chronic leukaemias of myeloid origin and in contrast to the myelodysplastic states, the great majority of the myeloid cells are morphologically normal.

The differential count and the blood film in CGL are so highly characteristic that atypical features should suggest either an alternative diagnosis or that transformation of CGL into the acute phase of the disease (see below) is occurring.

The NAP (see page 177) is useful in the differential diagnosis of CGL and other causes of neutrophilia. It is elevated in pregnancy and usually moderately to markedly elevated in reactive neutrophilia. On the other hand it is reduced in more than 90 percent of patients with uncomplicated CGL. It is elevated in a minority of patients with CGL, sometimes in association with pregnancy or the postoperative state (particularly postsplenectomy), or when the disease is transforming into the acute phase, but also in some patients in uncomplicated chronic phase.

Although in most patients the peripheral blood findings leave little doubt as to the diagnosis of CGL, definitive diagnosis requires examination of the bone marrow and cytogenetic analysis to detect the Philadelphia (Ph[1]) chromosome in myeloid cells. The Ph[1] chromosome is a chromosome 22 which has lost part of its long arm by translocation, usually to chromosome 9 (Fig. 8.6). Ph[1]

If the blood and bone marrow findings are characteristic of CGL but the Ph[1] chromosome is not found then the diagnosis of Ph[1]-negative CGL should be made. In some patients the same basic genetic events have occurred as in Ph[1]-positive CGL but the typical Ph[1] chromosome has been masked by other events, for example by translocation of further chromosomal material onto the Ph[1] chromosome. Patients with Ph[1]-negative CGL on average have a lower white cell count and platelet count at presentation than Ph[1]-positive patients, and thrombocytopenia is much commoner[29] but such differences do not allow prediction of chromosome status in an individual patient. Nor can Ph[1] status be predicted from the NAP score since activity is low or absent in the majority of patients with Ph[1]-negative as well as Ph[1]-positive disease.

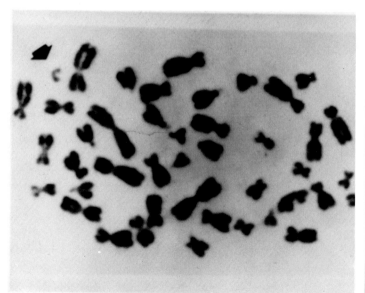

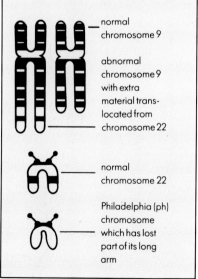

normal chromosome 9

abnormal chromosome 9 with extra material translocated from chromosome 22

normal chromosome 22

Philadelphia (ph) chromosome which has lost part of its long arm

Fig.8.6 (a) *Chromosomes of a bone marrow cell from a patient with chronic granulocytic leukaemia showing a Philadelphia (Ph¹) chromosome (arrowed); and a chromosome 9 with elongated long arm. Courtesy of Dr D. Coleman, St. Mary's Hospital, London.*

(b) *Diagrammatic representation of normal chromosomes 9 and 22, together with the abnormal chromosomes 9 and 22 (the Philadelphia chromosome).*

Occasionally patients with CGL have striking cyclical changes in the WBC with a periodicity of 50 to 70 days, and with the WBC varying from frankly leukaemic levels to almost normal. All myeloid cells participate in the cycles.

Most patients with CGL present with symptoms due to the disease and show all the usual peripheral blood features. Occasional patients who have developed the disease while being haematologically monitored have allowed the early stages of the disease to be defined.[91] The first detectable peripheral blood features are basophilia, thrombocytosis and a low NAP. Following this the neutrophil count and the total white cell count rise and small numbers of immature cells appear. With the progressive rise of the white cell count which follows, the percentage of immature cells steadily increases. In patients presenting with very high white cell counts blast cells may be as high as 15 percent, but while the patient remains in the chronic phase blast cells remain less numerous than promyelocytes and promyelocytes than myelocytes.

OTHER LEUKAEMIAS CHARACTERIZED BY NEUTROPHILIA

Atypical (Ph'-negative) chronic myeloid leukaemia

Some patients with a chronic leukaemia have clinical and haematological findings which are similar to those seen in patients with Ph'-positive CGL but with some haematological features being atypical. The monocyte count may be higher than expected in relation to the neutrophil count, and eosinophilia and basophilia may be lacking (Fig. 8.7). Neutrophils may be hypogranular or show other dysplastic features. Such laboratory findings are predictive of the absence of the Ph' chromo-

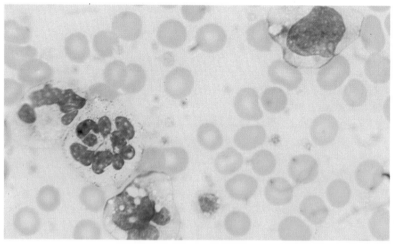

Fig.8.7 The blood film from a patient with Ph'−negative atypical chronic myeloid leukaemia showing

(a) a normal neutrophil[(1)], a macropolycyte[(2)], a monocyte[(3)] and a somewhat immature monocyte[(4)]; there is one large platelet[(5)];

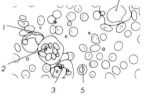

(b) numerous neutrophils[(1)], band forms[(2)], monocytes[(3)] and hypogranular myelocytes[(4)].

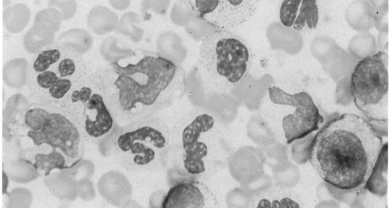

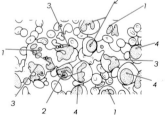

some. Patients with this condition on average have a lower haemoglobin concentration, white cell count and platelet count than patients with Ph¹-positive CGL. Confirmation of the diagnosis is by bone marrow examination and cytogenetic analysis. Monocytes are usually more prominent in the bone marrow than they are in CGL and eosinophil and basophil myelocytes are less prominent. Cytogenetic analysis may be normal or may disclose a clonal abnormality other than the Ph¹ chromosome. It is important for the laboratory to correctly distinguish between Ph¹-positive CGL and atypical Ph¹-negative CML since the latter condition is less responsive to treatment and survival is appreciably shorter.

Because the differential count is less characteristic and the white cell count is often lower (usually 50–100 × 10⁹/l) atypical Ph¹-negative CML can be harder to distinguish from a reactive condition than is CGL. The lack of toxic changes in the neutrophils is a helpful feature as is the NAP score which is low in the majority of patients and elevated in only a minority. If cytogenetic analysis discloses a clonal chromosomal abnormality strong support is given for the diagnosis of a leukaemic disorder.

Ph¹-negative chronic myeloid leukaemia may terminate by transformation into acute myeloid leukaemia.

Chronic myelomonocytic leukaemia (CMML)[70]

Chronic myelomonocytic leukaemia is a disease of the elderly. It is characterized by anaemia, monocytosis and neutrophilia with or without thrombocytopenia (Fig. 8.8). The patient may have splenomegaly or clinical features reflecting anaemia or thrombocytopenia, but

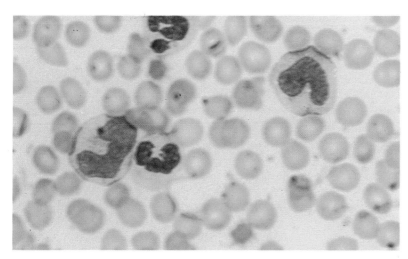

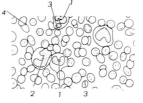

Fig.8.8 Blood films from two patients with chronic myelomonocytic leukaemia showing
(a) two neutrophils[1] and two mature monocytes[2]; two of the red cells are acanthocytic[3] and there is one tear-drop poikilocyte[4];

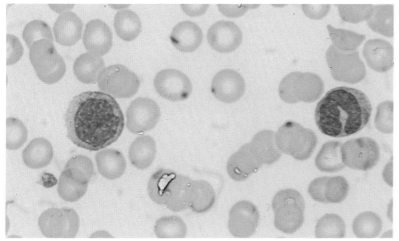

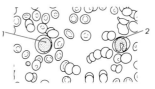

(b) a promonocyte[1] and a monocyte with increased cytoplasmic basophilia[2]; there is also macrocytosis and thrombocytopenia.

the haematological abnormalities may also be an unexpected incidental finding.

The WBC is usually moderately elevated, but ranges from 30 to 150 × 10⁹/l. Morphological abnormalities include anisocytosis, poikilocytosis, frequently macrocytosis, the presence of NRBC, hypogranularity and vacuolation of neutrophils, the presence of cells with characteristics intermediate between those of neutrophils and of monocytes, and the presence of occasional hypersegmented neutrophils or macropolycytes. CMML is classified as one of the myelodysplastic conditions (see page 214). Diagnosis requires the blood monocyte count to exceed 1 × 10⁹/l. Although neutrophilia is also characteristic, patients who have monocytosis without neutrophilia may also be included in this category. The diagnosis of CMML requires assessment of clinical features, and a bone marrow examination with careful consideration of the peripheral blood and bone marrow differential counts. If cytogenetic analysis shows a clonal cytogenetic abnormality, the diagnosis of a leukaemic disorder is strongly supported. When the diagnosis is not clear cut a period of observation and exclusion of other diagnoses, such as chronic infection, may be required. In some patients the differential diagnosis between CMML and a reactive condition is difficult. Helpful features are the lack of toxic changes in the neutrophils, the presence of dysplastic changes and the tendency for the monocytes to be large, or somewhat immature with features such as increased cytoplasmic basophilia or nucleoli; Döhle bodies may

occur in myelodysplastic conditions so their presence in the absence of other 'toxic' changes in neutrophils is not evidence of the haematological abnormalities being reactive.

It is usually easy to distinguish between CMML and CGL because of the characteristic features of the latter condition but the distinction between CMML and atypical CML is more difficult. The main distinguishing features are the greater degree of monocytosis and the lack of immature granulocytes (myeloblasts, promyelocytes and myelocytes) in the blood in CMML. CMML is largely confirmed to the elderly whereas atypical CML may also occur in younger subjects. Although the distinction between the two conditions may be difficult it is clinically important since CMML has a much better prognosis than atypical Ph¹-negative CML and patients may remain well, not requiring any treatment, for a period of years.

CMML may terminate by transforming into acute myeloid leukaemia, particularly into acute myelomonocytic leukaemia.⁶⁴

Juvenile chronic myeloid leukaemia

Children may develop typical Ph¹-positive CGL, although this is rare before adolescence. Children below 5 years of age may also develop a distinct Ph¹-negative condition designated juvenile chronic myeloid leukaemia. Clinical features are anaemia and splenomegaly and sometimes hepatomegaly and lymphadenopathy.

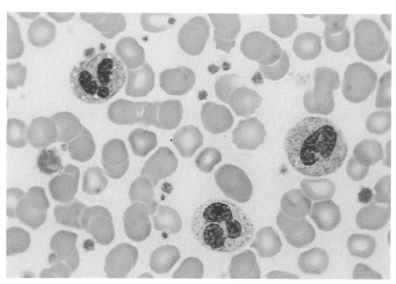

Fig.8.9 The blood film from a patient with chronic neutrophilic leukaemia. The neutrophils show 'toxic' granulation and vacuolation. One giant platelet is present. Other neutrophils showed Döhle bodies and macropolycytes were present.

The white cell count is usually lower than in CGL and myelocytes are less frequent, while monocytosis, thrombocytopenia and circulating NRBC are common features.[34] Monocytosis is particularly important in diagnosis since it is almost always present. The NAP score may be low, normal or high. The provisional diagnosis of a chronic myeloid leukaemia in infancy is an indication for a bone marrow aspiration and cytogenetic analysis to exclude the presence of the Ph[1] chromosome. Diagnosis may be aided by investigation for the abnormalities which are characteristic of this condition — a high level of fetal haemoglobin, a reduced percentage of haemoglobin A_2, reduced erythrocyte carbonic anhydrase, reduced expression of the erythrocyte I antigen, and elevated immunoglobulins.

The clinical course of juvenile myeloid leukaemia is quite variable. Termination by transformation into acute myeloblastic leukaemia may occur. Peripheral blood features which indicate a worse prognosis are a low platelet count, a high blast count and a high normoblast count.[34]

Neutrophilic leukaemia

Neutrophilic leukaemia is a rare condition characterized by anaemia and a marked neutrophilia with very few circulating immature cells (Fig. 8.9). Apart from the anaemia the major clinical feature is splenomegaly, with or without hepatomegaly.

The white cell count is usually of the order of 40–70 $\times 10^9$/l. Both toxic granules and Döhle bodies may be present in the neutrophils.[181] Ring neutrophils are relatively common.[92] Diagnosis is difficult and cannot be made on the peripheral blood features alone; it usually requires, in addition to consideration of the clinical features, bone marrow examination and cytogenetic analysis to exclude the presence of the Ph[1] chromosome, and a period of observation to exclude other conditions. The NAP is usually high which helps to make the distinction from CGL but does not help to distinguish between neutrophilic leukaemia and a reactive condition. Neutrophilic leukaemia may terminate by transforming into acute myeloid leukaemia.

CGL IN TRANSFORMATION

CGL continues a chronic course for a period of weeks, months or years before inevitably evolving into an acute phase. The first change may be an 'accelerated' phase in which the disease becomes refractory to treatment and features such as anaemia and persistent basophilia or neutrophilia are present. This is followed by a more acute blastic transformation. Blastic transformation may also supervene suddenly in the chronic phase of the disease. The acute phase takes many forms (Fig. 8.10). Not uncommonly blast transformation is of mixed cell types with there being more than one type of blast of myeloid lineage, or with both lymphoblasts and myeloid lineage blasts occurring together. A patient may also suffer two or more blast crises with cells of different morphology in succeeding crises. Myeloblasts and lymphoblasts are the commonest cell types in acute transformation, while early erythroblasts and megakaryoblasts are common as part of a mixed cell population. Other types of blast transformation are uncommon.

When blastic transformation occurs identification of the nature of the blast cells is important since lymphoblastic transformation has a better prognosis and the treatment is different. Cytochemistry, demonstration of terminal deoxynucleotidyl transferase and other cell marker studies will confirm the lymphoid nature of the blasts. The morphological characteristics of different types of blast cell are dealt with under AML and ALL (see below), but it should be noted that megakaryoblasts may be morphologically very similar to lymphoblasts and the application of cell marker studies may be necessary to make the distinction. When erythroblastic transformation occurs the blood may show macrocytosis, and when acute myelofibrosis occurs marked poikilocytosis is characteristic. Auer rods are considerably less common in myeloblastic transformation of CGL than in acute myeloblastic leukaemia.

EOSINOPHIL LEUCOCYTOSIS – EOSINOPHILIA

Eosinophilia is the elevation of the eosinophil count above levels observed in healthy subjects of the same age with no history of allergy. 0.35×10^9/l has been suggested as the upper limit of normal for an absolute eosinophil count performed in a haemocytometer;[8] a wider range has been found when the eosinophil count has been calculated from the total white cell count and the percentage of eosinophils (see Figs 6.4 and 6.5), although there is no reason why, if large numbers of cells are counted, these ranges should differ greatly. Eosinophil counts are higher in neonates (see Fig. 6.8) than in adults and a slow decline in the eosinophil count occurs with increasing age (see Fig. 6.10). Eosinophil counts are the same in males and females. The absolute eosinophil count is increased by vigorous exercise, but

not out of proportion to the increase in other leucocytes. Contrary to earlier reports there are no ethnic
differences in the eosinophil count[1] and subjects of all
ethnic origins should be assessed in relation to the same
reference intervals or normal ranges; high eosinophil
counts previously reported in Indians and Africans
appear to have been consequent on environmental influences.

Some of the causes of eosinophilia are shown in Figs
8.11 and 8.12, the commonest being allergic diseases
(particularly asthma, hayfever, and eczema) and, in
some parts of the world, parasitic infestations. Allergic
conditions causing eosinophilia are usually readily
apparent from the patient's medical history, but in the
case of parasitic infections the laboratory detection of
eosinophilia may be the finding which leads to the

correct diagnosis. In hospital patients eosinophilia can
be a useful sign of drug allergy.

When the eosinophil count is markedly elevated
(greater than 10×10^9/l) then the likely causes are far
fewer (Fig. 8.13).

Eosinophilia may be associated with pulmonary symptoms, often asthmatic in nature, together with pulmonary infiltrates detectable on chest X-ray. This combination of features suggests a range of diagnostic possibilities which are shown in Fig. 8.14. The laboratory detection of eosinophilia is important in indicating the relevant diagnostic possibilities. The finding of
eosinophilia helps to exclude other infiltrative lung conditions, such as Wegener's granulomatosis, which are
rarely associated with eosinophilia.

SOME HAEMATOLOGICAL ABNORMALITIES WHICH MAY BE DETECTED DURING THE ACCELERATED PHASE AND DURING ACUTE TRANSORMATION OF CHRONIC GRANULOCYTIC LEUKAEMIA	
Accelerated phase	**Blastic transformation**
red cells anaemia (including that due to red cell aplasia in which reticulocytes are very infrequent or absent), macrocytosis, marked poikilocytosis (may be consequent on bone marrow fibrosis), vacuolated erythroblasts (PAS positive), hypochromia and microcytosis. **white cells** refractory leucocytosis, increasing basophilia, disappearance of eosinophilia, increasing monocytosis, pseudo-Pelger and hypogranular neutrophils, pseudo-Chédiak–Higashi anomaly (giant granules), pseudo-Pelger eosinophils, increasing blast cell percentage with decreasing percentage of more mature cells, Auer rods in blast cells. **platelets** thrombocytopenia, thrombocytosis, micromegakaryocytes. **general** pancytopenia (may be consequent on refractory splenomegaly or, rarely, bone marrow necrosis).	myeloblastic transformation lymphoblastic transformation megakaryocytic transformation[125] megakaryoblastic transformation[23] (see Fig.3.69) erythroblastic transformation[156] monoblastic transformation[127] basophiloblastic transformation[138] mast cell transformation[152] eosinophil blast transformation[111] hypergranular promyelocytic transformation[84] various transformations with a mixture of cell types acute myelofibrosis

Fig.8.10 *Some haematological abnormalities which may be detected during the accelerated phase and during acute transformation of chronic granulocytic leukaemia.*

In patients with symptoms suggestive of obstructive airways disease the presence of eosinophilia usually indicates a reversible or asthmatic component to the airways obstruction, although it does not necessarily indicate allergic rather than other triggering factors.[141] In uncomplicated asthma the eosinophil count is rarely in excess of 2×10^9/l. Higher levels, often in association with deteriorating pulmonary function, may indicate either allergic aspergillosis or the Churg–Strauss syndrome. The Churg–Strauss syndrome is regarded as a variant of polyarteritis nodosa which is characterized by pulmonary infiltrates and eosinophilia, neither of which is characteristic of classical polyarteritis nodosa.[63] Some patients are also seen with some features of classic polyarteritis nodosa and some of the Churg–Strauss syndrome; they have been designated

---

SOME OF THE COMMONER CAUSES OF EOSINOPHILIA

parasitic infestations (particularly when tissue invasion has occurred)
schistosomiasis, trichinosis, strongyloidiasis, filariasis, cysticercosis, echinococcosis (hydatid cyst), visceral larva migrans (*Toxocara canis* and *catis*), Dirofilariasis (*Dirofilaria immitis* — dog heartworm)

allergic diseases
atopic eczema, asthma, allergic rhinitis (hayfever), acute urticaria, allergic bronchopulmonary aspergillosis and other allergic bronchopulmonary fungal infections

drug hypersensitivity
gold, suphonamides, penicillin

skin diseases
pemphigus, bullous pemphigoid, herpes gestationalis

Fig.8.11 *Some of the commoner causes of eosinophilia.*

SOME OF THE LESS COMMON AND RARE CAUSES OF EOSINOPHILIA

myeloid leukaemias
chronic granulocytic leukaemia, eosinophilic leukaemia, acute myelomonocytic leukaemia with eosinophilia

lymphoproliferative disorders
acute lymphoblastic leukaemia (cALL and T-ALL), non-Hodgkin's lymphoma (T-cell), Hodgkin's disease, mycosis fungoides and Sézary syndrome, angioimmunoblastic lymphadenopathy, angiolymphoid hyperplasia with eosinophilia

non-haematological malignant disease
carcinoma, sarcoma, glioma, mesothelioma, malignant melanoma, hepatoma, metastatic pituitary tumour[106]

bowel disease
eosinophilic gastroenteritis, Crohn's disease, ulcerative colitis

connective tissue disorders
Churg–Strauss variant of polyarteritis nodosa, systemic necrotizing vasculitis (variant of polyarteritis nodosa), rheumatoid arthritis, diffuse fasciitis with eosinophilia,[119] eosinophilic cellulitis,[171] progressive systemic sclerosis[57]

immune deficiency states and other conditions causing recurrent infections
Wiskott–Aldrich syndrome, Job's syndrome, infantile genetic agranulocytosis

cyclical neutropenia

cyclical eosinophilia with angioedema[73]

hereditary eosinophilia

miscellaneous
recovery from some bacterial and viral infections, scarlet fever, tuberculosis, coccidioidomycosis, *Pneumocystis pneumoniae* infection, disseminated histoplasmosis,[26] propranolol administration, haemodialysis,[118] drug abuse,[115] atheroembolic disease,[33] chronic graft-versus-host disease, chronic active hepatitis, thrombocytopenia with absent radii syndrome, chronic pancreatitis, systemic mastocytosis,[177] toxic oil syndrome[68]

Fig.8.12 *Some of the less common and rare causes of eosinophilia.*

as chronic necrotizing vasculitis or the 'overlap syndrome'. Eosinophilia of $1.5 \times 10^9/l$ or more is an important criterion in making the diagnosis of Churg–Strauss syndrome or the overlap syndrome.

In some patients with eosinophilia and pulmonary infiltration no underlying condition can be found. Many of these have a condition designated chronic eosinophilic pneumonia; the cause of this condition is unknown, but the chest X-ray shows distinctive peripheral infiltration and there is a predictable response to corticosteroid therapy. The combination of the characteristic X-ray appearance with eosinophilia has been considered sufficient to make the diagnosis[56] whereas in the minority of patients lacking eosinophilia a lung biopsy may be needed.

Eosinophilia is a rare manifestation of non-haemopoietic malignancy. It is usually associated with widespread malignant disease but rarely may provide a clue to a localized malignancy. Eosinophilia may be one feature of a myeloid leukaemia or may occur in association with lymphoid malignancy (Fig. 8.15a), particularly Hodgkin's disease or a T-cell malignancy. In the various myeloid leukaemias which may have eosinophilia as a feature the eosinophils appear to be part of the leukaemic clone of cells. In lymphoid malignancies it has generally been considered that the eosinophilia is reactive; this view was supported by the absence of eosinophil granules in association with clonally abnormal metaphases.[154] T lymphocytes have a role in eosinophilopoiesis and it could be that the malignant lympocytes secrete a lymphokine capable of stimulating eosinophilopoiesis. A recent report of a patient with eosinophilia in association with acute lymphoblastic leukaemia in whom eosinophil granules were associated with clonally abnormal metaphases[96] does, however, suggest that in some cases the eosinophils constitute

---

SOME CAUSES OF MARKED EOSINOPHILIA

parasitic infestations:
visceral larva migrans, trichinosis, tissue migration by larvae of ascaris, ankylostoma or strongyloides

drug hypersensitivity

Churg–Strauss variant of polyarteritis nodosa

Hodgkin's disease

idiopathic hypereosinophilic syndrome

eosinophilic leukaemia

Fig.8.13 *Some causes of marked eosinophilia.*

SOME CAUSES OF EOSINOPHILIA WITH PULMONARY INFILTRATION

parasitic infestations:
visceral larva migrans, filariasis, schistosomiasis, larval tissue migration stage of strongyloidiasis, ascariasis, ankylostomiasis

asthma

allergic bronchopulmonary aspergillosis

hypersensitivity reactions to drugs and chemicals

Churg–Strauss variant of polyarteritis nodosa and systemic necrotizing vasculitis[63]

tuberculosis (rarely)

coccidioidomycosis (rarely)

Pneumocystis pneumonia (rarely)

chronic idiopathic eosinophilic pneumonia

idiopathic hypereosinophilic syndrome

Fig.8.14 *Some causes of eosinophilia with pulmonary infiltration.*

part of the leukaemic population. When eosinophilia is associated with malignant disease it may be observed to remit and relapse with the underlying condition. Eosinophilia associated with lymphoid malignancy has been observed up to a year in advance of other evidence of the disease, and may recur some weeks before relapse can be detected.[36]

In reactive eosinophilia very high eosinophil counts may be reached. However, moderate to marked eosinophilia for which no cause can be found suggests the diagnosis of the *idiopathic hypereosinophilic syndrome* (HES) (Fig. 8.15b). This condition, commoner in males, is usually associated with tissue damage (to the heart and nervous system) which can be related to the release of constituents of eosinophil granules. Such tissue damage is not specific for the HES being seen sometimes in patients with a very high eosinophil count which is attributable to an underlying primary disease. The idiopathic hypereosinophilic syndrome has been arbitrarily defined as a peripheral blood eosinophil count of greater than $1.5 \times 10^9/l$ persisting for 6 months or more with no evidence of an underlying cause and with signs and symptoms of tissue damage.[44] The diagnosis of HES is thus to some extent a matter of exclusion of other conditions and it is also possible that the condition is heterogeneous. Diagnosis is aided, however, by certain laboratory features. Marked eosinophil vacuolation and degranulation (Fig. 8.15b and see also Figs 3.22 and 3.36) including even completely agranular eosinophils are common. Eosinophils may also be non-lobulated or hyperlobulated (up to 5 lobes) (see Fig. 3.35) and doughnut-shaped nuclei are sometimes seen. Some degree of eosinophil vacuolation and degranulation can also be seen in reactive eosinophilia but the more marked the changes the more likely it is that the diagnosis is HES. The number of degranulated cells is also of prognostic significance. If more than $1 \times 10^9/l$ degranulated cells are present then it is likely that cardiac damage is already present or will occur.[155] Abnormalities of eosinophil lobulation are likewise not specific to the HES although they are more common in it; they can be seen also in reactive eosinophilia and in myeloproliferative disorders. In reactive eosinophilia the most characteristic change is a slight increase in eosinophil nuclear lobulation and hypolobulated eosinophils are not usual. Other haematological abnormalities which may be detected in the HES are anaemia, anisocytosis, poikilocytosis (including tear drop poikilocytes), a leucoerythroblastic blood film, thrombocytopenia and the presence of neutrophils with heavy, rather basophilic granules (see Fig. 3.22). The latter abnormality may be so marked that the abnormal neutrophils are confused with basophils.

The diagnosis of *eosinophilic leukaemia* (Fig. 8.15c) needs to be considered when there is marked eosinophilia for which no cause can be found. The question as to whether or not the HES is a type of leukaemia is problematical but in the majority of cases there is no firm evidence of a leukaemic process. Eosinophilic leukaemia is very rare; the diagnosis should only be made when there is some clear evidence of leukaemia such as the presence of blast cells in the peripheral blood, an increased percentage of blasts in the bone marrow, the formation of soft tissue tumours composed of myeloblasts, or the presence of a clonal cytogenetic abnormality in myeloid cells. Eosinophils which are part of a clone of leukaemic cells occasionally contain Auer rods. A minority of patients with what appears to be the HES, who have no evidence of leukaemia at diagnosis, subsequently undergo a blast transformation thus providing evidence that the condition was leukaemic or at least preleukaemic in nature from the onset. A small minority of patients with eosinophilic leukaemia have been found to have the Ph[1] chromosome in myeloid cells and may thus be regarded as having a variant of chronic granulocytic leukaemia.[78] Some of these patients have also had basophilia[78] but as basophilia has similarly been observed in some patients with the HES and normal chromosomes[44] this feature is not particularly helpful in diagnosis.

When eosinophilia is detected for which no cause is readily apparent the blood film should be carefully examined for blast cells and lymphoma cells, for microfilariae (if the patient is from a relevant geographic area) and for morphologically abnormal eosinophils which may suggest the hypereosinophilic syndrome. The eosinophils should be quantified since the degree of elevation of the count is helpful in the differential diagnosis. If degranulated cells are present then they also should be quantified since large numbers may indicate the need for urgent treatment to prevent cardiac damage. Examination of the bone marrow is rarely helpful in elucidating the cause of eosinophilia but it is indicated if the differential diagnosis includes eosinophilic leukaemia or some other leukaemic or lymphomatous process. In the majority of patients, investigations seeking evidence of some systemic disease are more likely to allow a diagnosis than specifically haematological investigations.

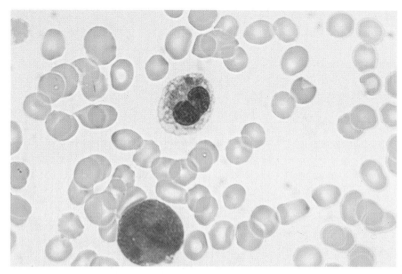

Fig.8.15 *Blood films from patients with eosinophilia* **(a)** *from a patient with acute lymphoblastic leukaemia showing a lymphoblast and a partly degranulated eosinophil;*

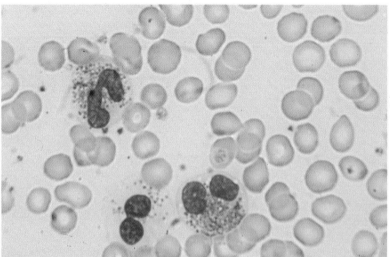

(b) *from a patient with the idiopathic hypereosinophilic syndrome; the three eosinophils show varying degrees of degranulation;*

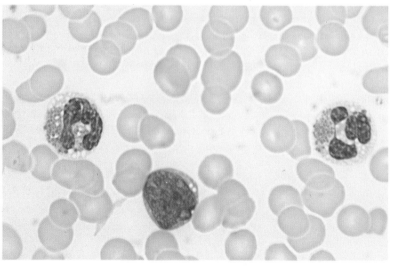

(c) *from a patient with eosinophilic leukaemia showing a blast cell and two vacuolated and partly degranulated eosinophils.*

BASOPHILIA

Some of the causes of basophilia are shown in Fig. 8.16. The detection of basophilia is useful in making the distinction between a myeloproliferative disorder and a reactive condition since only in myeloproliferative disorders and certain leukaemias is a marked increase in the basophil count at all common. A rising basophil count in CGL may indicate an accelerated phase of the disease and impending blast transformation. The occurrence of basophilia in association with ALL or AML may indicate that the patient is Ph[1] positive with the basophils and the leukaemic blast cells being derived from the same abnormal stem cell; this feature is an indication for cytogenetic analysis since prognosis is worse in Ph[1] positive patients and a variation in therapy may be indicated.

Abnormalities of basophil morphology are uncommon. Degranulation is seen during post-prandial hyperlipaemia and during acute allergic reactions such as acute urticaria and anaphylaxis.[7]

BASOPHILIC LEUKAEMIA

Basophilic leukaemia is extremely rare. The predominant cell in the peripheral blood is the basophil which constitutes 40 to 95 percent of cells. The majority of reported patients have had the Ph[1] chromosome so that the disease may be regarded as a variant of CGL.[75] Basophilic leukaemia needs to be distinguished from mast cell leukaemia and hypergranular promyelocytic leukaemia with which conditions it has certain morphological similarities. In basophilic leukaemia the predominant cell has the morphology of a mature basophil with a lobulated nucleus and dark purple granules overlying the nucleus; a few basophil myelocytes may also be present. In hypergranular promyelocytic leukaemia the cell is also heavily granulated and the nucleus may be lobulated (unlike that of a normal promyelocyte) hence the possibility of confusion with basophilic leukaemia. However the granules are purplish-red rather than purple and giant granules and stacks of Auer rods are usually present (see below). If there is any doubt as to the nature of the cells cytochemical stains will readily distinguish the basophil granule from the azurophilic granule of the promyelocyte (Fig. 8.17).

Rarely the blast cells in acute myeloid leukaemia (see below) can be demonstrated to be basophiloblasts.[172]

MAST CELL LEUKAEMIA

Mast cell leukaemia (Fig. 8.18 and see also Fig. 3.97) is a rare condition which may occur *de novo* or as a complication of systemic mastocytosis. A mast cell leukaemia or mixed basophil/mast cell leukaemia may also occur as the terminal phase of CGL.[152] Normal tissue mast cells have a small oval nucleus which is not obscured by the purple granules which pack the cytoplasm. In mast cell leukaemia some cells may resemble normal tissue mast cells, while others have bilobed or multilobed nuclei. Granules vary in colour from red to dark purple and may or may not obscure the nucleus. They may fuse into homogeneous masses. Less mature cells may have scanty granules and a nucleus which is oval or kidney shaped with nucleoli.[47,61] Mast cells may be distinguished from basophils by cytochemistry (Fig. 8.17) or by electron microscopy which shows basophils to have granules which are either uniform in consistency or contain finely particulate matter while mast cell granules are heterogeneous and contain whorled, scrolled, lamellate and crystalline structures.

SOME CAUSES OF BASOPHILIA[58,89,129,148]

Myeloproliferative and leukaemic disorders

chronic granulocytic leukaemia

polycythaemia rubra vera

myelofibrosis

essential thrombocytosis

basophilic leukaemia, eosinophil leukaemia and Ph[1]-positive acute leukaemia

Reactive

myxoedema

ulcerative colitis

idiopathic hypereosinophilic syndrome[44]

hypersensitivity states

oestrogen administration

hyperlipidaemia

Fig.8.16 *Some of the causes of basophilia.* [58,89,129,148]

SOME CYTOCHEMICAL TESTS USEFUL IN DISTINGUISHING BASOPHILS FROM CELLS WITH WHICH THEY MAY BE CONFUSED				
	Basophiloblast	Basophil	Mast cell	Hypergranular promyelocyte
myeloperoxidase	–	– or +*	–	+++
sudan black B	–	– or +	– or +	+++
chloroacetate esterase	–	– †	+++	+++
toluidine blue (metachromatic staining)	– or +	+++	+++	–

– = negative; + = weakly positive; +++ = strongly positive.
* Positive in basophil promyelocytes to metamyelocytes.
† Positive in basophil promyelocytes to metamyelocytes and may be positive in leukaemic basophils.[129]

Fig.8.17 *Some cytochemical tests useful in distinguishing basophils from cells with which they may be confused.*

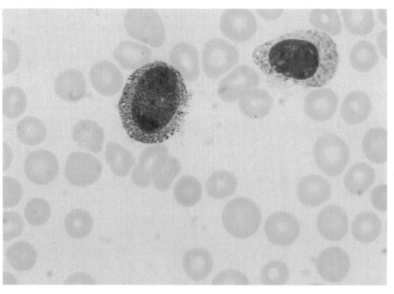

Fig.8.18 *The blood film of a patient with mast cell leukaemia.*

SOME OF THE CAUSES OF MONOCYTOSIS[72,108]

chronic infection including miliary tuberculosis

chronic inflammatory conditions:
Crohn's disease, ulcerative colitis, rheumatoid arthritis, systemic lupus erythematosus

carcinoma[6]

myeloproliferative and leukaemic conditions:
chronic myelomonocytic leukaemia and other myelodysplastic conditions, atypical Ph' negative chronic myeloid leukaemia, juvenile chronic myeloid leukaemia, chronic granulocytic leukaemia,* acute myeloid leukaemia, malignant histiocytosis

cyclical neutropenia, chronic idiopathic neutropenia

long term haemodialysis[133]

* Absolute but not relative monocytosis.

Fig.8.19 *Some causes of monocytosis.[72,108]*

It should be noted that not all leukaemias which occur in the course of systemic mastocytosis are mast cell leukaemia; acute monocytic and acute myeloblastic leukaemia may also develop, emphasizing the origin of the mast cell from a myeloid stem cell.

MONOCYTOSIS

The absolute monocyte count is higher in the neonate than at other stages of life (see Fig. 6.8). A physiological rise occurs in pregnancy (see Fig. 6.12), in parallel with the rise in the neutrophil count.

Some of the commoner causes of monocytosis are shown in Fig. 8.19. In examining a blood film showing monocytosis it is useful to look for other signs of chronic infection or inflammation which would support a reactive condition; it is also helpful to assess the maturity of the monocytes and whether or not promonocytes

or monoblasts are present. In chronic myelomonocytic leukaemia the monocytes may be somewhat larger and have more cytoplasmic basophilia than the monocytes in a reactive condition, and other features of myelodysplasia are usually detectable. In acute monocytic leukaemia or acute myelomonocytic leukaemia mature monocytes may be accompanied by promonocytes, monoblasts and immature granulocytic cells. In malignant histiocytosis the peripheral blood absolute monocyte count may or may not be elevated; the malignant cells vary in maturity from monoblasts to monocytes, and may have phagocytosed other myeloid cells (see page 211).

ACUTE MYELOID LEUKAEMIA

Acute myeloid leukaemia (AML) occurs at all ages but the incidence increases with increasing age. AML may occur *de novo* or may follow myelodysplasia, aplastic anaemia or myeloproliferative disorders such as chronic granulocytic leukaemia, polycythaemia rubra vera, essential thrombocythaemia and myelofibrosis. Major clinical features are anaemia, infection and haemorrhage; splenomegaly may occur but is slight in comparison with that which is usually seen in CGL. AML is most often manifest in the peripheral blood by anaemia, leucocytosis and thrombocytopenia with immature and morphologically abnormal myeloid cells being present.

In AML the absolute neutrophil count is most often reduced but in some patients it is normal or elevated. The differential count may show blast cells as the only major component or the 'hiatus leukaemicus' may be shown, that is there are blast cells and neutrophils with very few of the intervening cell types; this differential count is in striking contrast to that in CGL (see page 191). The presence of myeloblasts in the peripheral blood in the absence of appreciable numbers of promyelocytes and myelocytes is strongly suggestive of acute leukaemia or a related disorder even if the absolute number of blasts is not very high. If even an occasional blast contains an Auer rod (see Figs 3.58 and 7.17) there is little doubt that the diagnosis is acute myeloid leukaemia or myelodysplasia. The only other condition in which Auer rods have been described is the Chédiak–Higashi anomaly, and then in only a few cases.[107] When myeloblasts are present in the peripheral blood as part of a reactive process they are accompanied by promyelocytes and myelocytes, and Auer rods are not seen. In some patients with acute myeloid leukaemia the dominant cell type is not a myeloblast but is either an abnormal promyelocyte or a cell of the monocyte lineage — monoblast, promonocyte or monocyte. In acute myeloid leukaemia eosinophils and monocytes may be either reduced or elevated, depending on the specific type of leukaemia. Predominantly eosinophilic differentiation is rare and acute leukaemia with a basophilic component[172] is extremely rare.

A minority of patients with AML present with pancytopenia with few or no recognizable leukaemic cells in the peripheral blood. In these patients the diagnosis may be suspected because of morphological abnormalities in the remaining cells of the granulocytic series. This presentation is particularly common in acute megakaryoblastic leukaemia, which is often associated with the clinical and pathological features which have been designated acute myelofibrosis. The use of the terms subleukaemic and aleukaemic leukaemia is not helpful since there is a continuous spectrum from patients with no blasts in the peripheral blood to those with very high blast counts, and apart from the frequent presentation of acute megakaryoblastic leukaemia in this manner there is no particular significance in low peripheral blast counts. If the patient is observed without treatment the blast count usually rises rapidly.

The differential diagnosis between acute myeloid leukaemia and acute lymphoblastic leukaemia (ALL) is of vital importance since both the prognosis and the optimal treatment differ. The suspicion of AML or ALL requires examination of the bone marrow, but often the correct diagnosis can be deduced from the peripheral blood findings. In occasional patients in whom bone marrow fibrosis prevents successful aspiration the diagnosis is dependent on the blood findings supplemented by bone marrow trephine biopsy; this is particularly likely to be the case in acute megakaryoblastic leukaemia.

Acute myeloid leukaemia can be further divided into various categories. A French–American–British cooperative group (the FAB group) have defined criteria for the diagnosis of AML, and for distinguishing it from ALL and from the myelodysplastic syndromes (see below). They have classified AML into seven categories (M1 to M7) and ALL into three categories (L1 to L3).[9,10,12–14]

The FAB approach to the classification of AML is shown in Figs 8.20 and 8.21. Classification requires a differential count on 500 bone marrow cells and also a peripheral blood differential count. Typical peripheral blood features are shown in Figs 8.22–8.27. In general AML can be distinguished from ALL by the presence of Auer rods (see Figs 3.58 and 7.17) or the presence of more than 3 percent of bone marrow blasts which are sudan black B, myeloperoxidase or chloroacetate esterase positive (see Figs 7.16–7.18); these criteria may not, however, be met in the case of some monoblastic leukaemias, megakaryoblastic leukaemia and the rare leukaemia in which blasts have granules of basophil type.[172] Myeloblasts tend to have a finer chromatin pattern than lymphoblasts, larger pleomorphic nucleoli and more abundant cytoplasm, whereas lymphoblasts have a higher nucleocytoplasmic ratio, fewer and smaller nucleoli and a distinct nuclear membrane.

The definition of a myeloblast in the classification of the leukaemias is controversial. A myeloblast is a cell committed to the granulocytic pathway the definition of which often includes a lack of granules on Romanowsky staining. Since the maturation of leukaemic cells is abnormal and asynchrony between nuclear and cytoplasmic differentiation is common, very immature leukaemic cells may or may not have granules; their significance is not altered by whether or not a few granules are present. The FAB group have defined myeloblasts of two types, Type I having no granules and Type II having a few primary (azurophilic) granules; a cell falls into the promyelocyte rather than the myeloblast category if it has numerous granules, an eccentric nucleus, a low nucleocytoplasmic ratio, a lightly staining area in the cytoplasm indicating the presence of a Golgi zone or dense and/or clumped chromatin.[12] Type I and Type II myeloblasts are grouped together in assessing the number of blasts.

In reaching the diagnosis of AML and in categorizing it further it is also necessary to recognize a hypergranular promyelocyte, a variant promyelocyte, a monoblast, a promonocyte, a megakaryoblast and an early erythroblast.

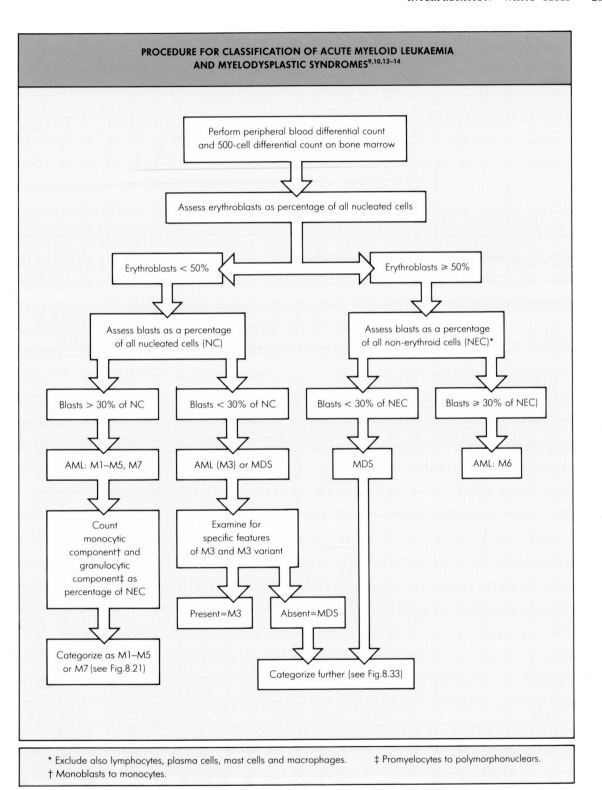

PROCEDURE FOR CLASSIFICATION OF ACUTE MYELOID LEUKAEMIA AND MYELODYSPLASTIC SYNDROMES[9,10,12–14]

Perform peripheral blood differential count and 500-cell differential count on bone marrow

Assess erythroblasts as percentage of all nucleated cells

Erythroblasts < 50%

Erythroblasts ≥ 50%

Assess blasts as a percentage of all nucleated cells (NC)

Assess blasts as a percentage of all non-erythroid cells (NEC)*

Blasts > 30% of NC

Blasts < 30% of NC

Blasts < 30% of NEC

Blasts ≥ 30% of NEC)

AML: M1–M5, M7

AML (M3) or MDS

MDS

AML: M6

Count monocytic component† and granulocytic component‡ as percentage of NEC

Examine for specific features of M3 and M3 variant

Present=M3

Absent=MDS

Categorize as M1–M5 or M7 (see Fig.8.21)

Categorize further (see Fig.8.33)

* Exclude also lymphocytes, plasma cells, mast cells and macrophages. ‡ Promyelocytes to polymorphonuclears.
† Monoblasts to monocytes.

Fig.8.20 *A procedure for the classification of acute myeloid leukaemia and the myelodysplastic syndromes.*[9,10,12–14] *The criteria apply to the bone marrow.*

THE FRENCH-AMERICAN-BRITISH (FAB) CLASSIFICATION OF ACUTE MYELOID LEUKAEMIA[9,10,12–14]

M1 (AML without maturation)

blasts $\geq$ 90 percent of NEC*; $\geq$ 3 percent of blasts positive for peroxidase or sudan black B; monocytic component $\leq$ 10 percent of NEC; granulocytic component $\leq$ 10 percent of NEC.

M2 (AML with granulocytic maturation)

blasts 30–89 percent of NEC; monocytic component <20 percent of NEC

M3 and M3 variant

characteristic morphology.

M4 (Acute myelomonocytic leukaemia)

blasts $\geq$ 30–89 percent of NEC; granulocytic component $\geq$ 20 percent of NEC; (including myeloblasts)

AND

EITHER	OR
BM monocytic component $\geq$ 20 percent AND PB monocyte count $\geq 5 \times 10^9/1$	BM resembling M2 but PB monocyte count $\geq 5 \times 10^9/1$ AND lysozyme elevated *
BM monocytic component $\geq$ 20 percent AND lysozyme elevated †	
BM monocytic component $\geq$ 20 percent AND cytochemical confirmation of monocyte component in BM ‡	BM resembling M2 but PB monocyte count $\geq 5 \times 10^9/1$ AND cytochemical demonstration of monocytic component

M5 (Acute monocytic leukaemia)

M5a without maturation or acute monoblastic leukaemia

monocytic component $\geq$ 80 percent of NEC

monoblasts $\geq$ 80 percent of monocytic component

M5b with maturation

monocytic component $\geq$ 80 percent of NEC

monoblasts $\geq$ 80 percent of monocytic component

M6 (Erythroleukaemia)

erythroblasts $\geq$ 50 percent, blasts $\geq$ 30 percent of NEC.

M7 (Megakaryoblastic leukaemia)

blasts demonstrated to be megakaryoblasts, for example by ultrastructural cytochemistry showing the presence of platelet peroxidase or by immunological cell marker studies showing the presence of platelet antigens

* NEC = non-erythroid cells.
† Lysozyme in serum or urine elevated threefold compared with normal.
‡ Positive for napthol AS-D acetate esterase activity, with activity being inhibited by fluoride.

Fig. 8.21 *The French-American-British (FAB) classification of acute myeloid leukaemia.*[9,10,12–14]
The criteria given apply to the bone marrow unless stated otherwise.

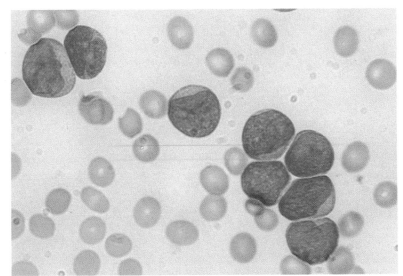

Fig.8.22 *The blood film of a patient with AML of M1 class: the blast cells have a fine chromatin pattern; they resemble lymphoblasts in having a few small nucleoli and a high nucleocytoplasmic ratio; in this patient only occasional blasts had fine azurophilic granules but myeloperoxidase, sudan black B and chloroacetate esterase were positive in a high percentage of blasts.*

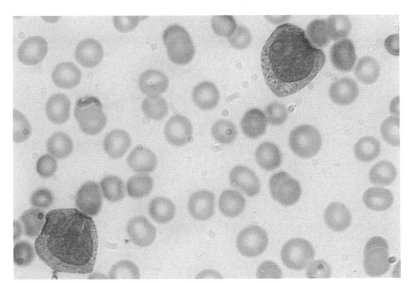

Fig.8.23 *The blood film of a patient with AML of M2 class: leukaemic cells are maturing beyond the blast stage, two promyelocytes have a single nucleolus and frequent azurophilic granules, one cell has a nucleus of bizarre shape.*

A hypergranular promyelocyte (Fig. 8.24a,b and see also Fig. 3.59) is larger than a normal myeloblast. Its nucleus may be oval, reniform (kidney shaped) or lobulated. Its cytoplasm is packed with azurophilic granules of varying size including giant granules (Fig. 8.24a). In some cells there are bundles or 'faggots' of needle-like Auer rods (Fig. 8.24b); these latter cells may have clear cytoplasm with few granules. The presence of hypergranular promyelocytes is required to categorize an acute leukaemia as M3. The variant promyelocyte is a large cell with a reniform, bilobed or multilobed nucleus

and with no granules or a few fine dust-like granules; bundles of Auer rods are less common than in the classical hypergranular promyelocyte. Patients with variant cells may have only a few typical hypergranular promyelocytes in the peripheral blood but larger numbers in the bone marrow. Unless the possibility of AML of M3 variant type[10] is considered and the characteristic cell is sought the patient may be misdiagnosed as having some type of monocytic leukaemia. Evidence that hypergranular promyelocytic leukaemia (M3) and M3 variant are part of the spectrum of the same disease type

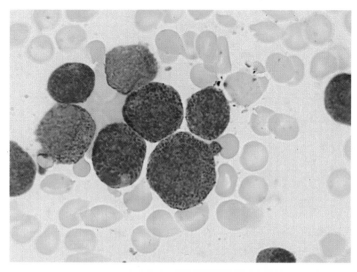

Fig.8.24 *The blood films of two patients with AML of M3 class:*
(a) *in this patient all the promyelocytes are hypergranular; one also contains a giant granule*[1]*;*

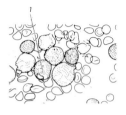

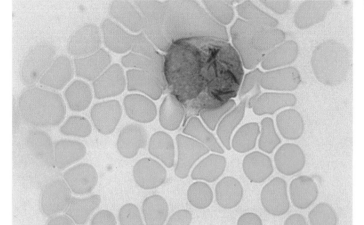

(b) *a cell showing few granules, but stacks of Auer rods*[1]*.*

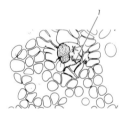

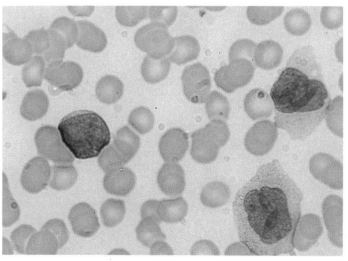

Fig.8.25 *The blood film of a patient with AML of M4 class showing one myeloblast and two monoblasts; the monoblasts are large with the lobulated nucleus having a fine lacy chromatin pattern and several nucleoli; the cytoplasm is voluminous with fine granulation and a vacuole in one of the cells.*

lies in the association of both with a high incidence of disseminated intravascular coagulation and with a characteristic chromosomal translocation, t(15;17), which is not associated with any other type of leukaemia. Cytochemical tests (Fig. 8.17) are important in confirming the nature of M3 variant since cytochemical reactions are strong despite the paucity of granules.

A monoblast (Fig. 8.28) is a large cell the diameter being up to 30 μm. The most immature monoblast is a round cell with a fine lacy chromatin pattern and a large vesicular nucleolus; there is a moderate amount of basophilic cytoplasm which may be vacuolated and may contain a few azurophil granules. A more mature

monoblast has more voluminous cytoplasm which is less basophilic and is often vacuolated. Pseudopodial projections may be present. The nucleus may show some indentation. Very occasional Auer rods may be seen in monoblasts. A promonocyte (Fig. 8.26) is a cell with characteristics intermediate between those of a monoblast and a monocyte. The nucleoli are smaller and less apparent than those of a monoblast, the nucleus is often indented, cytoplasmic granulation may be greater and cytoplasmic basophilia is intermediate between that of a monoblast and that of a mature monocyte with the cytoplasm often having a greyish ground-glass appearance. In AML with a monocytic component the

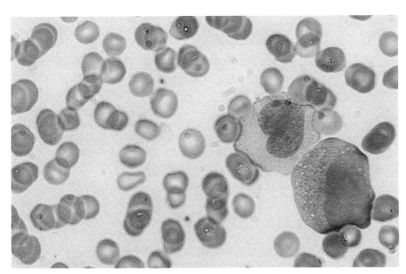

Fig.8.26 The blood film of a patient with AML of M5 class showing one promonocyte and one more mature cell of monocyte lineage; the promonocyte has moderately basophilic cytoplasm and cytoplasm which is granulated and vacuolated.

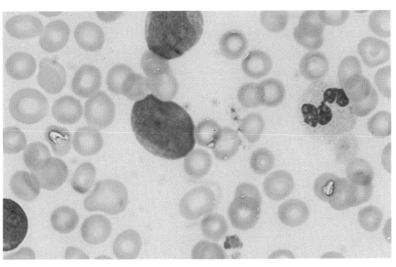

Fig.8.27 The blood film of a patient with AML of M7 class showing a neutrophil and three blast cells; the blasts are pleomorphic with no specific features to identify them as megakaryoblasts; their nature was demonstrated by immunological studies; the presence of a large hypogranular platelet adjacent to the neutrophil is the only clue that this leukaemia might be of megakaryocyte lineage (for other leukaemic cells of megakaryocyte lineage see Fig.3.69).

peripheral blood cells are often more mature than the bone marrow cells and their monocytic development is more obvious. It may therefore be the peripheral blood features which alert the haematologist to the monocytic element which might be missed if only the bone marrow features were considered.

Megakaryoblasts (Fig. 8.27) are highly variable in size, ranging from 10 to 25 μm, and quite variable in morphology. They often resemble L1 or L2 lymphoblasts (see below). Their true nature may be suggested by cytoplasmic blebs, by platelet shedding, or by the presence of bare nuclei to which platelets are adherent, but special techniques (see below) are often required for their identification.[13]

Early erythroblasts are medium to large in size with a high nucleocytoplasmic ratio, one to two nucleoli, and cytoplasm which is strongly basophilic except in the perinuclear region;[165] the cytoplasm may contain occasional small vacuoles or peroxidase-negative azurophilic granules.

In addition to the categorization of AML as M1 to M7 there are certain recognizable subtypes within these categories. Included within M2 is a subtype with heterogeneous blasts with the nucleoli often being large, the nucleus often being indented or cleft, and the cytoplasm basophilic and sometimes vacuolated.[159] A few cells contain giant granules (pseudo–Chédiak–Higashi phenomenon). A single large Auer rod is usual although occasional cells have two or three. This subtype of M2

has been found to be associated with soft tissue myeloid tumours and with a specific translocation, t(8;21) and to have a relatively good prognosis if this is the only karyotypic abnormality. Another subtype within M4 (or occasionally M2) is characterized by an increase of abnormal eosinophils in the bone marrow which is reflected by peripheral blood eosinophilia in about a third; a specific karyotypic abnormality, inversion of chromosome 16, is associated.[101]

In AML morphological abnormalities of myeloid cells are common (Fig. 8.29); the detection of such abnormalities helps to confirm the diagnosis of leukaemia and to distinguish AML from ALL.

The most important task of the laboratory when assessing the morphological features of a patient with acute leukaemia is to categorize the patient correctly as having either AML or ALL; in particular M1 and M7 need to be distinguished from ALL. It is also essential, because of the need for therapeutic measures to prevent or treat the associated coagulation abnormality, to recognize not only M3 but also the M3 variant. The correct categorization of patients into the other six categories of AML is useful in improving communication between haematologists and in assessing the treatment of patients in different centres in a uniform manner. It is likely that, with increasing knowledge of prognosis and appropriate treatment, assignment to the various categories will become increasingly relevant.

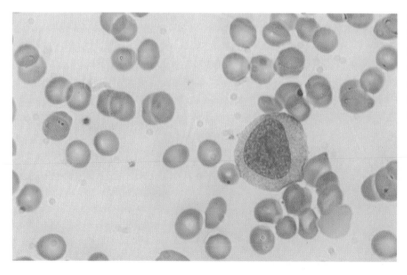

Fig.8.28 A monoblast in the blood film of a patient with AML of M5 class showing a large cell with voluminous cytoplasm and with the nucleus having a fine chromatin pattern and a large vesicular nucleolus.

ABNORMAL MORPHOLOGICAL FEATURES WHICH MAY OCCUR IN BLOOD CELLS IN AML

Leucocytes

blast cells

myeloblasts

cells larger or smaller than normal myeloblasts, very large (tetrapoid) blasts[164]

blasts of unusual shape including 'hand-mirror conformation' (lymphoblasts more often have this form)

nucleocytoplasmic asynchrony

indented or cleft nuclei, binuclearity, large nucleoli, detached nuclear fragments in the cytoplasm

Auer rods, giant granules, other cytoplasmic inclusions (rectangular, square, round, oval, irregular),[176] cytoplasmic vacuoles (sometimes lipid)

monoblasts

very large blasts: non-lobulated and hyperlobulated nuclei; giant nucleoli; multiple cytoplasmic projections; Auer rods (uncommon); heavy granulation which may be perinuclear.

promyelocytes

nucleocytoplasmic asynchrony

bilobed or multilobulated nuclei

hypergranularity, stacks of Auer rods, giant granules, flaming of peripheral cytoplasm,[158] hypogranularity

myelocytes

nucleocytoplasmic asynchrony, Auer rods (very rare); hypogranularity

polymorphonuclear neutrophils

hypolobulation (Pseudo-Pelger–Hüet anomaly), ring nuclei[157]

hypogranularity, giant granules, Auer rods (very rare)

macropolycytes

monocytes

very large monocytes, hyperlobulated nuclei, increased cytoplasmic basophilia or granulation

Erythrocytes

anisocytosis, poikilocytosis, macrocytosis

dimorphism with a population of microcytic, hypochromic cells

basophilic stippling

NRBC with megaloblastic, dyserythropoietic or sideroblastic features

Platelets

giant platelets

agranular platelets

circulating megakaryocytes which are generally mononuclear

General

increased necrobiotic cells

increased disintegrating forms (smear cells)

cells in mitosis

haemophagocytosis by leukaemic cells (myeloblasts, monoblasts, erythroblasts)

Fig.8.29 *Abnormal morphological features which may occur in blood cells in acute myeloid leukaemia.*

It is the morphological features which are of prime importance in diagnosing and categorizing AML but cytogenetic staining techniques are useful in differentiating between AML of M1 category and ALL of L2 category, and in distinguishing between M2 and M4 categories of AML. Immunological techniques to identify myeloid or lymphoid antigens are also of great use in this regard. In the diagnosis of acute megakaryoblastic leukaemia (M7) morphological features may suggest the diagnosis but ultrastructural cytochemistry or immunological cell marker studies are needed for confirmation. The common cytochemical techniques used in categorizing the acute leukaemias are shown in Fig. 8.30.

The distinction between AML and the myelodysplastic syndromes (see below) is also of critical importance since whether a patient is treated or merely observed is often determined by the precise diagnostic label which is attached. The therapeutic outcome may be affected greatly by inappropriate treatment or inappropriate lack of treatment.

In one particular circumstance the observation of morphological features suggestive of acute leukaemia may be misleading. This is in the case of infants with Down's syndrome. These infants have an increased incidence of acute leukaemia which may be either AML or ALL but they may also develop a transient proliferation of immature haemopoietic cells which is morphologically indistinguishable from acute leukaemia. It may be more correct to regard this syndrome as a transient or spontaneously remitting leukaemia rather than as a 'leukaemoid reaction' since not only may the infant have a very high blast count with bone marrow failure, but a cytogenetic abnormality (in addition to that associated with the Down's syndrome itself) may be present which disappears with the disappearance of the proliferating immature cells. Infants with Down's syndrome who have suffered a 'leukaemoid reaction' in the neonatal period appear at increased risk of developing acute leukaemia during infancy. Acute leukaemia of M7 morphology is particularly common in Down's syndrome and the 'leukaemoid reaction' may also involve proliferation of megakaryoblasts. Erythroleukaemia (M6) also appears to have a high incidence in Down's syndrome. It follows that if an infant is known to have Down's syndrome then the possibility that blasts are megakaryoblasts or erythroblasts should be considered and the finding of peripheral blood and bone marrow features which in other circumstances would be strongly suggestive or even diagnostic of acute leukaemia should not be taken as necessarily indicating a requirement for treatment.

BILINEAGE LEUKAEMIA

In a minority of patients, acute leukaemia can be categorized on morphology and/or cell marker studies as bilineage, that is, with some blasts being lymphoid and others being myeloid. (This phenomenon is more common in the acute phase of CGL than in acute leukaemia.) The bilineage leukaemias include some patients with Ph' positive acute leukaemia and some with the translocation t(4;11). The recognition of a bilineage leukaemia is important from both prognostic and therapeutic points of view. If it is suspected on morphological grounds it is an indication for cytochemical, cytogenetic and immunological cell marker studies.

THE MYELODYSPLASTIC SYNDROMES

The myelodysplastic syndromes are a group of morphologically heterogeneous conditions which are consequent on an acquired myeloid stem cell disorder leading to abnormal proliferation and disorderly maturation of one or more lineages of haemopoietic cells. There is a predilection for evolution into acute myeloid leukaemia for which reason the term 'preleukaemia' has also been used. 'Myelodysplastic syndromes' is a preferable designation for three reasons. Firstly, not all patients develop AML. Secondly, the term 'preleukaemia' cannot logically be applied to chronic myelomonocytic leukaemia (CMML) (see page 195), which nevertheless has many points of similarity with the other myelodysplastic syndromes. Thirdly, there are other conditions (such as aplastic anaemia and paroxysmal nocturnal haemoglobinuria) which may also be preleukaemic, but which are distinct from the myelodysplastic syndromes. The term 'dysmyelopoietic syndromes' is synonymous with 'myelodysplastic syndromes'.

The myelodysplastic syndromes may arise *de novo* or may be secondary to exposure to agents known to damage myeloid stem cells, such as ionizing radiation, benzene and drugs including alkylating agents, the nitrosoureas and procarbazine. Primary myelodysplasia is mainly a disease of the elderly but secondary myelodysplasia can occur at any age. Patients may present with clinical features consequent on bone marrow failure, or the diagnosis may be an incidental one in a patient suffering from another condition.

THE CYTOCHEMICAL REACTIONS OF LEUKAEMIC BLAST CELLS					
Cytochemical reaction	myeloblast*	monoblast	megakaryoblast	erythroblast	lymphoblast
myeloperoxidase	positive	negative or fine granular positivity	negative	negative†	negative
sudan black B	positive	negative or fine granular positivity	negative	negative	almost always negative (see page 182)
naphthol AS-D chloroacetate esterase (CAE)	positive	negative†	negative	negative†	negative
naphthol AS-D acetate esterase (NASDA)	variable weak positivity; fluoride resistant	strongly positive; fluoride sensitive	positive or negative; fluoride sensitive	may be positive in early erythroid cells	negative or weakly positive; fluoride resistant T-ALL may have focal positivity
α-naphthyl acetate esterase (ANAE)	usually negative; may be weakly positive	strongly positive‡	positive or negative; may be focal‡	positive or negative	strong focal positivity in blasts of T-ALL; occasional positive granules in cALL
acid phosphatase	positive – diffuse ± fine granular positivity	usually strongly positive – diffuse or granular; may be focal	positive; may be focal	positive; intense and focal	strong focal positivity in T-lymphoblasts; usually weak or negative in c-ALL and B-ALL
periodic acid-Schiff (PAS)	negative or weak diffuse positivity ± superimposed fine granular positivity	negative or weak diffuse ± superimposed fine to coarse granular positivity or occasionally block positivity	usually positive; may be granular, in cytoplasmic blebs	diffuse, or finely granular ± superimposed coarse granular or block positivity	may have coarse granular or block positivity on a negative background; often weak or negative in T-ALL and usually negative in B-ALL

* Auer rods have the same cytochemical reactions as the granules of myeloblasts; they are also PAS positive. Auer rods are more readily detected on a myeloperoxidase reaction or a sudan black B stain than on a Romanowsky stain. Hypergranular promyelocytes and their variant have the same pattern of reactivity as myeloblasts with the reactions being strongly positive; NASDA is positive and PAS usually shows moderately strong fine, dust-like positivity.
†Kass[94] states that positive reactions may occur.
‡Megakaryoblasts are much less likely to be positive for α-naphthyl butyrate esterase than for α-naphthyl acetate esterase, whereas monoblasts are strongly positive with both reactions.

Fig.8.30 The cytochemical reactions of leukaemic blast cells.

Myelodysplasia should be considered when a combination of features listed in Fig. 8.31 is observed. Characteristic morphological findings are shown in Fig. 8.32 and also Figs 3.17, 3.20, 3.30, 3.38, 3.41, 3.54 and 3.76. Among the features most commonly observed are hypogranular neutrophils with or without a pseudo-Pelger–Hüet anomaly of the neutrophil nuclei, and a macrocytic anaemia with or without a small population of hypochromic erythrocytes. A typical peripheral blood film allows a strong presumption of the diagnosis but bone marrow aspiration is required for definitive diagnosis and classification (Fig. 8.33). Cytochemical studies of peripheral blood, buffy coat or bone marrow cells may show abnormalities which support the diagnosis (Fig. 8.34). The presence of populations of neutrophils totally or partially deficient in myeloperoxidase may be detected on automated haematological counting instruments which employ the peroxidase reaction, as well as by cytochemical staining of blood films. Cytogenetic analysis is very useful since abnormalities are commonly found and the detection of an abnormal clone of cells gives strong support for the diagnosis. Certain cytogenetic abnormalities are strongly associated with specific morphological features. For example the 5q− abnormality (that is, the loss of part of the long arm of chomosome 5) is commonly associated with a combination of thrombocytosis and macrocytic anaemia, and monosomy 7 is commonly associated with pancytopenia.

SOME QUANTITATIVE AND QUALITATIVE ABNORMALITIES WHICH MAY BE PRESENT IN THE MYELODYSPLASTIC SYNDROMES

Granulopoiesis

neutropenia, neutrophilia, basophilia (rare)[163]

circulating blasts cells (with or without Auer rods) and other circulating immature cells, hypogranular promyelocytes and myelocytes

morphologically abnormal neutrophils: pseudo-Pelger nuclear anomaly, bizarre nuclear shapes including nuclear projections which sometimes resemble drumsticks, ring-shaped nuclei, dense chromatin clumping, hypersegmentation, hypogranularity, vacuolation, Döhle bodies

morphologically abnormal eosinophils: hypolobulated nuclei, nuclear projections, hypogranularity

Monocytopoiesis

monocytopenia, monocytosis, circulating promonocytes, monocytes with hyperlobulated nuclei, monocytes with increased cytoplasmic basophilia or granulation

Erythropoiesis

anaemia, reticulocytopenia

anisocytosis, poikilocytosis (including ovalocytes and tear drop cells and less commonly target cells, stomatocytes and schistocytes), macrocytosis, microcytosis or dimorphism with a population of microcytic cells,* polychromasia, basophilic stippling, Howell–Jolly bodies, Pappenheimer bodies

circulating erythroblasts (which may be binucleate or multinucleate or may show megaloblastic, sideroblastic or dyserythropoietic features)

Thrombopoiesis

thrombocytopenia, thrombocytosis

giant platelets, agranular platelets and platelets with a single large granule

circulating megakaryocytes and micromegakaryocytes

---

* Usually due to sideroblastic erythropoiesis but rarely due to acquired haemoglobin H disease.

Fig.8.31 *Some quantitative and qualitative abnormalities which may be present in the myelodysplastic syndromes.*

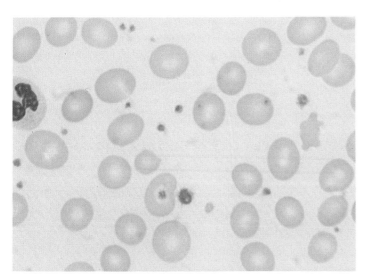

Fig.8.32 *Blood films from three patients showing typical morphological features of myelodysplasia:*

(a) *blood film from a patient with refractory anaemia showing anisocytosis, macrocytosis, and one poikilocyte[1]: the neutrophil has reduced granules[2];*

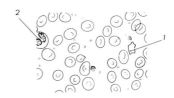

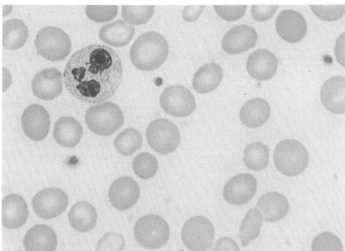

(b) *blood film from a patient with refractory anaemia with ringed sideroblasts[1] showing one target cell[1] and several hypochromic microcytes[2] – the remainder of the red cells are mainly normochromic macrocytes; the MCV was 103fl;*

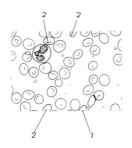

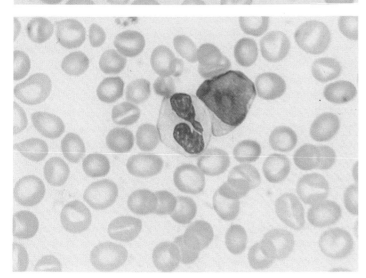

(c) *blood film from a patient with refractory anaemia with excess of blasts showing a myeloblast[1] and a hypogranular neutrophil[2]; the red cells show anisocytosis and poikilocytosis with the poikilocytes including teardrop[3] cells and stomatocytes[4]*

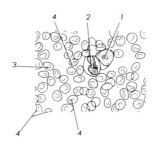

The haematology laboratory should be particularly alert to features suggestive of the myelodysplastic syndromes in patients who have been exposed to irradiation or alkylating agents (for example, patients with carcinoma, multiple myeloma or lymphoma). If such a patient develops cytopenia or a leucoerythroblastic anaemia the observation of features such as hypogranular, pseudo-Pelger neutrophils or a dimorphic blood film with Pappenheimer bodies, should suggest that the patient is not suffering from bone marrow infiltration by malignant cells representing the original disease process but rather is developing myelodysplasia.

Once the diagnosis of myelodysplasia has been made the blood film and count should be observed for features indicating further evolution of the disease. Any of the myelodysplastic syndromes may evolve into AML and the other myelodysplasias may evolve into RAEB-T (refractory anaemia with excess of blasts in transformation) and subsequently into AML. More rarely, particularly in children, ALL may supervene.[88]

LEUCOERYTHROBLASTIC ANAEMIA

A leucoerythroblastic blood film is one which shows both nucleated red blood cells and granulocyte precursors. If the patient is also anaemic, as the majority are, then the term 'leucoerythroblastic anaemia' is employed.

Fig.8.33 *FAB classification of the myelodysplastic syndromes.[12,14]*

FAB CLASSIFICATION OF THE MYELODYSPLASTIC SYNDROMES[12,14]		
Syndrome	**Peripheral blood**	**Bone Marrow***
refractory anaemia or refractory cytopenia†		blasts <5 percent, ringed sideroblasts <15 percent of nucleated cells
refractory anaemia with ringed sideroblasts or idiopathic acquired sideroblastic anaemia	anaemia, reticulocytopenia	blasts <5 percent, ringed sideroblasts >15 percent of nucleated cells
refractory anaemia with excess of blasts (RAEB)	anaemia, reticulocytopenia, blasts <5 percent	blasts 5–20 percent
chronic myelomonocytic leukaemia (CMML)	monocyte count > 1×10^9/l, granulocytes often increased, blasts <5 percent	blasts <20 percent
refractory anemia with excess of blasts in transformation (RAEB-t)	blasts >5 percent or Auer rods present	blasts 20–30 percent or Auer rods present

* The blast percentage is calculated as shown in Fig. 8.20 and patients meeting the criteria for AML are excluded.
† Refractory neutropenia or refractory thrombocytopenia due to myelodysplasia may be classified with refractory anaemia and the designation refractory cytopenia may therefore be preferred.

CYTOCHEMICAL ABNORMALITIES WHICH MAY BE DETECTED IN PERIPHERAL BLOOD CELLS IN THE MYELODYSPLASTIC SYNDROMES[142]

Granulopoiesis

myeloperoxidase:
decreased, coarse granules or clusters, Auer rods

chloroacetate esterase:
decreased

neutrophil alkaline phosphatase:
increased, decreased or absent

periodic acid-Schiff (PAS):
coarse PAS positive granules

α-naphthyl acetate esterase:
increased[144]

Monocytopoiesis

naphthol AS-D acetate esterase:
decreased

Erythropoiesis

circulating NRBC:
ring sideroblasts and other abnormal sideroblasts; strong perinuclear positivity for α-napthyl acetate esterase in some NRBC; strong perinuclear or focal positivity for acid phosphatase in some NRBC: cytoplasmic positivity (block or strong diffuse positivity) with the periodic acid-Schiff (PAS) stain in some NRBC.

erythrocytes:
some cells show PAS positivity; granules may be demonstrated with Perls' stain; haemoglobin H preparation may be positive[167] (rare); haemoglobin F-containing cells may be demonstrated by a Kleihauer test.

Fig.8.34 *Cytochemical abnormalities which may be detected in peripheral blood cells in the myelodysplastic syndromes.[142]*

Leucoerythroblastosis is physiological in the neonatal period. During pregnancy granulocyte precursors are commonly present in the peripheral blood but circulating erythroblasts are less commonly detected. In other circumstances a pathological process is indicated.

Some of the causes of leucoerythroblastosis are shown in Fig. 8.35. The majority of examples are consequent on haemopoietic malignancy or bone marrow infiltration.[27,168] The laboratory detection of a leucoerythroblastic anaemia is often an important indication of metastatic malignancy, although bone marrow metastases may be present without there being any such abnormality; in one study half of a group of patients in whom bone marrow metastases were detected had no haematological abnormalities.[24]

SOME OF THE CAUSES OF A LEUCOERYTHROBLASTIC BLOOD FILM[27,168]

bone marrow infiltration and haemopoietic malignancy: carcinoma, lymphoma (Hodgkin's disease, non-Hodgkin's lymphoma), multiple myeloma, AML, ALL, CGL, CLL, CMML and other myelodysplasias, idiopathic myelofibrosis, polycythaemia rubra vera, tuberculosis and other granulomatous conditions, storage diseases

acute haemolysis

severe infection

severe haemorrhage and shock

rebound following bone marrow failure or suppression

crisis of sickle cell anaemia

thalassaemia major

megaloblastic anaemia

systemic lupus erythematosus[100]

severe nutritional rickets[179]

marble bone disease (osteopetrosis)

Fig.8.35 *Some of the causes of a leucoerythroblastic blood film.[27,168]*

Leucoerythroblastosis is commonly associated with polychromasia, and sometimes with the presence of very basophilic macrocytes; these represent 'shift reticulocytes', that is reticulocytes which have been prematurely released from the bone marrow.

In many patients with a leucoerythroblastic anaemia the cause is readily apparent from consideration of the clinical features. When this is not so, careful assessment of the blood film may aid in the differential diagnosis. Features suggestive of haemolysis, infection or megaloblastic haemopoiesis may be present. The presence of micromegakaryocytes, megakaryocyte fragments, or a number of blasts out of proportion to the number of myelocytes is strongly suggestive of a myeloproliferative, myelodysplastic or leukaemic disorder. Neutrophils which are hypogranular or show the pseudo–Pelger–Hüet anomaly indicate myelodysplasia or leukaemia. Marked poikilocytosis including tear-drop poikilocytes is suggestive of either idiopathic myelofibrosis or an infiltrative condition with increased reticulin and collagen deposition; in contrast, little poikilocytosis is seen when leucoerythroblastosis is secondary to haemolysis, infection or haemorrhage.

The detection of leucoerythroblastic anaemia for which no explanation is apparent is an indication for a bone marrow aspiration. If the blood film shows striking poikilocytosis there is usually reticulin and collagen deposition in the bone marrow which leads to a dry tap (that is, no marrow is aspirated), a blood tap, or a non-diagnostic aspirate; a trephine biopsy is then essential for diagnosis.

IDIOPATHIC MYELOFIBROSIS

Idiopathic myelofibrosis is a disease of the elderly. It is characterized by deposition of excess reticulin and collagen in the marrow as a consequence of a myeloproliferative disorder. Pallor and splenomegaly are the only notable clinical features.

The name 'idiopathic myelofibrosis' was coined before it was known that a clonal disorder of myelopoiesis underlay the fibrosis of the marrow. An alternative name, agnogenic myeloid metaplasia, reflects the occurrence of extramedullary haemopoiesis which is also a feature of the disease. This disease is also known as myelosclerosis. 'Idiopathic' myelofibrosis develops de novo but an essentially identical condition occurs as a complication of other myeloproliferative disorders such as polycythaemia rubra vera and essential thrombocythaemia. The bone marrow fibrosis which can occur as a

complication of chronic granulocytic leukaemia is also essentially similar, since in all these conditions there is proliferation of an abnormal clone of myeloid cells with a secondary, reactive proliferation of fibroblasts. When myelofibrosis develops as a complication of another identifiable myeloproliferative disorder the haematological features of myelofibrosis are superimposed on or replace those of the original condition.

Early in the development of idiopathic myelofibrosis the haemoglobin may be normal and leucocytosis and thrombocytosis may be present. The white cell count rarely exceeds $50 \times 10^9/l$. The leucocytosis is due mainly to neutrophilia; basophilia may occur and occasionally eosinophilia. With disease progression anaemia, leucopenia and thrombocytopenia supervene. Very rarely, in early cases, leucoerythroblastosis is absent, but in the great majority of patients the blood film shows both leucoerythroblastosis and extreme poikilocytosis. Among the poikilocytes tear drop cells (Fig. 8.36) are particularly characteristic. Ovalocytes and oval macrocytes are also common. Occasionally elliptocytosis is a dominant feature.

The blood film in idiopathic myelofibrosis is highly characteristic but very similar findings may be present when the bone marrow is infiltrated, for example by carcinoma cells, and reactive fibrosis has occurred. Certain features strengthen the suspicion of idiopathic myelofibrosis. Circulating micromegakaryocytes (see Fig. 3.68) provide very strong evidence of a myeloid stem cell disorder. Other circulating megakaryocytes or megakaryocyte fragments, giant platelets, basophilia and a disproportionate number of myeloblasts are also highly suggestive of idiopathic myelofibrosis rather than fibrosis secondary to a non-haemopoietic malignancy.

Patients with idiopathic myelofibrosis may require splenectomy, which leads to a modification of haematological features. In addition to the superimposition of the usual features of hyposplenism there is also a reduction in poikilocytes, particularly a reduction in the number of tear drop poikilocytes.[55] This indicates that the spleen plays a role in the production of poikilocytosis in this condition.

The haematology laboratory should be alert to the development of the features of myelofibrosis in patients with other myeloproliferative disorders and to the development of acute myeloid leukaemia which may be the termination of idiopathic myelofibrosis.

ACUTE MYELOFIBROSIS

The blood film in acute myelofibrosis, which is a variant of acute myeloid leukaemia (see page 205), is dissimilar to that in chronic idiopathic myelofibrosis. The major feature is pancytopenia. Small numbers of blasts are present; often these can be demonstrated to be megakaryoblasts. Poikilocytosis is very minor in extent and very few NRBC and granulocyte precursors are seen. This condition therefore enters into the differential diagnosis of pancytopenia, rather than being likely to be confused with chronic idiopathic myelofibrosis.

LEUKAEMOID REACTIONS

A leukaemoid reaction is a haematological abnormality which simulates leukaemia and thus may be confused with it, but which is, in fact, reactive to some other disease. In a leukaemoid reaction the abnormalities reverse when the underlying condition is corrected. In many of the early reports of leukaemoid reactions the patient did not recover from the primary disease and correction of the haematological abnormalities did not occur. In such cases it is difficult to be sure that the patient did not have leukaemia coexisting with some other disease. This is so in many of the earlier reports of an apparent leukaemoid reaction with tuberculosis. Leukaemoid reaction may be myeloid or lymphoid.

MYELOID LEUKAEMOID REACTIONS

Leukaemoid reactions rarely simulate chronic granulocytic leukaemia since the characteristic spectrum of changes is virtually never seen in reactive conditions. The differential diagnosis of CGL and reactive conditions is discussed on page 191 and tabulated in Fig. 8.3. The myeloid leukaemias which are most likely to be simulated in a leukaemoid reaction are neutrophilic leukaemia, atypical Ph[1] negative chronic myeloid leukaemia, CMML (Fig. 8.37) and AML. Causes of myeloid leukaemoid reactions include any strong stimulus to bone marrow activity such as severe bacterial infection (particularly if complicated by megaloblastic anaemia, alcohol-induced bone marrow damage or prior agranulocytosis), tuberculosis, and carcinoma or other malignant disease (with or without bone marrow metastases).

Useful features in making the distinction between leukaemia and a leukaemoid reaction include toxic changes such as toxic granulation and vacuolation and a preponderance of more mature cells in a leukaemoid reaction, and hypogranular neutrophils and the presence of a disproportionate number of myeloblasts in many leukaemias. A low NAP score is strongly in favour of a diagnosis of leukaemia since it is almost invariably raised in a leukaemoid reaction. If Auer rods are seen in myeloblasts then a confident diagnosis of leukaemia or of myelodysplasia can be made.

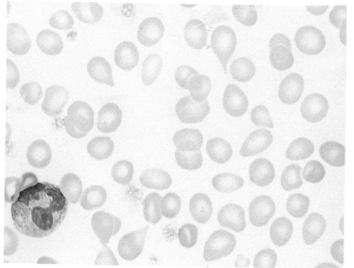

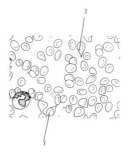

Fig.8.36 *The blood film of a patient with idiopathic myelofibrosis showing anisocytosis and poikilocytosis with prominent teardrop poikilocytes[1].*

The particular problems in distinguishing between leukaemia and a leukaemoid reaction in infants with Down's syndrome have been discussed above (see page 214). Infants with the syndrome of thrombocytopenia with absent radii may have a leukaemoid reaction following haemorrhage.[174]

If clinical and haematological features do not permit the distinction between leukaemia and a leukaemoid reaction then a bone marrow aspiration is indicated; this should include cytogenetic analysis and culture and direct microscopy for *Mycobacterium tuberculosis*.

LYMPHOID LEUKAEMOID REACTIONS

The blood films of whooping cough (Fig. 8.38) and of acute infectious lymphocytosis (see page 223) may simulate chronic lymphocytic leukaemia. Since the clinical features and the age range affected are totally different from CLL no problem occurs in practice. CLL has been misdiagnosed in patients with post-splenectomy lymphocytosis; knowledge of the levels which the lymphocyte count may sometimes reach following splenectomy, and careful examination of the blood film for postsplenectomy features will avoid this

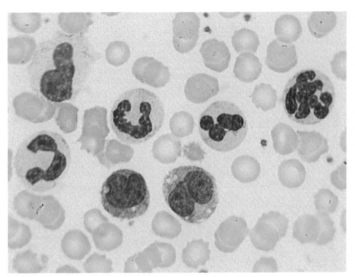

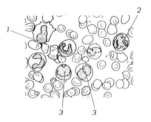

Fig.8.37 *The blood film of a patient with leukaemoid reaction consequent on severe postoperative sepsis due to a Gram-negative organism; the WBC was 92×10⁹/ l with a neutrophil count of 74×10⁹/l and a monocyte count of 16×10⁹/l; the film shows a band form[1], neutrophils including a macropolycyte[2], and monocytes with increased cytoplasmic basophilia[3].*

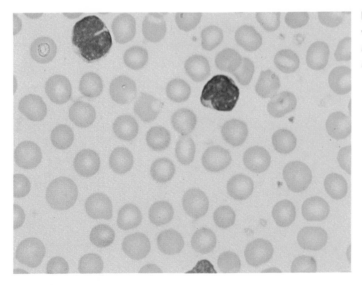

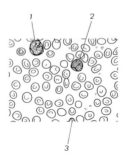

Fig.8.38 *The blood film of a child with whooping cough showing a cleft lymphocyte[1], a lymphocyte of normal morphology[2] and a smear cell[3].*

problem. Acute lymphoblastic leukaemia may be simulated by infectious mononucleosis and other viral infections which cause atypical lymphocytes, and by tuberculosis and congenital syphilis. When a test for heterophile antibody is negative and clinical and peripheral blood features do not allow the distinction between ALL and a leukaemoid reaction a bone marrow aspiration should be performed, and if necessary, immunological cell marker studies carried out on any population of immature lymphoid cells.

SOME CAUSES OF A LYMPHOCYTOSIS

many viral infections including measles (rubeola), german measles (rubella), mumps, chicken pox (varicella), influenza, infectious hepatitis (hepatitis A), infectious mononucleosis (EB virus), infectious lymphocytosis (certain Coxsackie viruses, adenovirus types 2, 5 and 12, echovirus 7),[60,85,110,124,126] cytomegalovirus infection, human immunodeficiency virus infection (HIV)

certain bacterial infections including whooping cough (Bordetella pertussis), brucellosis, tuberculosis, syphilis, plague (Pasteurella pestis)[137]

bacterial infections in infants and young children

rickettsial infections such as scrub typhus (Rickettsia tsutsugamushi)[15]

allergic reactions to drugs

serum sickness

splenectomy

Addison's disease, hypopituitarism, hyperthyroidism[99]

cigarette smoking[31]

acute severe illness including trauma, status epilepticus and cardiac arrest[161]

ß-thalassaemia intermedia[93]

lymphoproliferative disorders including chronic lymphocytic leukaemia (CLL), non-Hodgkin's lymphoma, Waldenström's macroglobulinaemia, heavy chain disease, mycosis fungoides and Sézary syndrome, Hodgkin's disease (rarely)

Fig.8.39 *Some causes of a lymphocytosis.*

LYMPHOCYTOSIS AND ABNORMAL LYMPHOCYTE MORPHOLOGY

Lymphocytosis is an increase of the absolute lymphocyte count above that which would be expected in a healthy subject of the same age. In an adult a lymphocyte count in excess of 3.5×10^9/l may be taken as indicating lymphocytosis. Since the lymphocyte count of infants and children is considerably higher than that of adults it is particularly important to use age adjusted reference limits for this parameter (see Figs 6.8 and 6.10). The lymphocyte count is increased by vigorous exercise and also by the injection of or endogenous release of adrenaline. Some pathological causes of a lymphocytosis are shown in Fig. 8.39.

In assessing the peripheral blood lymphocytes it is necessary to consider both morphology and numbers.

Lymphocytosis may occur with there being little morphological abnormality. This is so in the case of whooping cough (*Bordetella pertussis* infection) (Fig. 8.38) and in the group of conditions designated 'acute infectious lymphocytosis' now known to represent infection by a number of different viruses. The lymphocytes of chronic lymphocytic leukaemia are often said to be morphologically normal but in fact subtle abnormalities are frequently present. The lymphocytosis which is seen postsplenectomy is usually of modest degree (for example, $3.5–4.5 \times 10^9$/l) and the lymphocyte morphology is close to normal; occasional patients show a more marked lymphocytosis (up to 10×10^9/l) and in some such patients confusion with chronic lymphocytic leukaemia has occurred.

If a lymphocytosis is observed the morphology of the lymphocytes should be carefully assessed since certain morphological abnormalities are diagnostically useful. The most important distinction to be made is between lymphocytosis which is reactive to another disease and lymphocytosis which is due to a lymphoproliferative disorder such as leukaemia or lymphoma. The most striking reactive changes are those of infectious mononucleosis which are highly characteristic (see below) but not pathognomonic; identical changes sometimes occur in response to infection by cytomegalovirus or other viruses or as part of a hypersensitivity reaction to a drug. More often viral infections and a variety of other conditions produce changes which are similar to those of infectious mononucleosis but much less marked. Children develop such reactive changes much more readily than do adults and even apparently healthy children may have some lymphocytes of this type. No consistent terminology has been applied to the morphologically abnormal lymphocytes seen in infectious mononucleosis and other conditions. The term 'atypical mononuclear cells' has frequently been used, but since such cells are now known to be lymphoid it seems more appropriate that the name applied should indicate this. The term now most commonly applied in Britain is probably 'atypical lymphocyte', but recently in the USA the designation 'variant lymphocyte' has been encouraged. The term 'virocyte' is better avoided since such cells may be produced in response to stimuli other than viral infections. The description 'reactive changes' should be used with circumspection since it can sometimes be difficult to distinguish on morphology alone between reactive changes and a pleomorphic lymphoma.

A variety of abnormalities of lymphocyte morphology occur in patients with lymphoproliferative disorders, sometimes without the total lymphocyte count being elevated. Typical features will be described in the following pages.

INFECTIOUS MONONUCLEOSIS

Infectious mononucleosis is an acute illness due to a primary infection by the EB (Epstein–Barr) virus which haematologically is characterized by an absolute lymphocytosis with many large, pleomorphic, highly abnormal lymphocytes — cells so atypical that they were initially called 'atypical mononuclear cells'. The term 'infectious mononucleosis' derives from these cells. Common clinical manifestations are fever and lymphadenopathy (from which the designation 'glandular fever' derives), pharyngitis, and hepatitis. Infectious mononucleosis is predominantly a disease of adolescents and young adults.

The majority of the morphologically abnormal cells in infectious mononucleosis are T lymphocytes which are reacting to virus-infected B lymphocytes; a minority of the abnormal cells are B lymphocytes. It is the degree of pleomorphism which is the most characteristic feature of the abnormal cells (Fig. 8.40). Many are very large with diameters of 15–30 μm and with abundant strongly basophilic cytoplasm. Some have large, central nucleoli and resemble immunoblasts (that is, they have the same morphology as cells stimulated *in vitro* by mitogens); others resemble the blasts of acute lymphoblastic leukaemia. Nuclei may be round, oval, reniform or lobulated. The chromatin may be diffuse with nucleoli, or partly condensed. The cytoplasm may be vacuolated, foamy or granulated, and moderately or strongly basophilic; the basophilia may be confined to the cytoplasmic margins. Where the atypical cells come into contact with other cells the cytoplasmic margins sometimes appear scalloped (Fig. 8.40c). Some cells have the conformation of hand-mirrors. Some plasma cells and plasmacytoid lymphocytes are usually present. Binucleate cells and cells in mitosis can occur. The atypical cells may have cytochemical abnormalities such as block-positivity on a periodic acid–Schiff stain (usually a feature of ALL) and the presence of tartrate-resistant acid phosphatase (usually a feature of hairy cell leukaemia); however cytochemistry is not important in the diagnosis of infectious mononucleosis. Rare patients with primary infection by the EB virus have severe lymphopenia rather than lymphocytosis.[4]

Changes in other cell lines are quite common although they tend to be overshadowed by the changes in the lymphocytes. In one series 10 percent of neutrophil counts were less than 1×10^9/l.[30] Neutrophilia may also occur. Neutrophils commonly show toxic granulation, left shift and Döhle bodies; despite these toxic changes the neutrophil alkaline phosphatase score is usually reduced. Agranulocytosis may occur. Neutrophil agglutination is a rare finding.[79] Reduction of the eosinophil count is usual; during recovery eosinophilia supervenes. Thrombocytopenia is not uncommon, the platelet count being less than 150×10^9/l in about a third of patients. Severe thrombocytopenia sometimes occurs, probably consequent on peripheral destruction of platelets. Haemolytic anaemia due to a cold antibody, usually but not always with anti-i specificity, can occur and the blood film then shows red cell agglutination (which is absent in films made in warm conditions), some spherocytes and, later, the development of polychromasia. The direct antiglobulin test is positive due to the presence of complement on the red cells. A larger number of patients show cold-induced agglutination of the red cells without overt haemolysis. Subjects with hereditary spherocytosis appear particularly prone to haemolysis during infectious mononucleosis. Aplastic anaemia is a rare complication of infectious mononucleosis, developing 1 to 6 weeks after presentation. Another rare complication is pancytopenia consequent on virus-induced haemophagocytosis.

Automated differential counters show abnormalities in patients with infectious mononucleosis. In Technicon instruments there is an increase of large unstained cells. In Coulter instruments there is an abnormality of the lymphocyte component of the white cell histogram with expansion into the mononuclear area. In young children primary EB virus infection may be

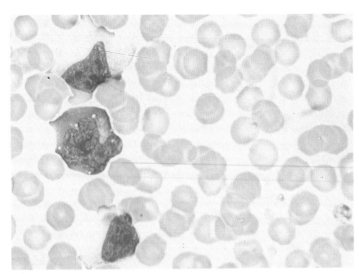

Fig.8.40 *The blood film of a patient with infectious mononucleosis:*
(a) *pleomorphic cells, one of which has voluminous cytoplasm[1] and another of which has vacuolated, basophilic cytoplasm and a lobulated nucleus[2];*

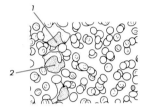

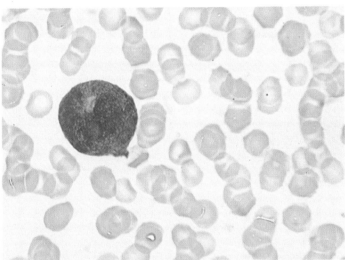

(b) *large lymphoid cell with intensely basophilic cytoplasm, a prominent Golgi zone and a large nucleolus;*

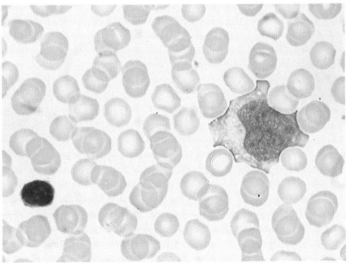

(c) *a normal small lymphocyte and a large abnormal lymphocyte with voluminous cytoplasm which has scalloped edges.*

clinically silent and some of those who do have a clinical illness do not have the large numbers of atypical lymphocytes which characterize the illness in young adults; nevertheless clinically and morphologically typical cases do occur even in children less than 2 years of age.

In older patients with infectious mononucleosis the degree of lymphocytosis and the percentage of atypical lymphocytes may be less than is usually observed in younger subjects.[32]

The finding of morphological features suggestive of infectious mononucleosis is an indication to test for heterophile antibodies against sheep or horse red cells. The heterphile antibodies which are commonly produced in infectious mononucleosis are not absorbed by guinea pig kidney whereas such absorption does occur with heterophile antibodies occurring in other conditions. A titre of 1:28 with sheep cells after guinea pig kidney absorption is regarded as positive. Rapid slide tests for heterophile antibodies are sensitive and very convenient with a false positive rate of 1–2 percent. At presentation 60 percent of patients with infectious mononucleosis have a positive heterophile antibody test and up to 90 percent become positive if closely followed. 'Heterophile-negative mononucleosis' most often represents infection by cytomegalovirus (70 percent in one series[86]) but a minority (16 percent in the same series) can be demonstrated by specific serological tests for antiviral antibodies to be due to primary infection by the EB virus. Specific tests for antiviral antibody are, however, too complex to be of use for routine diagnostic purposes and tests for heterophile antibody remain the mainstay of confirmation of the diagnosis.

OTHER CAUSE OF ATYPICAL LYMPHOCYTES

Only a small number of conditions are likely to produce a sufficient number of highly abnormal lymphocytes to simulate infectious mononucleosis. Of these by far the commonest is infection by cytomegalovirus. Other causes of atypical lymphocytes are shown in Fig. 8.41.

SOME CAUSES OF ATYPICAL LYMPHOCYTES

viral infections
infectious mononucleosis (EB virus), cytomegalovirus infection,* infectious hepatitis (hepatitis A),* measles (rubeola), german measles (rubella), echovirus, adenovirus,* chicken pox (varicella), herpes simplex, herpes zoster, influenza, mumps, lymphocytic meningitis (lymphocytic choriomeningitis virus), human immunodeficiency virus (HIV) infection[49]

bacterial infections
brucellosis, tuberculosis, syphilis

Mycoplasma pneumoniale infection

protozoan infections
toxoplasmosis,* malaria, babesiosis

immunizations

serum sickness (rarely)

hypersensitivity to drugs*
para-aminosalicylic acid, sulphasalazine, sodium phenytoin, mesantoin, dapsone, phenothiazines

angioimmunoblastic lymphadenopathy[51]

systemic lupus erythematosus[54]

sarcoidosis[52]

graft-versus-host disease

graft rejection

Hodgkin's disease

* Conditions which may cause sufficiently large numbers of atypical lymphocytes to be confused with infectious mononucleosis.

Fig.8.41 *Some causes of atypical lymphocytes.*

LYMPHOPROLIFERATIVE DISORDERS

By convention the term 'lymphoproliferative disorder' is generally used to mean a proliferation of a clone of malignant lymphocytes, although certain conditions with abnormal lymphoid proliferation of uncertain nature are also sometimes included under this general heading. Lymphoproliferative disorders may be divided broadly into lymphomas, which have their initial manifestations in tissues, and lymphoid leukaemias, which have their initial manifestations in the blood and bone marrow. This distinction is generally useful although there is some overlap between the two categories. Chronic lymphocytic leukaemia and well differentiated lymphocytic lymphoma, for example, have cells of very similar morphology and immunological phenotye which are present respectively in the blood and bone marrow, or in other tissues. Similarly, the cells of T-ALL and of T-lymphoblastic lymphoma are very similar.

Individual lymphoproliferative disorders have distinctive morphological features which will be discussed under the individual disease types.

Acute lymphoblastic leukaemia (ALL)

Acute lymphoblastic leukaemia (ALL) can occur at any age but is predominantly a disease of children. The clinical features often include pallor, a bleeding tendency, hepatomegaly, splenomegaly and lymphadenopathy. Haematologically it is characterized by infiltration of the bone marrow by malignant lymphoblasts which are usually also present in the peripheral blood.

Patients with ALL commonly have anaemia, thrombocytopenia and neutropenia. The total WBC is elevated in about two-thirds of patients and is low in about a third. The great majority have leukaemic lymphoblasts in the peripheral blood. If leukaemic cells are infrequent they may be more readily detected along the edges of the blood film or in a buffy coat preparation. Immature granulocytes and NRBC may be present. Rare patients have marked eosinophilia. The absolute reticulocyte count is low. Rare patients with ALL suffer an episode of transient pancytopenia due to bone marrow aplasia several months prior to the onset of the ALL.[150]

The features most useful in distinguishing ALL from AML are: the high nucleocytoplasmic ratio of the blasts; the presence of some chromatin condensation, particularly in the smaller blasts; the small, often indistinct nucleoli; the distinct nuclear membranes and the usual lack of any dysplastic features in granulocytic cells. The presence of azurophilic granules or inclusions in leukaemic cells does not exclude a diagnosis of ALL as long as a specific cytochemical stains for myeloid cells are negative (Fig. 8.30).

Uncommon morphological features in ALL include blasts with phagocytic properties[65] or with large cytoplasmic inclusions.[66] In the majority of patients with ALL the neutrophils are morphologically normal. The presence of basophilia or of morphologically abnormal neutrophils suggests that a multipotent stem cell is involved in the leukaemic process; some such patients are Ph' positive so this observation is an indication for cytogenetic analysis. However many Ph' positive patients cannot be suspected from the morphology.

ALL has been divided by the FAB group into three morphological catgories — L1, L2 and L3[9] (Figs 8.42–8.45). Other classifications also exist. There is some correlation between morphology and cell lineage, and between morphology and prognosis. Approximately 80 percent of cases of ALL are L1 and only 1–2 percent are L3. ALL of L3 morphology is quite distinctive (Fig. 8.45), the cytological features being identical to those of Burkitt's lymphoma cells. L3 ALL may occur as a *de novo* leukaemia or as a leukaemic phase of Burkitt's lymphoma. The differentiation between L1 and L2 morphology (Figs 8.43 and 8.44) is more difficult than the identification of L3 and a scoring system has been devised to help improve consistency.[11] Various modifications of the classification have also been suggested. Patients with L1 morphology may, on relapse, have L2 morphology whereas L2 will relapse as L2.

ALL is a heterogeneous disease. Cases differ not only morphologically but in the immunological phenotype of the cells. In the majority of patients the lymphoblasts resemble the precursors of B lymphocytes and share an antigen which has been designated the common ALL (cALL) antigen. This type of leukaemia is referred to as common ALL (cALL). Included within the common ALL group are a subset in whom leukaemia cells have cytoplasmic μ chains; they are designated pre-B ALL. In a minority of patients (10–25 percent) the leukaemic cells are phenotypically the same as precursors of T lymphocytes and this may be designated T-ALL. In a smaller minority of patients the leukaemic cells either are B lymphoblasts (B-ALL), or cannot be caterogized as belonging to either T or B lymphocyte lineages. Although cases of B-ALL constitute only 1–2 percent of childhood ALL they may constitute as many as 10–12 percent of adult ALL.[39] It is important that ALL should be classified immunologically as well as morphological-ly since whether patients have cALL, T-ALL, B-ALL or unclassifiable ALL influences both prognosis and treat-ment. ALL with L3 morphology is almost always found to be B-ALL. However, not all B-ALL can be recognized morphologically since some fall into the L2 category. T-ALL can sometimes be suspected on haematological and clinical grounds since a proportion have a high white cell count and a mediastinal mass on chest X-ray. Certain morphological features which can suggest T-ALL include the presence of blasts with a convoluted nucleus, the presence of a minor population of small lymphoid cells with a markedly hyperchromatic convo-luted nucleus[40] and the presence of nuclear radial segmentation.[122] The morphological variant, 'hand-mirror cell leukaemia' is commonly of early T phenotype.[77] Cytochemistry can be useful since T-ALL often lacks PAS block-positivity (see Fig. 7.20) and is much more likely than non-T ALL to show strong focal positivity for acid phosphatase (see Fig. 7.21). Although useful, clinical and haematological features cannot predict the nature of the cells with certainty and for detailed classification immunological cell markers should also be studied.

The suspicion of the diagnosis of ALL thus requires confirmation of the diagnosis followed by morphologic-al and immunological classification. Ideally cytogenetic analysis should also be performed. A bone marrow aspiration is required for definitive diagnosis and classi-fication but when there are appreciable numbers of cir-culating blast cells cytochemical and immunological studies are readily performed on the peripheral blood.

Chronic lymphocytic leukaemia (B cell type, B-CLL)

Chronic lymphocytic leukaemia (CLL) is a disease of middle-aged and elderly persons characterized clinically by hepatomegaly, splenomegaly and lymphadenopathy and haematologically by a proliferation of mature lym-phocytes which have a B lymphocyte phenotype in the majority of patients. CLL with T lymphocyte is discus-sed on page 232.

In CLL the lymphocytes are small, although often somewhat larger than normal peripheral blood lympho-cytes, with a high nucleocytoplasmic ratio and with round nuclei having clumped chromatin (Fig. 8.46 and see also Fig. 3.60). Although a nucleolus is apparent on electron microscopy it is usually inapparent or barely apparent on light microscopy. The scanty cytoplasm is weakly basophilic.

Category	Morphological features	Correlates
THE FAB CLASSIFICATION OF ACUTE LYMPHOBLASTIC LEUKAEMIA[9]		
L1	A relatively homogeneous cell population with the predominant cell being relatively small (up to twice the diameter of a lymphocyte) with scanty cytoplasm and a nucleus of regular shape with homogenous nuclear chromatin (usually finely dispersed but may be clumped in the smaller cells) and inconspicuous nucleoli; some cytoplasmic vacuoles may be present.	The majority of children have L1 morphology. Prognosis is better than for L2.
L2	Cells are larger and more heterogeneous with regard to size, chromatin pattern and nuclear shape. Cytoplasm is more abundant and sometimes moderately basophilic; azurophilic granules or vacuoles may be present. Nuclei are irregular and may be indented, clefted or convoluted. Nucleoli are usually present and may be large with perinuclear chromatin condensation.	The majority of adults have L2 morphology, particularly adults with B-ALL. cALL antigen is less often positive than when morphology is L1.[103]
L3	Cells are large and relatively homogeneous with cytoplasm being moderately abundant, strongly basophilic and usually vacuolated. Nuclei are regular in shape, round or oval, with dense finely stippled chromatin and prominent vesicular nucleoli. The mitotic rate is high.	almost always B-ALL. worse prognosis than L1 or L2.

Fig.8.42 The FAB classification of acute lymphoblastic leukaemia.[9]

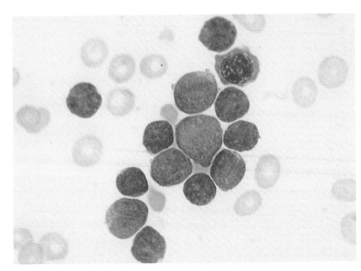

Fig.8.43 Blood film of a patient with ALL of L1 subclass. The film shows lymphoblasts[1] and one nucleated red blood cell[2]. The blasts vary in size but are relatively uniform in morphology; the smaller blasts show some chromatin condensation, which can be a feature of lymphoblasts but not of myeloblasts.

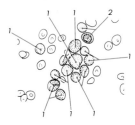

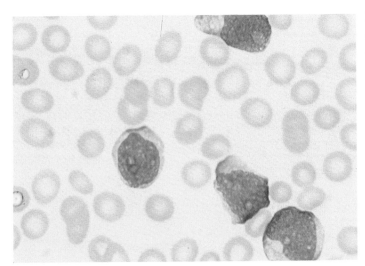

Fig.8.44 The blood film of a patient with ALL of L2 class; the blasts are larger and more pleomorphic than those of L1 ALL and have a more diffuse chromatin pattern; one of the blasts has a hand-mirror conformation; immunologically the cells were T cells.

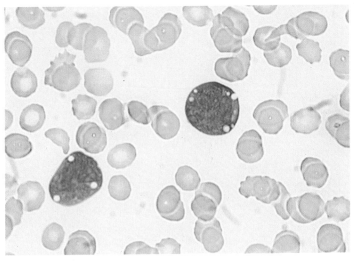

Fig.8.45 The blood film of a patient with ALL of L3 class; the blasts have strongly basophilic vacuolated cytoplasm.

CLL lymphocytes are mechanically fragile so that many of them disintegrate on the spreading of the blood film to form 'smear cells' (see Fig. 3.60). Although smear cells may be seen in other lymphoproliferative conditions and in some cases of reactive lymphocytosis they are particularly characteristic of CLL and in patients in whom the peripheral blood lymphocyte count is not yet greatly elevated they are a useful diagnostic feature. Smear cells are not formed if a blood film is prepared by centrifugation. The lymphocyte morphology varies between different patients with CLL but in an individual patient is characteristically fairly uniform, more uniform than the morphology of normal lymphocytes. In some cases of CLL the nuclei have coarse blocks of clumped chromatin while in others there is a diffuse chromatin pattern; in some cases there are detectable nucleoli; some have scanty cytoplasm, some have cytoplasm with increased basophilia and a paranuclear pale area representing the Golgi zone while yet others have plentiful pale cytoplasm; some patients have somewhat pleomorphic cells. A few vacuoles in a small percentage of cells are commonly seen but in a minority of patients vacuoles are numerous. In addition to vacuoles, other cytoplasmic inclusions which may be detected on a Romanowsky-stained blood film and which are characteristic of an individual patient include non-staining cytoplasmic rods or crystals, faintly basophilic globules and azurophilic granules or crystals.

Most such inclusions have been demonstrated to be within the endoplasmic reticulum and to be composed of immunoglobulin. Other morphological abnormalities which may occur are cleft nuclei, detached nuclear fragments and binucleate lymphocytes. Many patients have a small proportion of less mature cells (nucleolated or with prolymphocyte morphology). The presence of a small number of such cells does not have any prognostic significance but if more than 10 percent of cells are prolymphocytes this is indicative of advanced disease and a worse prognosis[59] The presence of inclusions has also been associated with a worse prognosis.[134] as has nuclear clefting in some[132] but not in other studies.[71]

Various arbitrary levels of lymphocyte count (for example, >4, >10 or $>15 \times 10^9/l$), together with more than 40 percent of lymphocytes in the bone marrow, have been suggested as necessary for the diagnosis of CLL. The characteristic morphology (a fairly uniform population of lymphocytes with an increase of smear cells) is of more importance in making the diagnosis than any particular lymphocyte count. If there is diagnostic difficulty then immunological cell markers are helpful (Fig. 8.47). The lymphocyte count in CLL ranges from just above the normal range to levels of 500 $\times 10^9/l$ or more. A lymphocytopenic preleukaemic phase may precede the development of CLL.[21] When corticosteroids are administered the absolute lymphocyte count may, in early CLL, show the

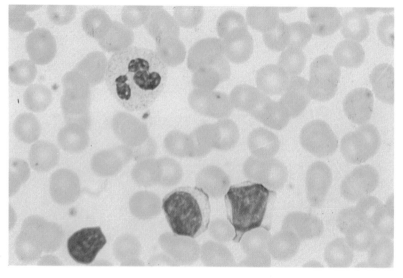

Fig.8.46 The blood film of a patient with CLL of B cell type.

normal response which is a fall, but in the majority of patients there is a sharp increase with the count remaining elevated for 2 to 4 weeks. This is not a cause for concern, but rather is the expected result and is compatible with a beneficial response to therapy.

As CLL advances, the peripheral blood also shows a normocytic, normochromic anaemia and thrombocytopenia. Neutropenia is not common in the untreated patient. In the minority of patients who have a paraprotein, rouleaux may be increased. CLL may be complicated by autoimmune haemolytic anaemia in which case the blood film shows spherocytes and the direct antiglobulin test is positive. There may be polychromasia and an elevation of the reticulocyte count but because of the diminished bone marrow reserve this may not be proportionate to the degree of anaemia. Autoimmune thrombocytopenic purpura may also develop and is suspected when the platelet count is reduced out of proportion to other indicators of disease severity. When anaemia or thrombocytopenia is due to an autoantibody it does not have the same grave significance as when it is due to heavy bone marrow infiltration. Autoimmune anaemia and thrombocytopenia may coexist. Pure red cell aplasia, which may also have an immunological

MEMBRANE MARKERS IN SOME LEUKAEMIAS OF B LYMPHOCYTES[37,38,41,145]					
	Smlg*	MRFC†	CALLA‡ (CD 10)	T1§ (CD 5)	FMC7§
chronic lymphocytic leukaemia	Positive in 85–90 percent, weak, usually IgM and IgD**	high percentage of cells positive	negative	positive	usually negative
follicular lymphoma	moderately strongly positive	lower percentage of cells positive than in CLL	often positive	most cases positive[145]	sometimes positive– weak to moderate
prolymphocytic leukaemia	strongly positive	lower percentage of cells positive than in CLL	negative	most cases positive[145]	moderately strongly positive
HCL	moderately strongly positive	lower percentage of cells positive than in CLL	negative	negative	strongly positive

* Smlg = surface membrane immunoglobulin.
† MRFC = mouse rosette forming cells.
‡ CALLA = common ALL antigen.

§ T1 and FMC7 – antigens detected by monoclonal antibodies.
** A minority of patients with B-CLL have no detectable Smlg; they can be identified as B-CLL by their having a high percentage of MRFC.[35]

Fig.8.47 *Membrane markers of some leukaemias of B lymphocytes.*[37,38,41,145]

basis, is a rare complication of B-CLL; [180] it is suspected when there is a severe normocytic, normochromic anaemia with reticulocytes being either absent or very infrequent. Some patients with pure red cell aplasia have had macrocytosis.

The diagnosis of CLL may be aided by histograms of cell size produced by various current models of Coulter counter. The cell residues of CLL lymphocytes are commonly smaller than those of normal lymphocytes though size distribution may also be normal.[2] This is in contrast to other lymphoproliferative disorders in which the size of the cell residues is normal or increased. On Technicon instruments, CLL is characterized by an increase of lymphocytes with a lesser increase of LUC (large unstained cells). A marked increase of LUC has been associated with a worse prognosis.[16] CLL can be associatd with erroneous measurements of the WBC on some Ortho instruments[50] and erroneous measurements of the lymphocyte percentage and absolute lymphocyte count occur on the Coulter S Plus IV and related instruments. Other erroneous test results which may be occur in CLL are discussed in Chapter 5.

There are three aspects to examining the blood film in a patient with suspected CLL — diagnosis, staging, and detection of complications. Diagnosis has been discussed above. With regard to staging, there have been several systems devised for the clinicopathological staging of CLL, with the aim of giving more prognostic information than can be obtained from the WBC alone.[17,131] Staging is particularly important in comparing the results of different forms of treatment since CLL is a disease which is often detected as an incidental finding in an asymptomatic patient, and the proportion of patients with early stage disease differs greatly between different centres. Staging systems generally include consideration of the haemoglobin concentration and the platelet count.

Complications of CLL which may be detected by examination of the blood film include not only immune cytopenias, which have been discussed above, but also prolymphocytic transformation and Richter's syndrome.

When CLL undergoes a prolymphocytic transformation cells with the morphology of prolymphocytes (see page 235) appear in the blood in increasing numbers.[62] Two distinct populations may be discernible. This alteration of morphology indicates a worse prognosis.

Rarely transformation into a large cell lymphoma occurs in lymph nodes or other tissues (Richter's syndrome). These more malignant cells do not necessarily appear in the peripheral blood but when they do so they have the morphology of lymphoblasts or of B-immunoblasts (large cells with a moderate amount of cytoplasm which is often basophilic, and with a large central nucleolus); this may be termed blast transformation of CLL. When Richter's syndrome develops the peripheral blood lymphocyte count may rise, fall (rarely) or be unchanged.

The peripheral blood in μ heavy chain disease may be identical with that of CLL. The specific morphological features which allow other lymphoproliferative disorders to be distinguished from CLL are discussed under the individual disease types.

Chronic lymphocytic leukaemia of T cell type (T-CLL)

In a small minority of patients with CLL leukaemic cells are found to be T lymphocytes (Fig. 8.48). CLL is more likely to be of T-cell type if the patient is relatively young, if there is skin infiltration, marked splenomegaly with little lymphadenopathy, central nervous system infiltration, or severe cytopenia out of proportion to the degree of lymphocytosis. There is also an association between T-CLL and rheumatoid arthritis.[3,123]

T-CLL is clinically, morphologically and immunologically heterogeneous. It can be more difficult than in the case of B-CLL to be certain that a T lymphocyte proliferation is leukaemic in nature. This is because of the lack of a readily available marker of monoclonality equivalent to the surface membrane immunoglobulin in a population of B lymphocytes. In the case of the T lymphocyte, proof of monoclonality usually depends on the demonstration either of a cytogenetic abnormality confined to the proliferating T lymphocytes, or of a clonal rearrangement of T cell receptor genes. In some patients it is difficult to be certain whether a T lymphocyte proliferation is leukaemic or reactive to an unknown stimulus; in this circumstance the term T cell lymphocytosis is preferred.

The lymphocyte count in T-CLL tends to be lower than that in B-CLL. In some patients the cells are morphologically indistinguishable from those of B-CLL but in others there are atypical features. The abnormal T cells may be pleomorphic. Other atypical features may include: larger size; deeply basophilic cytoplasm; indented, cleft or lobulated nuclei; and cytoplasmic granules. In comparison with B-CLL, smear cells are usually infrequent. The most characteristic feature of T-CLL is the presence of azurophilic cytoplasmic granules, these being much commoner than in B-CLL. Cells may have the morphology of large granular lymphocytes with voluminous, weakly basophilic cytoplasm and prominent azurophilic granules; on electron microscopy the azurophilic granules are found to represent either electron dense granules or parallel tubular arrays. When the cells are large granular lymphocytes the term 'large granular lymphocyte leukaemia' has been used. In the majority of such cases the cells have both T cell and natural killer cell markers but included within this group are a minority whose cells have natural killer cell markers but are negative for T-cell markers[43] (Fig. 8.49).

If T-CLL is suspected cytochemical studies may support the diagnosis and immunological studies of cell surface markers will allow a definitive diagnosis (Fig. 8.50). T-CLL cells are positive for acid phosphatase; B-CLL cells are weak or negative. The positivity may be focal (localized to the Golgi zone) or there may be cytoplasmic granules which are positive. Electron microscopy may be diagnostically useful since parallel tubular arrays are highly characteristic of large granular lymphocytes. Immunological markers are very variable. Cells may be CD4 positive (helper phenotype), CD8 positive (suppressor phenotype) or neither. When the cells are large granular lymphocytes they usually have the markers characteristic of natural killer cells (HNK1 and OKM1 (CD 11) positive).

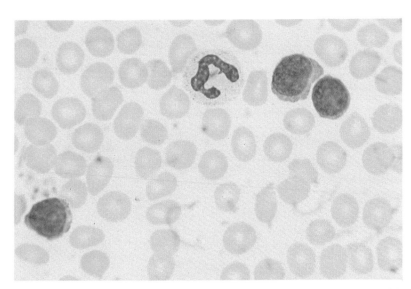

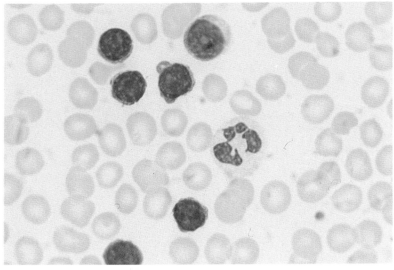

Fig.8.48 *The blood films of two patients with CLL of T cell type; in neither patient was the cell type predictable from the morphology.*

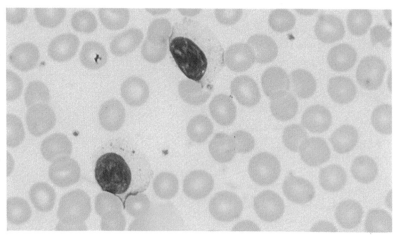

Fig.8.49 *The blood film of a patient with large granular lymphocyte leukaemia; the cells had the markers of natural killer cells and T cell markers.*

MEMBRANE MARKERS IN SOME LEUKAEMIAS OF T-LYMPHOCYTES					
	E Rosettes* T11† (CD 2)	**T3† (CD 3)**	**T6† (CD 1)**	**T4† and T8† (CD 4 and CD 8)**	**TDT‡**
T chronic lymphocytic leukaemia	positive	positive	negative	most often T8 positive, T4 negative; sometimes T4 positive, T8 negative	negative
T prolymphocytic leukaemia	positive	positive	negative	usually T4 positive, T8 negative; sometimes T8 positive, T4 negative or T8 positive, T4 positive	negative
Adult T-cell leukaemia lymphoma§	positive	positive	negative	usually T4 positive, T8 negative but may be T4 negative, T8 negative	negative
Sézary syndrome/ mycosis fungoides	positive or negative	positive	negative	usually T4 positive, T8 negative but may be T8 positive, T4 negative, positive for both T4 and T8 or negative for both T4 and T8	negative
T acute lymphoblastic leukaemia	positive or negative	positive or negative	positive or negative	may be negative for both T4 and T8 or positive for both	positive

* Forming rosettes with sheep red blood cells.
† Various antigens detected by monoclonal antibodies: T11 (CD2), T3 (CD3), T6 (CD1), T4 (CD4), T8 (CD8).
‡ Terminal deoxynucleotidyl transferase.
§ CD25 (anti-Tac) positive.

Fig.8.50 *Some cell membrane markers in T cell leukaemias.*

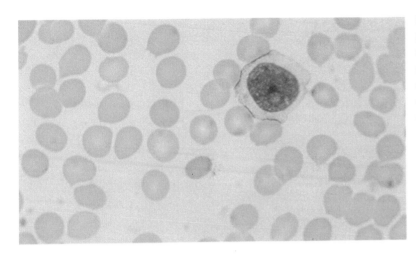

Fig.8.51 *The blood film of a patient with prolymphocytic leukaemia; the prolymphocyte has plentiful cytoplasm the nucleus has a vesicular nucleolus around which some chromatin condensation has occurred.*

T-CLL is often complicated by severe cytopenias, particularly neutropenia, but also thrombocytopenia and anaemia, which may be normocytic and normochromic, or macrocytic. Megaloblastic erythropoiesis has been described[83] and pure red cell aplasia may occur. Adult onset cyclical neutropenia has also been associated with a proliferation of large granular lymphocytes.[105] It is likely that at least some of the cytopenias seen in T-CLL are immunologically mediated, being due to an interaction between the T lymphocyte and myeloid cells.

It is probable that further study of patients with T-CLL will reveal subtypes with different biological behaviour. Those who have CD4-positive cells usually have a more aggressive clinical course than those with CD8-positive cells. The latter group may not require therapy and spontaneous remissions have occurred, even in those with evidence of a proliferating clone of presumed neoplastic cells.[175] The observation of clinical or laboratory features which would be atypical in B-CLL but consistent with T-CLL is an indication for cell marker studies both to determine the true nature of the disease in the individual patient and also to help clarify the usual features of this group of conditions.

The various clinicopathological staging systems which have been devised for B-CLL are not applicable to T-CLL.

Prolymphocytic leukaemia (B cell type)

Prolymphocytic leukaemia (PLL) is a disease of the elderly characterized by marked hepatomegaly and splenomegaly with a proliferation of abnormal lymphoid cells which have been given the designation prolymphocytes.[69] PLL is generally a B lymphocyte proliferation. T-PLL is described separately below.

Prolymphocytes (Fig. 8.51) are larger than normal lymphocytes and the lymphocytes of CLL. The amount of cytoplasm is variable, but more abundant than in CLL. The nucleus has a prominent vesicular nucleolus. Prolymphocytes differ from lymphoblasts in having a greater degree of chromatin condensation, particularly around the nucleolus and beneath the nuclear membrane. In the majority of cases the nucleus is round and regular, but in a minority it is cleft.[114] Uncommonly the cytoplasm contains vacuoles, azurophilic granules or inclusions of needle, rod or rectangular form.[135] Erythrophagocytosis by PLL cells has been reported.[112] In PLL the majority of cells have the characteristic morphology but there is an admixture with smaller, less characteristic cells.

The WBC in PLL is characteristically higher than in CLL with counts occasionally as high as $1000 \times 10^9/l$. Anaemia and thrombocytopenia are common. (Because of the often very marked splenomegaly cytopenias may often be partly consequent on hypersplenism.)

The diagnosis of PLL is usually straightforward because of the very distinctive morphology. Cell marker studies (Fig. 8.47) confirm the diagnosis and distinguish between B-PLL and T-PLL

T-prolymphocytic leukaemia (T-PLL)

About 20 percent of PLL are of T cell type. T-PLL should be suspected when the morphology of PLL is found in a patient with lymphadenopathy or skin infiltration, both of which are common in T-PLL and very uncommon in B-PLL. T-PLL may be morphologically indistinguishable from B-PLL. In other cases there are perceptible differences such as some irregularity of the nuclear shape or, less often, marked nuclear irregularity with clefting, lobulation or convolution of the nucleus; a minority of cells may resemble either those of adult T-cell leukaemia/lymphoma or those of the Sézary syndrome.[48,114] In a minority of patients with T-PLL the leukaemic cells are relatively small with less cytoplasm; such cases can be difficult to recognize on light microscopy but on electron microscopy their characteristics are similar to those of other cases of either B- or T-PLL.

Cytochemistry shows focal positivity for acid phosphatase although the reaction may be weak. α-naphthyl acetate esterase also shows focal positivity. Neither of these acid hydrolases is detected in B-PLL. Cell marker studies (Fig. 8.50) allow a definitive diagnosis.

Lymphoma

Lymphoma is distinguished from leukaemia by the pathological process being predominantly in the lymph node or other tissues rather than in the peripheral blood and bone marrow. Lymphomas are a heterogeneous group of conditions divided broadly into Hodgkin's disease — characterized by specific malignant cells known as Reed–Sternberg cells — and non-Hodgkin's lymphoma. Non-Hodgkin's lymphoma not uncommonly has a leukaemic phase, sometimes at disease onset, sometimes during the course of the disease. This is not the case in Hodgkin's disease in which a leukaemic phase with circulation of Reed–Sternberg cells is recognized (see page 83) but is extremely rare. The term 'lymphosarcoma cell leukaemia' has been used to describe the leukaemic phase of non-Hodgkin's lympoma, particularly the leukaemic phase of follicular lymphoma in which the morphology of the cells is distinctive.

The morphology of circulating lymphoma cells is dependent on the histological type of the lymphoma (Fig. 8.52). In some circumstances a proliferation of cells which are morphologically and phenotypically the same may be designated lymphoma in one patient and leukaemia in another, depending on the initial predominant manifestation. Thus Burkitt's lymphoma may have a leukaemic phase with cells which are identical to those of *de novo* ALL of L3 type; T-lymphoblastic lymphoma may have cells which are identical to those of T-ALL; small lymphocytic cell lymphoma, if it enters a leukaemic phase, has cells which are identical to those of CLL. However, the circulating lymphoma cell most commonly observed is that of follicular lymphoma (Fig.

8.53) and this differs from the CLL cell both morphologically and in immunological phenotype. If there is any difficulty in making a firm diagnosis on morphology alone then cell marker studies will help to differentiate the two conditions (Fig. 8.47).

The likelihood of a leukaemic phase differs between the different histological types of lymphoma. Dissemination of malignant cells into the peripheral blood is very common in lymphoblastic lymphoma, this condition being closely akin to ALL. In follicular lymphoma a leukaemic phase is quite common, being seen — either at onset or during the course of the disease — in 20 to 30

MORPHOLOGY OF CIRCULATING LYMPHOMA CELLS

small lymphocytic lymphoma
identical to chronic lymphocytic leukaemia

lympho-plasmacytic lymphoma
similar morphology to CLL but with more cytoplasm which is more basophilic and may have a Golgi zone; the nucleus may be eccentric

follicular, mainly small cleaved cell
more pleomorphic than CLL; small cells with scanty cytoplasm; nuclei often oval, angular, notched, or cleft with more homogeneous chromatin pattern; occasional binucleate cells

follicular, mixed small cleaved cell and large cell
some cells as in the above category but with an admixture of larger cells with a more diffuse chromatin pattern and nucleoli*

follicular, predominantly large cell
large cells with a high nucleocytoplasmic ratio; nuclei round or cleft with a diffuse chromatin pattern and multiple prominent nucleoli; moderate cytoplasmic basophilia*

large cell, diffuse
large, pleomorphic blast-like cells; may have multiple nucleoli and basophilic cytoplasm

large cell, immunoblastic
large cells with basophilic cytoplasm and a single large central nucleolus; basophilic cytoplasm

lymphoblastic
morphology identical to ALL of L1 or L2 type

Burkitt's lymphoma
identical to ALL of L3 morphology

* Commonly only small cells are seen in the peripheral blood although large cells are present in tissues.

Fig.8.52 *The morphology of circulating lymphoma cells.*

percent of patients, or even more frequently if cell marker studies are employed rather than morphology alone. In follicular lymphoma, the lymphoma cells may be sufficiently numerous to cause a lymphocytosis, or they may be detected by their characteristic morphology, even in the absence of a lymphocytosis. In diffuse large cell lymphoma and in Burkitt's lymphoma a leukaemic phase is quite uncommon.

The significance of a leukaemic phase varies with the histological type of lymphoma. In lymphoblastic lymphoma and in Burkitt's lymphoma a leukaemic conversion is indicative of a poor prognosis. In diffuse large cell lymphoma leukaemic conversion is usually a pre-terminal event with death occurring within a matter of months. In follicular lymphoma, however, the occurrence of a leukaemic phase is of less serious import. Nevertheless it is of some importance that the laboratory detects these cells since their presence indicates that the disease is widespread (Stage IV) and intensive local treatment with curative intent (as is applicable in Stage I and Stage II disease) is therefore not indicated. Follicular lymphoma is sometimes diagnosed first from the peripheral blood findings when the nature of an illness is not otherwise clear. The number of lymphoma

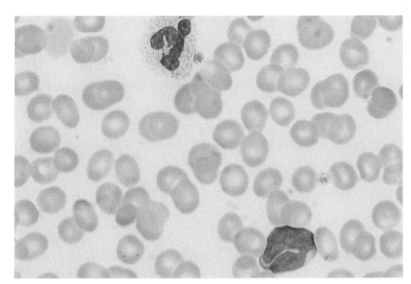

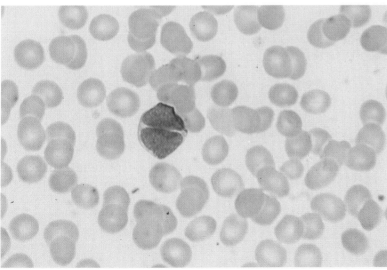

Fig.8.53 *The blood film of a patient with non-Hodgkin's lymphoma of follicular, small cleaved cell type showing two cleaved lymphoma cells.*

cells in the peripheral blood may fluctuate during the course of the disease and may fall spontaneously, even in the absence of therapy. In a minority of patients with follicular lymphoma the cells which appear in the blood are not typical small follicle centre cells but are large blast-like cells. In this particular circumstance a worse prognosis is indicated since the morphology of the cells shows that the disease has evolved into a more malignant phase.

Mycosis fungoides and Sézary syndrome

Mycosis fungoides is a T cell lymphoma characterized by lymphoma cells with highly convoluted nuclei which infiltrate not only the dermis but also, focally, the epidermis. Sézary syndrome indicates circulation in the blood of T cells with the same cytological features and immunological phenotype as the cells of mycosis fungoides; this syndrome is best regarded as a variant of mycosis fungoides with the two conditions being grouped together under the designation 'cutaneous T cell lymphomas'. The syndrome originally described by Sézary was the triad of erythroderma, lymphadenopathy and the presence in the peripheral blood of the large, highly abnormal cells which he termed 'cellules monstreuses'. By definition the Sézary syndrome has recognizable circulating lymphoma cells. Mycosis fungoides may not have such cells detectable in the early stages of the disease but does have when the disease is advanced.

Mycosis fungoides cells or Sézary cells may be similar in size to normal peripheral blood lymphocytes (8–10 μm — small cell variant) (Fig. 8.54a) or may be two or more times normal size (15–20 μm — large cell variant) (Fig. 8.54b). It was the large cell variant which Sézary initially described. Cytogenetic analysis shows that the small cell is diploid or near diploid whereas the large cell is tetraploid. Individual patients may have mainly small Sézary cells, mainly large Sézary cells, or a mixture. Both large and small cells have a high nucleocytoplasmic ratio. The nuclei are highly infolded — described as convoluted or cerebriform — and may be hyperchromatic. Nucleoli are barely visible. The nuclear convolution is more apparent on electron microscopy, when the outline is serpentine, than on light microscopy. The scanty to moderate amount of cytoplasm is weakly basophilic. Peripheral cytoplasmic vacuoles stain with a periodic acid-Schiff (PAS) stain to produce an appearance of 'beading' around the nucleus. Morphologically abnormal cells may be recognized when the total lymphocyte count is still normal, but late in the disease a frankly leukaemic phase occurs with the white cell count sometimes reaching $200 \times 10^9/l$ or more. Early in the disease, when abnormal cells are infrequent, examination of a buffy coat preparation may aid in their detection and therefore help in making the diagnosis.

Associated haematological features may include eosinophilia and monocytopenia. Since bone marrow infiltration is slight other cytopenias are uncommon.

The diagnosis of mycosis fungoides and the Sézary syndrome rest on clinical features, skin biopsy and morphology of the peripheral blood lymphocytes. Morphology may be supplemented by electron microscopy and cell marker studies (Fig. 8.50). Diagnosis of the small cell variant of the Sézary syndrome may be difficult since normal peripheral blood lymphocytes may develop highly infolded nuclei in various inflammatory disorders and occasional such cells are even seen in a proportion of healthy subjects.[166] When diagnosis is difficult the PAS stain, electron microscopy, and cytogenetic analysis to detect cytogenetically abnormal cells are helpful. Cells having both a cerebriform nucleus and a diameter of greater than 14 μm have been considered as being specific for cutaneous T cell lymphoma.[166]

Hairy cell leukaemia

Hairy cell leukaemia[18,76] is a disease of middle age characterized by splenomegaly and anaemia with splenic and bone marrow infiltration by an unusual B cell designated a hairy cell (Fig. 8.55). In a small minority of patients the malignant hairy cell is a T cell or a cell with both T and B markers. The number of hairy cells in the peripheral blood varies from numerous to very infrequent.

The hairy cell is up to twice the diameter of a normal peripheral blood lymphocyte, with a diameter of 10–20 μm. The nucleus is round to oval, or, rarely, dumbbell-shaped; it may be central or eccentric. The chromatin pattern is more diffuse than that of a normal lymphocyte and there is a distinct nuclear membrane. A few cells have a single pale nucleolus. The cytoplasm is moderately abundant and weakly basophilic with the cell outline being quite irregular — villous or serrated with frequent 'hairy' projections. The cell outline may be very indistinct. The cytoplasm may contain a few small azurophilic granules which are either round or cigar-shaped.

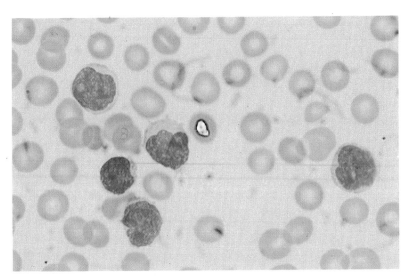

Fig.8.54 *The blood films of two patients with the Sézary syndrome:*
(a) *small cell variant showing nuclear folding;*

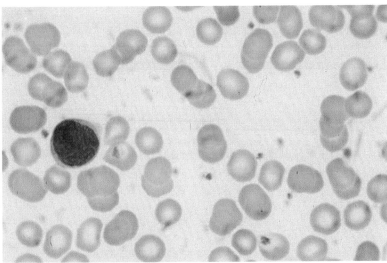

(b) *two fields with the large cell variant showing folded, hyperchromatic nuclei.*

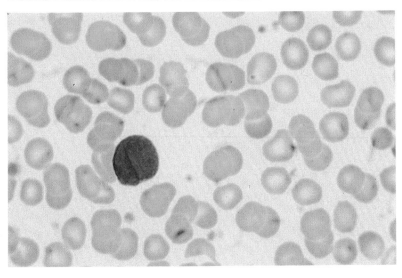

Hairy cell leukaemia is usually associated with anaemia, neutropenia, monocytopenia and thrombocytopenia. Red cells can be macrocytic with erythropoiesis being dyserythropoietic. Platelets are sometimes hypogranular and poorly functioning. The total white cell count is elevated in only 10–20 percent of patients. Because attempts at bone marrow aspiration often result in a 'dry tap' examination of the peripheral blood is very important in the diagnosis of hairy cell leukaemia. When hairy cells are very infrequent examination of a buffy coat preparation is useful. Patients with pancytopenia and a dry tap have sometimes been misdiagnosed as suffering from aplastic anaemia when the presence of infrequent hairy cells in the blood has not been appreciated. Uncommon haematological complications of hairy cell leukaemia are sideroblastic anaemia[113] and autoimmune haemolytic anaemia with spherocytes and a positive direct antiglobulin test.

Hairy cells are so distinctive in their morphological features that the diagnosis is usually straightforward as long as the condition is considered. Immunological markers are shown in Fig. 8.47. Confirmation of the diagnosis is by cytochemical studies since the great majority of patients with hairy cell leukaemia have tartrate-resistant acid phosphatase in their leukaemic cells; this isoenzyme of acid phosphatase is very uncommon in other lymphoproliferative disorders. Electron microscopy is also useful in that a characteristic structure, the ribosomal lamellar complex, is seen in about half of patients with hairy cell leukaemia; it may also be seen, however, in 5–10 percent of patients with chronic lymphocytic leukaemia and occasionally in patients with other lymphoproliferative disorders.

In a variant of hairy cell leukaemia[42] the cytoplasm is more basophilic than in classical hairy cell leukaemia and there is a prominent nucleolus. Monocytopenia is not a feature. The white cell count is usually higher.

Adult T cell leukaemia/lymphoma (ATLL)

Adult T cell leukaemia/lymphoma (ATLL) is a disease of adults originating mainly in Japan[146] and the Caribbean who have been previously infected with the HTLV I virus (the human T cell lymphotropic virus I). It may manifest itself clinically either as leukaemia or as lymphoma, with skin infiltration and hypercalcaemia being common features. During the leukaemic phase which may occur at onset or during the course of the disease, large pleomorphic lymphoid cells, often with polylobulated nuclei, are present (Fig. 8.56). A minority of cells resemble those of the Sézary syndrome. Anaemia occurs in a minority of patients. Neutrophilia may occur.

The diagnosis requires demonstration of antibodies to the HTLV I virus, and is supported by cell marker studies (Fig. 8.50) and by electron microscopy which demonstrates clearly the complex lobulation of the nucleus.

In general the prognosis of ATLL is poor with a median survival of less than 2 years. However some patients with high counts of characteristic abnormal cells

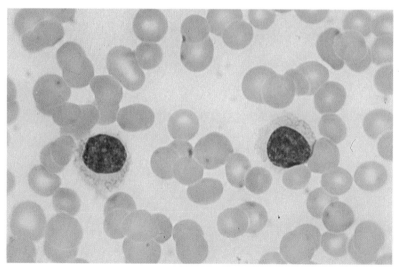

Fig.8.55 The blood film of a patient with hairy cell leukaemia showing two hairy cells; both have plentiful cytoplasm with irregular margins and in one fine hair-like projections are present.

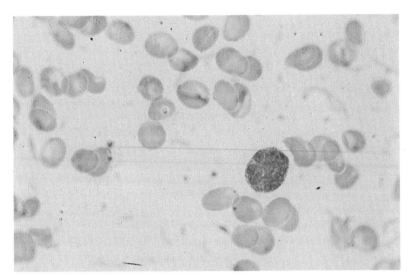
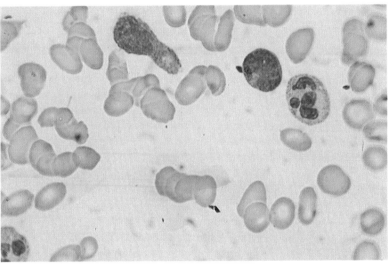
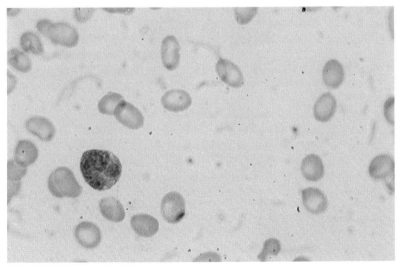

Fig. 8.56 *Three fields from the blood film of a patient with adult T cell leukaemia-lymphoma (ATLL); the malignant cells are pleomorphic with several of them showing the clover leaf nuclear formation characteristic of this condition.*

have had a chronic course, or have had spontaneous remissions and relapses.[95] Other seropositive subjects have had smaller numbers of abnormal cells for some years before progressing to typical ATLL. This latter group may be regarded as having a pre-leukaemic state, or smouldering ATLL.[97,178]

Other lymphoproliferative disorders

Chronic cold haemagglutinin disease (CHAD)

Chronic cold haemagglutinin disease is a chronic cold haemolytic anaemia occurring in elderly people which is consequent on the presence of a cold agglutinin produced by a clone of abnormal lymphoid cells. Clinical features are peripheral cyanosis on exposure to cold, and episodic cold-related haemolysis. The peripheral blood film shows agglutination of red blood cells, particularly in films prepared in cool conditions (see Figs 3.1 and 3.7). A few spherocytes and polychromasia are usually present and there may also be macrocytosis consequent on the haemolysis. A lymphocytosis may or may not be present. The morphology of the lymphocytes may be similar to that in CLL but more often the cells have some plasmacytoid features, that is they have somewhat more cytoplasm, the nucleus is eccentric, the cytoplasm is basophilic, and a pale-staining area representing the Golgi zone is present at one edge of the nucleus.

The haematology laboratory should be alert to the erroneous results produced by automated counters in patients with a cold agglutinin (see page 132).

Multiple myeloma

Multiple myeloma is a disease consequent on the proliferation of a clone of malignant plasma cells, which are called myeloma cells. It occurs mainly in the elderly. Clinically the condition is characterized by bone pain and anaemia.

The most striking haematological abnormalities are those due to the presence of an abnormal immunoglobulin produced by the malignant plasma cells; this is designated a paraprotein and is usually immunoglobulin G or immunoglobulin A. The presence of the paraprotein leads to increased bluish background staining due to affinity of the protein for the azure B or methylene blue of the stain (see Fig. 3.2), increased rouleaux formation by red cells (see Fig. 3.94) and an increased erythrocyte sedimentation rate (ESR). Very occasionally the abnormal protein forms crystals or precipitates in the peripheral blood film. This is particularly likely if the paraprotein is a cryoprotein and the blood

film is made in cool conditions (Fig.3.28). A cryoprotein may form amorphous or globular masses or irregular branching and aggregating threads. Cryoglobulins are weakly basophilic so stain pale blue or grey. Rarely a precipitated cryoprotein may be ingested by peripheral blood neutrophils or monocytes (see Figs 3.28 and 3.53). It should be noted that in a substantial minority of patients with multiple myeloma there is either no paraprotein secreted or the paraprotein, rather than being a complete immunoglobulin, is a Bence–Jones protein (the light chain only of an immunoglobulin which being of low molecular weight is excreted in the urine). In such patients the characteristic rouleaux and staining abnormalities are not seen and the ESR is not elevated; the diagnosis of multiple myeloma is sometimes missed because this is not realized.

Patients with multiple myeloma commonly have anaemia, which is most often normocytic and normochromic, but macrocytosis, of uncertain aetiology, is also seen. Leucopenia and thrombocytopenia can occur; a minority of patients have thrombocytosis. The blood film may be leucoerythroblastic . Usually a few plasmacytoid lymphocytes or a small number of plasma cells are seen (see Fig. 3.94). In a minority of patients the number of myeloma cells in the peripheral blood is sufficiently high that the designation 'plasma cell leukaemia' is applied (see page 244).

The development of myelodysplasia which may be followed by acute myeloblastic leukaemia is not uncommon in patients with multiple myeloma. In at least some patients this is a complication of therapy with alkylating agents such as melphalan. The appearance of a population of hypochromic, microcytic cells is often the first warning of this.

The laboratory should also be alert to the erroneous results which may be produced by automated counters consequent on the presence of the paraprotein; artefactual results are most likely if the paraprotein is a cryoprotein (see Chapter 5).

Waldenström's macroglobulinaemia

Waldenström's macroglobulinaemia is a lymphoproliferative disorder, occurring in the elderly, in which a clone of abnormal lymphoid cells produce an immunoglobulin M paraprotein which causes hyperviscosity of the blood. Clinical features are due either to hyperviscosity or are those due directly to the lymphoid proliferation such as hepatomegaly, splenomegaly and lymphadenopathy.

The haematological features of Waldenström's macroglobulinaemia are anaemia, increased rouleaux formation, increased background staining and sometimes a peripheral blood lymphocytosis. In those without lymphocytosis the white cell count may be low. The ESR may be elevated, but when the viscosity is very high the ESR is paradoxically low. The lymphocytes may be morphologically very similar to those of CLL or may have plasmacytoid features. Cytoplasmic inclusions or vacuoles can be present. The IgM paraprotein is sometimes a cold agglutinin or a cryoprotein in which case the abnormalities described above will occur.

Heavy chain diseases
The heavy chain diseases are lymphoproliferative disorders in which the proliferating cells secrete the heavy chain of immunoglobulin, that is the γ, α or μ heavy chain. All the heavy chain diseases are rare.

In α heavy chain disease the malignant cells characteristically infiltrate the bowel wall and the peripheral blood is usually normal. In γ and μ heavy chain diseases the clinical features are similar to those of CLL. In μ heavy chain disease the peripheral blood findings are also very often identical to those of CLL and demonstration of the abnormal heavy chain in the serum is

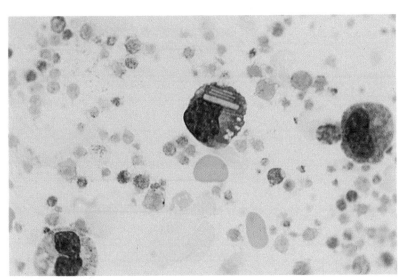

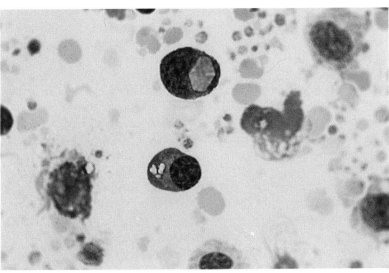

Fig. 8.57 *Two fields showing plasma cells containing either crystals or vacuoles from the peripheral blood (buffy-coat preparation) of a patient who had bacterial sepsis and no evidence of multiple myeloma.*

necessary to distinguish between the two conditions. In γ heavy chain disease anaemia, leucopenia, neutropenia and eosinophilia have been observed. Some patients have been lymphopenic. Atypical plasma cells can appear in the blood and several cases of overt plasma cell leukaemia have been described. Demonstration of the abnormal γ chains is serum or urine is necessary to make the diagnosis.

Splenic lymphoma with villous lymphocytes

The circulating lymphoma cells of splenic lymphoma with villous lymphocytes are larger than CLL lymphocytes and often nucleolated; cytoplasm is moderately basophilic with thread-like projections.[116]

Essential cryoglobulinaemia

The paraprotein of multiple myeloma or Waldenström's macroglobulinaemia may be a cryoglobulin. When a monoclonal immunoglobulin with cryoprotein properties is produced in a patient who does not have multiple myeloma or Waldenström's macroglobulinaemia the condition is designated essential cryoglobulinaemia.

The blood film in essential cryoglobulinaemia may show precipitated cryoglobulin and rouleaux formation and the ESR may be increased. The cryoprotein may interfere with the functioning of automated blood counters (see Chapter 5). Although recognition of a cryoglobulin precipitate in a blood film may lead to the diagnosis of cryoglobulinaemia only a small proportion of cryoglobulins are in fact detected in this way, and if this diagnosis is suspected on clinical grounds, serum should be inspected after being held at 4°C for at least some days and preferably one week.

BLOOD PLASMACYTOSIS AND PLASMA CELL LEUKAEMIA

Plasmacytosis is the appearance in the peripheral blood of appreciable numbers of plasma cells. Peripheral blood plasmacytosis may be reactive (see Figs 3.49 and 3.50), or may be part of a plasma cell dyscrasia (see Fig. 3.94).

Conditions which may cause a reactive plasmacytosis include bacterial and viral infections, immunizations, hypersensitivity reactions to drugs, systemic lupus erythematosus and angioimmunoblastic lymphadenopathy. In reactive plasmacytosis the number of circulating plasma cells is usually low but occasionally quite considerable numbers are present; a case of serum sickness due to tetanus antitoxin, for example, was found to have 3.2×10^9/l plasma cells.[117] In reactive

plasmacytosis the plasma cells are usually mature, although occasional plasmablasts may be seen and atypical lymphocytes may also be present. The plasma cells may have cytoplasmic vacuoles which contain their secretory product, or, rarely, they may contain crystals (Fig. 8.57).

In multiple myeloma abnormal plasma cells designated myeloma cells may circulate in the peripheral blood (see Fig. 3.94). In some patients they are undetectable or rare while in others they are present in such numbers as to be designated plasma cell leukaemia. This latter term has been arbitrarily defined as the presence of an absolute plasma cell count of more than 2×10^9/l with plasma cells also being more than 20 percent of nucleated cells in the blood.[98] Plasma cell leukaemia is particularly a feature of IgD myeloma. In multiple myeloma the circulating cells in some patients are very similar in morphology to normal plasma cells, whereas in other patients they are grossly abnormal with a diffuse chromatin pattern, nucleoli, dissociation of cytoplasmic and nuclear maturation, binuclearity, mitotic figures and cytoplasmic vacuolation. Plasma cell leukaemia also occurs in some cases of γ heavy chain disease and rarely in Waldenström's macroglobulinaemia.

When plasmacytosis is consequent on multiple myeloma the other features of this condition will be apparent in the blood (see page 242). In reactive plasmacytosis increased rouleaux and an elevated ESR may also occur, but the extent of the abnormality is generally less than in multiple myeloma. Reactive plasmacytosis is commonly associated with other reactive changes such as a left shift, neutrophilia, toxic granulation, Döhle bodies and thrombocytosis, whereas plasmacytosis due to multiple myeloma is more likely to be accompanied by anaemia and thrombocytopenia with occasional immature granulocytes and NRBC. The peripheral blood findings of angioimmunoblastic lymphadenopathy may, however, be quite similar to those of multiple myeloma. It is frequently possible to make a diagnosis of reactive plasmacytosis by consideration of the clinical and morphological features together. When this is not possible a bone marrow examination is indicated.

NEUTROPENIA

Neutropenia is a reduction of the absolute neutrophil count below what would be expected in a healthy subject of the same age, sex and ethnic origin. It may be an isolated phenomenon or part of a pancytopenia. An apparent neutropenia on an automated screening differential count should always be confirmed on a blood film since it may be consequent on ageing of the blood sample or, less often, white cell agglutination. Some of the causes of neutropenia are shown in Fig. 8.58.

The detection of unexpected neutropenia by the laboratory can be of vital importance, since drug-induced agranulocytosis can be rapidly fatal. In many circumstances the likely cause of neutropenia will be readily apparent from the clinical history, including the

SOME CAUSES OF NEUTROPENIA

infections:
viral:
measles, mumps, rubella, influenza, infectious hepatitis, infectious mononucleosis, yellow fever, dengue, Colorado tick fever, parvovirus,[140] acquired immune deficiency syndrome (end-stage HIV infection)

bacterial:
typhoid, paratyphoid, brucellosis, some Gram negative infections (early in disease process), overwhelming bacterial infection, bacterial infection in neonates, tularaemia[130]

rickettsial:
typhus fever (some cases), scrub typhus,[147] rickettsial pox[22]

protozoal:
malaria, kala azar, trypanosomiasis

fungal:
histoplasmosis[74]

drugs:
cytotoxic chemotherapy, idiosyncratic reactions (most commonly to antithyroid drugs, sulphonamides, chlorpromazine, gold), interferon therapy

irradiation

bone marrow replacement:
AML, ALL, multiple myeloma, carcinoma

myelodysplastic syndromes and idiopathic myelofibrosis

megaloblastic anaemia

aplastic anaemia:
Fanconi's anaemia, acquired aplastic anaemia, paroxysmal nocturnal haemoglobinuria

acute anaphylaxis

hypersplenism

autoimmune neutropenia:
isolated immune neutropenia
immune neutropenia associated with systemic lupus erythematosus, rheumatoid arthritis (Felty's syndrome), scleroderma, hyperthyroidism, chronic active hepatitis, polyarteritis nodosa, thymoma, Hodgkin's disease,[170] angioimmunoblastic lymphadenopathy[151]
autoimmune panleukopenia[45]
neutropenia associated with T-CLL

alloimmune neutropenia (in neonates)

cyclical neutropenia, including adult onset cyclical neutropenia associated with proliferation of large granular lymphocytes[105]

haemodialysis (during the first few hours) and early in filtration leukopheresis

hypopituitarism, Addison's disease, hyperthyroidism[99]

paroxysmal cold haemoglobinuria (during attacks)

alcoholism[104]

anorexia nervosa and starvation

haemophagocytic syndromes including malignant histiocytosis and virally-induced haemophagocytic syndromes

Kawasaki disease

copper deficiency[46]

hypercarotenaemia[149]

Certain rare congenital neutropenias:[174]
congenital aleukocytosis (reticular agenesis), infantile genetic agranulocytosis, neutropenia with pancreatic insufficiency, familial benign neutropenia, familial severe neutropenia, congenital dysgranulopoietic neutropenia,[128] lazy leucocyte syndrome, Chédiak–Higashi syndrome, dyskeratosis congenita with neutropenia, associated with X-linked agammaglobulinaemia (a third of cases), associated with cartilage-hair hypoplasia, associated with certain inborn errors of metabolism (idiopathic hyperglycinaemia, isovaleric acidaemia, methylmalonic acidaemia)

Fig.8.58 *Some of the causes of neutropenia.*

history of drug intake. When the neutropenia is unexplained, examination of the blood film may be very useful. It should be specifically examined for features suggestive of infection, leukaemia, myelodysplasia, alcohol abuse or bone marrow infiltration. When the medical history and blood film examination do not disclose the cause of neutropenia bone marrow examination becomes necessary.

EOSINOPENIA

Eosinopenia is a reduction of the absolute eosinophil count below what would be expected in a healthy subject of the same age. Eosinopenia is rarely noted on a routine blood film; since the eosinophil is a relatively infrequent cell type none may be seen in a routine 100-cell differential count and it is necessary either to perform an absolute eosinophil count or to count a larger number of cells in order to establish that eosinopenia is present. Eosinopenia is more likely to be observed with an automated differential count on an instrument which categorizes eosinophils separately, such as the various Technicon instruments.

Some of the commoner causes of a low eosinophil count are shown in Fig. 8.59. Rare causes of eosinopenia include thymoma, pure eosinophil aplasia,[121] apparent autoimmune destruction of eosinophils and basophils,[90] and autoimmune panleukopenia.[45] Eosinophils are also usually reduced, together with other granulocytes, in pancytopenia from a variety of causes.

Eosinopenia is a common non-specific response and is rarely of diagnostic significance. Its detection therefore does not generally require any comment or investigation. Whether new clinical relevance will emerge with the more widespread introduction of automated counters capable of reliably identifying eosinopenia remains to be established.

BASOPENIA

Basopenia is a reduction of the absolute basophil count below that which would be expected in a healthy subject. Basopenia is never detected in a routine blood count. Since basophils are a very low percentage of normal blood cells there are commonly none detected in

---

SOME CAUSES OF EOSINOPENIA

acute stress including trauma and surgery, burns, epileptic convulsions, acute infections, acute inflammation, myocardial infarction, anoxia and exposure to cold

Cushing's syndrome

drugs including corticosteroids and ACTH, adrenaline and other ß-agonists, histamine and aminophylline

pregnancy and, in particular, labour

haemodialysis (during actual procedure)

Fig.8.59 *Some of the causes of eosinopenia.*

SOME CAUSES OF BASOPENIA

acute stress including infection and haemorrhage

Cushing's syndrome, ACTH and corticosteroids

anaphylaxis, acute urticaria and other acute allergic reactions

hyperthyroidism

progesterone administration

Fig.8.60 *Some of the causes of basopenia.*

a routine 100-cell differential count, and there may be still none seen if 200 or even 500 cells are counted. To establish that basopenia exists therefore requires either the counting of a very large number of cells, an absolute basophil count or an automated differential count on an instrument which categorizes basophils separately. Some of the known causes of basopenia are shown in Fig. 8.60. It is possible that with the more widespread introduction of automated differential counters capable of recognizing basophils new diagnostic significance and clinical usefulness will emerge.

MONOCYTOPENIA

Monocytopenia is the reduction of the absolute monocyte count below that which would be expected in a healthy subject. Monocytopenia may be seen as part of a pancytopenia. It is rarely an isolated phenomenon. The monocyte count falls following corticosteroid administration. It is reduced out of proportion to other cells in hairy cell leukaemia.

LYMPHOPENIA (LYMPHOCYTOPENIA)

Lymphopenia or, more correctly, lymphocytopenia is a reduction of the lymphocyte count below what would be expected in a healthy subject of the same age. Lymphopenia is extremely common as part of the response to acute stress, although it is often overshadowed by the coexisting neutrophil leucocytosis and toxic changes. With the increasing importance of the diagnosis of the acquired immunodeficiency syndrome it is important to realize how very common lymphopenia is in acutely ill patients, regardless of the nature of the illness. The frequency of its occurrence has been more appreciated with the introduction of automated differential counters.

Some of the causes of lymphocytopenia are shown in Fig. 8.61.

PANCYTOPENIA

Pancytopenia is a reduction of the red cell count (with consequent anaemia), associated with leukopenia and thrombocytopenia. Leukopenia mainly reflects a reduction in the absolute neutrophil count, although other granulocytes and also monocytes and lymphocytes are commonly reduced.

Some of the causes of pancytopenia are shown in Fig. 8.62. In hospital practice the commonest cause of pancytopenia is cytotoxic or immunosuppressive chemotherapy.

When the aetiology is not readily apparent from the clinical history, the blood film should be carefully examined for evidence of bone marrow infiltration, multiple myeloma, lymphoma, leukaemia and myelodysplasia. The edges and tail of the film should be examined for hairy cells, blast cells and malignant histiocytes. The finding of a leucoerythroblastic blood film suggests the range of possibilities shown in Fig. 8.35 but the lack of leucoerythroblastic features does not exclude bone marrow infiltration as a cause of pancytopenia. In aplastic and hypoplastic anaemias the lack of leucoerythroblastic features, the lack of polychromasia, and the low absolute reticulocyte count are helpful features. Macrocytosis may be seen in hypoplastic and aplastic anaemias and also in the myelodysplasias so is not very helpful in the differential diagnosis. A combination of macrocytes with target cells and stomatocytes suggests that the pancytopenia may be due to alcohol toxicity or liver disease with hypersplenism. When pancytopenia is due to bone marrow infiltration by Hodgkin's disease hypochromia and microcytosis, increased rouleaux or eosinophilia may also be present. Severe lymphopenia will be present when pancytopenia is due to the HIV virus, but quite marked lymphopenia can also occur with a variety of other serious illnesses.

When pancytopenia is due to severe chronic megaloblastic anaemia the diagnosis is readily suspected from the usual blood film features but the diagnosis of pancytopenia due to the acute onset of megaloblastic erythropoiesis is more difficult. A few macrocytes and hypersegmented neutrophils may be present and are of diagnostic importance if found; in some patients, because of the acute onset and the sudden failure of bone marrow output of cells, the MCV is normal and no macrocytes or hypersegmented neutrophils are present. The absolute reticulocyte count is very low. Such 'megaloblastic arrest' is seen in acutely ill patients, often in association with pregnancy, surgery or sepsis. Because of the lack of the usual blood features of a megaloblastic anaemia a high index of suspicion leading to a readiness to do a bone marrow aspiration is essential if this important diagnosis is not to be missed. Delay in diagnosis and consequent delay in instituting treatment may otherwise lead to fatal complications of a potentially curable condition.

In general, a bone marrow examination is indicated in any patient with pancytopenia in whom the cause cannot be reliably determined from the clinical history and the peripheral blood findings.

SOME OF THE CAUSES OF LYMPHOCYTOPENIA

acute stress including trauma, surgery, burns, acute infection, fulminant hepatic failure

Cushing's syndrome and administration of corticosteroids and ACTH

carcinoma (particularly with advanced disease)

Hodgkin's disease (particularly with advanced disease)

uraemia (acute and chronic)

acquired immune deficiency syndrome

cytotoxic and immunosuppressive chemotherapy, antilymphocyte and antithymocyte globulin

irradiation

alcoholism[104]

coeliac disease[20]

systemic lupus erythematosus[25]

sarcoidosis[52]

angioimmunoblastic lymphadenopathy[51]

aplastic anaemia and agranulocytosis

myelodysplasia[28]

anorexia nervosa[19]

intestinal lymphangiectasia and Whipple's disease

graft-versus-host disease[5]

certain rare congenital syndromes including reticular agenesis, severe combined immune deficiency, Swiss type agammaglobulinaemia, some cases of thymic hypoplasia (di George syndrome) and ataxia telangiectasia

Fig.8.61 *Some of the causes of lymphocytopenia.*

SOME CAUSES OF PANCYTOPENIA

bone marrow infiltration including ALL, AML, carcinoma, lymphoma, multiple myeloma and hairy cell leukaemia

aplastic and hypoplastic anaemias including paroxysmal nocturnal haemoglobinuria

myelodysplastic syndromes

myelofibrosis (both idiopathic and secondary myelofibrosis), acute myelofibrosis

cytotoxic chemotherapy and irradiation

acute or severe megaloblastic anaemia

drug-induced immune pancytopenia (for example due to phenacetin, para-aminosalicylic acid, sulphonamides and rifampicin)

combined immunocytopenia[173]

systemic lupus erythematosus

thymoma[53]

graft-versus-host disease[5]

hypersplenism

acquired immune deficiency syndrome (end-stage HIV infection)

haemophagocytic syndromes including malignant histiocytosis and virus-induced haemophagocytosis

fusariosis (infection with the fungus *Fusarium*)[99]

anorexia nervosa[19]

Wilson's disease[82]

hyperthyroidism (rarely)[160]

alcohol toxicity[104]

copper deficiency[139]

marble bone disease (osteopetrosis)

Fig.8.62 *Some of the causes of pancytopenia.*

References

1. Bain BJ, Seed M & Godsland I (1985) Normal values for the peripheral blood white cell counts in women of four different ethnic groups. *Journal of Clinical Pathology*, **37**, 188–193.

2. Bain BJ (1986) An assessment of the three-population differential count on the Coulter Counter Model S Plus IV. *Clinical and Laboratory Haematology*, **8**, 347–359

3. Bakri KM (1986) Polyarthritis and neutropenia. *Annals of Internal Medicine*, **104**, 127 (letter).

4. Bar RS, Adlard J & Thomas FB (1975) Lymphopenic infectious mononucleosis. *Archives of Internal Medicine*, **135**, 334–337.

5. Barrett AJ (1987) Graft-versus-host disease: a review. *Journal of the Royal Society of Medicine*, **80**, 368–373.

6. Barrett O (1970) Monocytosis in malignant disease. *Annals of Internal Medicine*, **73**, 991–992.

7. Beerman H & Nicholas L (1967) The basophil degranulation test — a review of the literature. *American Journal of Medical Science*, **253**, 473–492.

8. Beeson PB & Bass DA (1977) The eosinophil. Volume XIV in the series *Major problems in internal medicine*. Edited by LH Smith. Philadelphia: WB Saunders Co.

9. Bennett JM, Catovsky D, Daniel MT, Flandrin G, Galton DAG, Gralnick HR & Sultan-C (1976) Proposals for the classification of the acute leukaemias (FAB cooperative group). *British Journal of Haematology*, **33**, 451–458.

10. Bennett JM, Catovsky D, Daniel MT, Flandrin G, Galton DAG, Gralnick HR & Sultan-C (1980) A variant form of acute hypergranular promyelocytic leukaemia (M3). *British Journal of Haematology*, **44**, 169–170.

11. Bennett JM, Catovsky D, Daniel MT, Flandrin G, Galton DAG, Gralnick HR & Sultan-C (1981) The morphological classification of acute lymphoblastic leukaemia: concordance among observers and clinical correlations. *British Journal of Haematology*, **47**, 553–561.

12. Bennett JM, Catovsky D, Daniel MT, Flandrin G, Galton DAG, Gralnick HR & Sultan-C (1982) Proposals for the classification of the myelodysplastic syndromes. *British Journal of Haematology*, **51**, 189–199.

13. Bennett JM, Catovsky D & Daniel MT (1985) Criteria for the diagnosis of acute leukaemia of megakaryocytic lineage (M7): a report of the French–American–British cooperative group. *Annals of Internal Medicine*, **103**, 460–462.

14. Bennett JM, Catovsky D, Daniel MT, Flandrin G, Galton DAG, Gralnick HR & Sultan-C (1985) Proposed revised criteria for the classification of acute myeloid leukaemia. *Annals of Internal Medicine*, **103**, 620–629.

15. Berman SJ & Kundin WD (1973) Scrub typhus in South Vietnam. *Annals of Internal Medicine*, **79**, 26–30.

16. Binet JL, Vaugier G, Dighiero G, d'Athis P & Charron D (1977) Investigation of a new parameter in chronic lymphocytic leukemia: the percentage of large peripheral lymphocytes determined by the Hemalog D. *American Journal of Medicine*, **63**, 683–688.

17. Binet JL, Auquier A, Dighiero G et al. (1981) A new prognostic classification of chronic lymphocytic leukaemia derived from a multivariate survival analysis. *Cancer*, **48**, 198–206.

18. Bouroncle BA, Wiseman BK & Doan CA (1958) Leukemic reticuloendotheliosis. *Blood*, **13**, 609–630.

19. Bowers TK & Eckert E (1978) Leukopenia in anorexia nervosa. *Archives of Internal Medicine*, **138**, 1520–1523.

20. Brandt L & Stensam M (1975) Subnormal lymphocyte counts in adult coeliac disease. *Lancet*, **i**, 978–979 (letter).

21. Brandt L & Nilsson PG (1980) Lymphocytopenia preceding chronic lymphocytic leukemia. *Acta Medica Scandinavica*, **208**, 13–16.

22. Brettman LR, Lewin S, Holzman RS, Goldman WD, Marr JS, Kechijian P & Schinella R (1981) Rickettsial pox: report of an outbreak and a contemporary review. *Medicine*, **60**, 363–372.

23. Breton–Gorius J, Reyes F, Vernant JP, Tulliez M & Dreyfus B (1978) The blast crisis of chronic granulocytic leukaemia: megakaryoblastic nature of cells revealed by the presence of platelet-peroxidase — a cytochemical study. *British Journal of Haematology*, **39**, 295–303.

24. Broghamer WL & Keeling MM (1977) The bone marrow biopsy, osteoscan, and peripheral blood in non-hemopoietic cancer. *Cancer*, **40**, 836–840.

25. Budman DR & Steinberg AD (1977) Hematologic aspects of systemic lupus erythematosus. *Annals of Internal Medicine*, **86**, 220–229.

26. Bullock WE, Artz RP, Bhathena D & Tung SK (1979) Histoplasmosis. *Archives of Internal Medicine*, **139**, 700–702.

27. Burkett LL, Cox ML & Fields ML (1965) Leukoerythroblastosis in the adult. *American Journal of Clinical Pathology*, **44**, 494–498.

28. Bynoe AG, Scott CS, Ford P & Roberts BE (1983) Decreased T helper cells in the myelodysplastic syndromes. *British Journal of Haematology*, **54**, 97–102.

29. Canellos GP, Whang-Peng J & deVita VT (1976) Chronic granulocytic leukemia without the Philadelphia chromosome. *American Journal of Clinical Pathology*, **65**, 467–470.

30. Cantow EF & Kostinas JE (1966) Studies on infectious mononucleosis IV. Changes in the granulocyte series. *American Journal of Clinical Pathology*, **46**, 43–47.

31. Carstairs KC, Francombe WH, Scott JG & Gelfand EW (1985) Persistent B polyclonal lymphocytosis, induced by cigarette smoking? *Lancet*, **i**, 1094 (letter).

32. Carter JW, Edson RS & Kennedy CC (1978) Infectious mononucleosis in the older patient. *Mayo Clinic Proceedings*, **53**, 146–150.

33. Carvajal JA, Anderson R, Weiss L, Grismer J & Berman R (1967) Atheroembolism. An etiologic factor in renal insufficiency, gastrointestinal haemorrhages and peripheral vascular disease. *Archives of Internal Medicine*, **119**, 593–599.

34. Castro-Malapina H, Schaison G, Passe S, Pasquier A, Berger R, Bayle-Weisgerber C, Miller D, Seligman M & Bernard J (1984) Subacute and chronic myelomonocytic leukemia in children (Juvenile chronic myeloid leukemia). *Cancer*, **54**, 675–686.

35. Catorsky D, Pittman S, O'Brien M, Cherchi M, Costello C, Foa R, Pearce E, Hoffbrand AV, Janossy G, Ganeshaguru K & Greaves MF (1979) Multiparameter studies in lymphoid leukaemias. *American Journal of Clinical Pathology*, **72**, 736–745.

36. Catovsky D, Bernasconi C, Verdonck PJ, Postma A, Hows J, Van der Does-Van den Berg A, Rees JKH, Castelli G, Morra E & Galton DAG (1980) The association of eosinophilia with lymphoblastic leukaemia of lymphoma: a study of seven patients. *British Journal of Haematology*, **45**, 523–534.

37. Catovsky D, Cherchi M, Brooks D, Bradley J & Zola H (1981) Heterogeneity of B-cell leukemias demonstrated by the monoclonal antibody FMC7. *Blood*, **58**, 406–409.

38. Catovsky D, Wechsler A & Cherchi M (1981) Correspondence. *Blood*, **58**, 410 (letter).

39. Catovsky D (1981) In *The leukaemic cell*. Edited by D Catovsky. Edinburgh: Churchill Livingstone.

40. Catovsky D, Linch DC & Beverley PC (1982) T-cell disorders in haematological diseases. *Clinics in Haematology*, **11**, 661–695.

41. Catovsky D (1984) Chronic lymphocytic, prolymphocytic and hairy cell leukaemias. In Butterworths International Medical Reviews. *Haematology 1. Leukemias*. Edited by JM Goldman & HD Preisler. London: Butterworths.

42. Catovsky D, O'Brien M, Melo JV, Wardle J & Brozovic M (1984) Hairy cell leukemia (HCL) variant: an intermediate disease between HCL and B-prolymphocytic leukemia. *Seminars in Oncology*, **11**, 362–369.

43. Chan WC, Link S, Mawle A, Check I, Brynes RK & Winton EF (1986) Heterogeneity of large granular lymphocyte proliferations: delineation of two major subtypes. *Blood*, **68**, 1142–1153.

44. Chusid MJ, Dale DC, West BC & Wolff SM (1975) The hypereosinophilic syndrome. *Medicine*, **54**, 1–27.

45. Cline MJ, Opelz G, Saxon A, Fahey JL & Golde DW (1977) Autoimmune panleukopenia. *New England Journal of Medicine*, **295**, 1489–1493.

46. Cordano A, Placko RP & Graham GG (1966) Hypocupremia and neutropenia in copper deficiency. *Blood*, **28**, 280–283.

47. Coser P, Quaglino D, de Pasquale A, Colombetti V & Prinoth O (1980) Cytobiological and clinical aspects of tissue mast cell leukaemia. *British Journal of Haematology*, **45**, 5–12.

48. Costello C, Catovsky D, O'Brien M, Morilla R & Varadi S (1980) Chronic T-cell leukaemias I Morphology, cytochemistry and ultrastructure. *Leukaemia Research*, **4**, 463–476.

49. Craig A, Tucker J, Ludlam CA, Philp ID, Tedder RS, Macnicol MF & Steel CM (1985) Severe glandular fever like illness following infection by HTLV-III virus. *British Journal of Haematology*, **61**, 568 (abstract).

50. Cross J & Strange CA (1987) Erroneous Ortho ELT800/WS WBC in chronic lymphatic leukaemia. *Clinical and Laboratory Haematology*, **9**, 371–376.

51. Cullen MH, Stansfeld AG, Oliver RTD, Lister TA & Malpas JS (1979) Angioimmunoblastic lymphadenopathy: report of ten cases and review of the literature. *Quarterly Journal of Medicine*, **48**, 151–177.

52. Daniele RP & Rowlands DT (1976) Lymphocyte subpopulations in sarcoidosis: correlations with disease activity and duration. *Annals of Internal Medicine*, **85**, 593–600.

53. Dawson MA (1972) Thymoma associated with pancytopenia and Hashimoto's thyroiditis. *American Journal of Medicine*, **52**, 533–537.

54. Delbarre F, Go AL & Kahan A (1975) Hyperbasophilic immunoblasts in the circulating blood in chronic inflammatory rheumatic and collagen diseases. *Annals of Rheumatic Diseases*, **34**, 422–430.

55. diBella NJ, Silverstein MN & Hoagland C (1977) Effect of splenectomy on tear-drop shaped erythrocytes in agnogenic myeloid metaplasia. *Archives of Internal Medicine*, **137**, 380–381.

56. Dines DE (1978) Chronic eosinophilic pneumonia. *Mayo Clinic Proceedings*, **53**, 129–130.

57. Don IJ, Khettry U & Canoso JJ (1978) Progressive systemic sclerosis with eosinophilia and a fulminant course. *American Journal of Medicine*, **65**, 346–348.

58. Dvorak AM & Dvorak HF (1979) The basophil. *Archives of Pathology and Laboratory Medicine*, **103**, 551–557.

59. Economopoulos T, Fotopoulos S, Hatzioannou J & Gardikas C (1982) 'Prolymphocytoid' cells in chronic lymphatic leukemia and their prognostic significance. *Scandinavian Journal of Haematology*, **28**, 238–242.

60. Editorial (1968) Lymphocytopoietic viruses. *New England Journal of Medicine*, **279**, 432–433.

61. Efrati P, Klajman A & Spitz H (1957) Mast cell leukemia? — Malignant mastocytosis with leukemia-like manifestations. *Blood*, **12**, 869–882.

62. Enno A, Catovsky D, O'Brien M, Cherchi M, Kumaran TO & Galton DAG (1979) Prolymphocytoid transformation of chronic lymphocytic leukaemia. *British Journal of Haematology*, **41**, 9–18.

63. Fauci AS, Harley JB, Roberts WC, Ferrans VJ, Gralnick HR & Bjornson BH (1982) NIH Conference. The idiopathic hypereosinophilic syndrome. *Annals of Internal Medicine*, **97**, 78–92.

64. Fenaux P, Jouet JP, Zandecki M, Lai JL, Simon M, Pollet JP & Bauters F (1987) Chronic and subacute myelomonocytic leukaemia in the adult: a report of 60 cases with special reference to prognostic factors. *British Journal of Haematology*, **65**, 101–106.

65. Foadi MD, Slater AM & Pegrum GD (1978) Erythrophagocytosis by acute lymphoblastic leukaemic cells. *Scandinavian Journal of Haematology*, **20**, 85–88.

66. Fradera J, Vélez-Garcia E & White JC (1986) Acute lymphoblastic leukaemia with unusual cytoplasmic granulation: a morphological, cytochemical and ultrastructural study. *Blood*, **68**, 406–411.

67. Frayha RA, Shulman LE & Stevens MB (1980) Haematological abnormalities in scleroderma. A study of 180 cases. *Acta Haematologica*, **64**, 25–30.

68. Gabriel LC, Escribano LM, Villa E, Leira C & Valdes MD (1986) Ultrastructural study of blood cells in toxic oil syndrome. *Acta Haematologica*, **75**, 165–170.

69. Galton DAG, Goldman JM, Wiltshaw E, Catovsky D, Henry K & Goldenberg J (1974) Prolymphocytic leukaemia. *British Journal of Haematology*, **27**, 7–23.

70. Geary CG, Catovsky D, Wiltshaw E, Milner GR, Scholes MC, Van Noorden S, Wadsworth LD, Muldal S, MacIver JE & Galton DAG (1975) Chronic myelomonocytic leukaemia. British Journal of Haematology, **30,** 289–302.

71. Ghani AM & Krause JR (1986) Investigations of cell size and nuclear clefts as prognostic parameters in chronic lymphocytic leukemia. Cancer, **58,** 2233–2238.

72. Glaser RM, Walker RI & Herrion JC (1970) The significance of hematologic abnormalities in patients with tuberculosis. Archives of Internal Medicine, **125,** 691–695.

73. Gleich GJ, Schroeter AL, Marcoux JP, Sachs MI, O'Connell EJ & Kohler PF (1984) Episodic angioedema associated with eosinophilia. New England Journal of Medicine, **310,** 1621–1626.

74. Goodwin RA, Shapiro JL, Thurman GH, Thurman SS & des Prez RM (1980) Disseminated histoplasmosis: clinical and pathologic correlations. Medicine, **59,** 1–33.

75. Goh K-o & Anderson FW (1979) Cytogenetic studies in basophilic chronic myelocytic leukemia. Archives of Pathology and Laboratory Medicine, **103,** 288–290.

76. Golomb HM, Vardiman J, Sweet DL, Simon D & Variakojis D (1978) Hairy cell leukaemia: evidence for the existence of a spectrum of functional characteristics. British Journal of Haematology, **38,** 161–170.

77. Gramatzki M, Strong DM, Duval-Arnould B, Morstyn A & Schumacher HR (1985) Hand-mirror variant of acute lymphoblastic leukemia. Cancer, **55,** 77–83.

78. Gruenwald H, Kiossoglou KA, Mitus WJ & Dameshek W (1965) Philadelphia chromosome in eosinophilic leukemia. American Journal of Medicine, **39,** 1003–1010.

79. Guibaud S, Plumet-Leger A & Frobert Y (1983) Transient neutrophil aggregation in a patient with acute mononucleosis. American Journal of Clinical Pathology, **80,** 883–884.

80. Hayhoe FGJ & Quaglino D (1980) Haematological Cytochemistry. New York: Churchill Livingstone.

81. Herring WB, Smith LG, Walker RI & Herion JC (1974) Hereditary neutrophilia. American Journal of Medicine, **56,** 729–734.

82. Hoagland HC & Goldstein NP (1978) Hematologic (cytopenic) manifestations of Wilson's Disease. Mayo Clinic Proceedings, **53,** 498–500.

83. Hocking WG, Singh R, Schroff R & Golde DW (1983) Cell mediated inhibition of erythropoiesis and megaloblastic anemia in T-cell chronic lymphocytic leukemia. Cancer, **51,** 631–636.

84. Hogge DE, Misawa S, Schiffer CA & Testa JR (1984) Promyelocytic blast crisis in chronic granulocytic leukaemia. Leukaemia Research, **8,** 1019–1023.

85. Horwitz MS & Moore CT (1968) Acute infectious lymphocytosis. New England Journal of Medicine, **279,** 399–404.

86. Horwitz CA, Henle W, Henle G, Polesky H, Balfour HH, Siem RA, Borken S & Ward PCJ (1977) Heterophil-negative infectious mononucleosis and mononucleosis-like illnesses. American Journal of Medicine, **63,** 947–957.

87. International working formulation for clinical use (1984) Non-Hodgkins lymphoma: managment strategies. New England Journal of Medicine, **311,** 1506.

88. Jacobs A & Clark RE (1986) Pathogenesis and clinical variations in the myelodysplastic syndromes. In Clinics in Haematology, volume 15. Edited by JD Griffin. pp.925–951. London: WB Saunders.

89. Juhlin L (1963) Basophil and eosinophil leucocytes in various internal disorders. Acta Medica Scandinavica, **174,** 249–255.

90. Juhlin LL & Michaëlsson G (1977) A new syndrome characterised by absence of eosinophils and basophils. Lancet, **i,** 1233–1235.

91. Kamada N & Uchino H (1978) Chronologic sequence in the appearance of clinical and laboratory findings characteristic of chronic myelocytic leukemia. Blood, **51,** 843–850.

92. Kanoh T, Saigo K & Yamagishi M (1986) Neutrophils with ring-shaped nuclei in chronic neutrophilic leukemia. American Journal of Clinical Pathology, **86,** 748–751.

93. Kapadia A, de Sousa M, Markenson AL, Miller DR, Good RA & Gupta S (1980) Lymphoid cell sets and serum immunoglobulins in patients with thalassaemia intermedia. British Journal of Haematology, **45,** 405–416.

94. Kass L (1982) Leukemia, cytology and cytochemistry, Philadelphia: JB Lippincott.

95. Kawano F, Tsuda H, Yamaguchi K, Nishimura H, Sanada I, Matsuzaki H, Ishii M & Takatsuki K (1984) Unusual clinical courses of adult T cell leukemia in siblings. Cancer, **54,** 131–134.

96. Keene B, Mendelow B, Pinto MR, Bezwoda W, MacDougall L, Falkson G, Ruff P & Bernstein R (1987) Abnormalities of chromosome 12p13 and malignant proliferation of eosinophils: a nonrandom association. British Journal of Haematology, **67,** 25–31.

97. Kinoshita K, Amagasaki T, Ikeda S et al. (1985) Preleukemic state of adult T cell leukemia: abnormal T lymphocytosis induced by human adult T cell leukemia-lymphoma virus. Blood, **66,** 120–127.

98. Kyle RA, Maldonado JE & Bayrd ED (1974) Plasma cell leukemia. Report on 17 cases. Archives of Internal Medicine, **133,** 813–818.

99. Lascari AD (1984) Hematologic manifestations of childhood diseases. New York: Theme-Stratton Inc.

100. Lau KS & White JC (1969) Myelosclerosis associated with systemic lupus erythematosus in patients in West Malaysia. Journal of Clinical Pathology. **22,** 433–438.

101. Le Beau MM, Larson RA, Bitter MA, Vardiman JW, Golomb HM & Rowley JD (1983) Association of an inversion of chromosome 16 with abnormal marrow eosinophils in acute myelomonocytic leukemia. New England Journal of Medicine, **309,** 630–636.

102. Lilleyman JS, Britton JA & Laycock BJ (1981) Morphological metamorphosis in relapsing lymphoblastic leukaemia. Journal of Clinical Pathology, **34,** 60–62.

103. Lilleyman JS, Hann IM, Stevens RF, Eden OB & Richards SM (1986) French–American–British (FAB) morphological classification of childhood lymphoblastic leukaemia and its clinical importance. Journal of Clinical Pathology, **39,** 998–1002.

104. Liu YK (1973) Leukopenia in alcoholics. American Journal of Medicine, **54,** 605–610.

105. Loughran TP, Kadin ME, Starkebaum G, Abkowitz JL, Clark EA, Disteche C & Lum LG (1985) Leukemia of large granular lymphocytes: association with clonal chromosomal abnormalities and autoimmune neutropenia, thrombocytopenia and hemolytic anemia. *Annals of Internal Medicine,* **102,** 169–175.

106. Lowe D, Jorizzo J & Hutt MSR (1981) Tumour-associated eosinophilia: a review *Journal of Clinical Pathology,* **34,** 1343–1348.

107. Maier M & Buriot D (1978) Maladie de Chediak–Higashi. Significance nosologique de la presence de corps d'Auer dans les myeloblastes. *Nouvelle Presse Medicale,* **7,** 286.

108. Maldonado JE & Hanlon DG (1965) Monocytosis: a current appraisal. *Mayo Clinic Proceedings,* **40,** 248–259.

109. Malech HL & Gallin JI (1987) Current concepts immunology: neutrophils in human diseases. *New England Journal of Medicine,* **317,** 687–694.

110. Mandall BK & Stokes KJ (1973) Acute infectious lymphocytosis and enteroviruses. *Lancet,* **i,** 1392–1393.

111. Marinone G, Rossi G & Verzura P (1983) Eosinophilic blast crisis in a case of chronic myeloid leukaemia. *British Journal of Haematology,* **55,** 251–256.

112. Martelli MF, Falini B, Tabilio A, Velardi A & Rossodivita M (1980) Prolymphocytic leukemia with erythrophagocytic activity. *British Journal of Haematology,* **46,** 141–142.

113. Martelli MF, Falini B, Rambotti P, Tonato M & Davis S (1981) Sideroblastic anemia associated with hairy cell leukemia. *Cancer,* **48,** 762–767.

114. Matutes E, Talavera JG, O'Brien M & Catovsky D (1986) The morphological spectrum of T-prolymphocytic leukaemia. *British Journal of Haematology,* **64,** 111–124.

115. Mayron LW, Alling S & Kaplan E (1972) Eosinophilia and drug abuse. *Annals of Allergy,* **30,** 632–637.

116. Melo JV, Hegde U, Parreira A, Thompson I, Lampert IA & Catovsky D (1987) Splenic B cell lymphoma with circulating villous lymphocytes: differential diagnosis of B cell leukaemias with large spleens. *Journal of Clinical Pathology,* **40,** 642–651.

117. Moake JL, Landry PR, Oren ME, Sayer BL & Heffner LT (1974) Transient peripheral plasmacytosis. *American Journal of Clinical Pathology,* **62,** 8–15.

118. Montoliu J, López-Pedret J, Andreu L & Revert L (1981) Eosinophilia in patients undergoing dialysis. *British Medical Journal,* **282,** 2098.

119. Moutsopoulos HM, Webber BL, Fostiropoulos G, Goules D & Shulman LE (1980) Diffuse fasciitis with eosinophilia. *American Journal of Medicine,* **68,** 701–709.

120. Munt PW (1971) Miliary tuberculosis in the chemotherapy era: with a clinical review in 69 American adults. *Medicine,* **51,** 139–155.

121. Nakahate T, Spicer SS, Leary AG, Ogawa M, Franklin W & Goetzl EJ (1984) Circulating eosinophil colony-forming cells in pure eosinophil aplasia. *Annals of Internal Medicine,* **101,** 321–324.

122. Neftel KA, Stahel R, Müller OM, Morell A & Arrenbrecht S (1983) Radial segmentation of nuclei (Reider cells): a morphological marker of T-cell neoplasms. *Acta Haematologica,* **70,** 213–219.

123. Newland AC, Catovsky D, Linch D, Cawley JC, Beverley P, San Miguel JF, Gordon-Smith EC, Blecher TE, Shahriari S & Varadi S (1984) Chronic T cell lymphocytosis: a review of 21 cases. *British Journal of Haematology,* **58,** 433–446.

124. Nkrumah FK & Addy PAK (1973) Acute infectious lymphocytosis. *Lancet,* **i,** 1257–1258 (letter).

125. Ogawa M, Fried J, Sakai Y, Strife A & Clarkson BD (1970) Studies of cellular proliferation in human leukaemia. *Cancer,* **25,** 1031–1049.

126. Olson LC, Miller G & Hanshaw JB (1964) Acute infectious lymphocytosis. *Lancet,* **i,** 200–201.

127. Ondreyco SM, Kjeldsberg CR, Fineman RM, Vaninetti S & Kushner JP (1981) Monoblastic transformation in chronic myelogenous leukaemia. *Cancer,* **48,** 957–963.

128. Parmley RT, Crist WM, Ragab AH, Boxer LA, Malluh A, Lui VK & Derby CP (1980) Congenital dysgranulopoeitic neutropenia: clinical, serologic, ultrastructural and in vitro proliferative characteristics *Blood,* **56,** 465–475.

129. Parwaresch MR (1976) The human blood basophil. Morphology, origin, kinetics, function and pathology. Berlin: Springer-Verlag.

130. Pullen RL & Stuart BM (1945) Tularemia. *Journal of the American Medical Association,* **129,** 495–500.

131. Rai KR, Sawitsky A, Cronkite EP, Chanana AD, Levy PN & Pasternack BS (1975) Clinical staging of chronic lymphocytic leukaemia. *Blood,* **46,** 219–234.

132. Ralfklær E, Geisler C, Hansen MM & Hou-Jensen K (1983) Nuclear clefts in chronic lymphocytic leukaemia. *Scandinavian Journal of Haematology,* **30,** 5–12.

133. Raska K, Raskova J, Shea SM, Frankel RM, Wood RH, Lifter J, Ghobrial I, Eisinger RP & Homer L (1983) T cell subsets and cellular immunity in end-stage renal disease. *American Journal of Medicine,* **75,** 734–740.

134. Rilke F, Pilotti S, Carbone A & Lombardi L (1978) Morphology of lymphatic cells and their derived tumours. *Journal of Clinical Pathology,* **31,** 1009–1056.

135. Robinson DSF, Melo JV, Andrews C, Schey SA & Catovsky D (1985) Intracytoplasmic inclusions in B prolymphocytic leukaemia: ultrastructural, cytochemical and immunological studies. *Journal of Clinical Pathology,* **38,** 897–903.

136. Robinson WA (1974) Granulocytosis in neoplasia. *Annals of the New York Academy of Science,* **230,** 212–218.

137. Rogers L (1905) The blood changes in plague. *Journal of Pathology,* **10,** 291–295.

138. Rosenthal S, Schwartz JKH & Canellos GP (1977) Basophilic chronic granulocytic leukaemia with hyperhistaminaemia. *British Journal of Haematology,* **36,** 367–372.

139. Ruocco L, Baldi N, Cecconi A, Marini A, Azzarà A, Ambrogi F & Grassi B (1986) Severe pancytopenia due to copper deficiency. *Acta Haematologica,* **76,** 224–226.

140. Saunders PWG, Reid MM & Cohen BJ (1986) Human parvovirus induced cytopenias: a report of five cases. *British Journal of Haematology,* **63,** 407–410.

141. Schatz M, Wasserman S & Patterson R (1982) The eosinophil and the lung. *Archives of Internal Medicine,* **142,** 1515–1519.

142. Schmalzl F, Konwalinka G, Michlmayr G, Abbrederis K & Braunsteiner H (1978) Detection of cytochemical and morphological abnormalities in 'Preleukaemia'. *Acta Haematologica,* **59,** 1–18.

143. Schwabe AD & Peters RS (1974) Familial mediterranean fever in Armenians. Analysis of 100 cases. *Medicine,* **53,** 453–462.

144. Scott CS, Cahill A, Bynoe AG, Ainley MJ, Hough D & Roberts BE (1983) Esterase cytochemistry in myelodysplastic syndromes and megaloblastic anaemias: demonstration of abnormal staining patterns associated with dysmyelopoiesis. *British Journal of Haematology*, **55**, 411–418.

145. Scott CS, Limbert HJ, Mackarill ID & Roberts BE (1985) Membrane phenotypes in B-cell lymphoproliferative disorders. *Journal of Clinical Pathology*, **38**, 995–1001.

146. Shamoto M, Murakami S & Zenke T (1981) Adult T-cell leukaemia in Japan. *Cancer*, **47**, 1804–1811.

147. Sheehy TW, Birmingham A, Hazlett D & Turk RE (1973) Scrub typhus. *Archives of Internal Medicine*, **132**, 77–80.

148. Shelley WB & Parnes HM (1965) The absolute basophil count. *Journal of the American Medical Association*, **192**, 368–370.

149. Shoenfeld Y, Shaklai M, Ben-Baruch N, Hirschorn M & Pinkhaus J (1982) Neutropenia induced by hypercarotenaemia. *Lancet*, **i**, 1245 (letter).

150. Sills RH & Stockman JA (1981) Preleukemic states in children with acute lymphoblastic leukaemia. *Cancer*, **48**, 110–112.

151. Snustad DG, Koss W & Fontana JA (1984) Angioimmunoblastic lymphadenopathy and associated selective myeloid hypoplasia. *Cancer*, **53**, 2129–2134.

152. Soler J, O'Brien M, Tavares de Castro J, San Miguel JF, Kearney L, Goldman JM & Catovsky D (1985) Blast crisis of chronic granulocytic leukemia with mast cell and basophil precursors. *American Journal of Clinical Pathology*, **83**, 254–259.

153. Spiers ASD, Bain BJ & Turner JE (1977) The peripheral blood in chronic granulocytic leukaemia. *Scandinavian Journal of Haematology*, **18**, 25–38.

154. Spitzer G & Garson OM (1973) Lymphoblastic leukaemia with marked eosinophilia: a report of two cases. *Blood*, **42**, 377–384.

155. Spry C (1980) in *The eosinophil in health and disease* Edited by AAF Mahmoud, KP Austin & AS Simon, New York: Grune & Stratton.

156. Srodes CH, Hyde EH & Boggs DR (1973) Autonomous erythropoiesis during erythroblastic crisis of chronic myelocytic leukaemia. *Journal of Clinical Investigation*, **52**, 512–515.

157. Stavem P, Hjort PF, Vogt E, van der Hagen CB (1969) Ring-shaped nuclei of granulocytes in a patient with acute erythroleukaemia. *Scandinavian Journal of Haematology*, **6**, 31–32.

158. Stavem P, Ly B, Egeberg O & Bull O (1977) Flaming promyelocytes in acute promyelocytic leukaemia. Light and electron microscopic study. *Scandinavian Journal of Haematology*, **19**, 99–105.

159. Swirsky DM, Li YS, Matthews JG, Flemans RJ, Rees JHK & Hayhoe FGJ (1984) 8;21 translocation in acute granulocytic leukaemia: cytological, cytochemical and clinical features. *British Journal of Haematology*, **56**, 199–213.

160. Talansky AL, Schulman P, Vinciguerra VP, Margouleff D, Budman DR & Degman TJ (1981) Pancytopenia complicating Graves' disease and drug-induced hyperthyroidism. *Archives of Internal Medicine*, **141**, 544–545.

161. Teggatz JR, Peterson L & Parkin J (1985) Transient absolute lymphocytosis in adults presenting in critical emergency situations. *American Journal of Clinical Pathology*, **84**, 557

162. Tindall JP, Beeker SK & Rosse WF (1969) Familial cold urticaria. *Archives of Internal Medicine*, **124**, 129–134.

163. Tinegate HN & Chetty MN (1986) Basophilia as a feature of the myelodysplastic syndrome. *Clinical and Laboratory Haematology*, **8**, 269–271.

164. Trujillo JM, Cork A, Drewinko B, Hart JS & Freireich EJ (1971) Case report: tetraploid leukaemia. *Blood*, **38**, 632–637.

165. Villeval JL, Cramer F, Lemoine A, Henri A, Bettaieb A, Bernaudin F, Beuzard Y, Berger R, Flandrin G, Breton-Gorius J & Vainchenker W (1986) Phenotype of early erythroblastic leukaemias. *Blood*, **68**, 1167–1174.

166. Vonderheid EC, Sobel EL, Nowell PC, Finan JB, Helfrich MK & Whipple S (1985) Diagnostic and prognostic significance of Sézary cells in the peripheral blood. *Blood*, **66**, 358–366.

167. Weatherall DJ, Old J, Longley J, Wood WG, Clegg JB, Pollock A & Lewis MJ (1978) Acquired haemoglobin H disease in leukaemia: pathophysiology and molecular basis. *British Journal of Haematology*, **38**, 305–322.

168. Weick JK, Hagedorn AB & Linman JW (1974) Leukoerythroblastosis. Diagnostic and prognostic significance. *Mayo Clinic Proceedings*, **49**, 110–113.

169. Weil SC & Hrisinko MA (1987) A hybrid eosinophilic-basophilic granulocyte in chronic granulocytic leukaemia. *American Journal of Clinical Pathology*, **87**, 66–70.

170. Weitberg AB & Harmon DC (1984) Autoimmune neutropenia. *Annals of Internal Medicine*, **100**, 702–703.

171. Wells GC & Smith NP (1979) Eosinophilic cellulitis. *British Journal of Dermatology*, **100**, 101–109.

172. Wick MR, Li C-Y & Pierre RV (1982) Acute nonlymphocytic leukaemia with basophilic differentiation. *Blood*, **60**, 38–45.

173. Wiesneth M, Pflieger H, Frickhofen N & Heimpel H (1985) Idiopathic combined immunocytopenia. *British Journal of Haematology*, **61**, 339–348.

174. Willoughby MLN (1977) *Paediatric Haematology.* Edinburgh: Churchill Livingstone.

175. Winton EF, Chan WC, Check I, Colenda KW, Bongiovanni KF & Waldmann TA (1986) Spontaneous regression of a monoclonal proliferation of large granular lymphocytes associated with a reversal of anemia and neutropenia. *Blood*, **67**, 1427–1432.

176. Wolf DJ, Fialk MA, Mouradian J, Gottfried EL & Pasmantier MW (1980) Unusual intracytoplasmic inclusions in acute myeloblastic leukaemia. *American Journal of Haematology*, **9**, 413–420.

177. Yam LT, Yam C-F & Li CY (1980) Eosinophilia in systemic mastocytosis. *American Journal of Clinical Pathology*, **73**, 48–54.

178. Yamaguchi K, Nishimura H, Kohrogi H, Jono M, Miyamoto Y & Takatsuki K (1983) A proposal for smouldering adult T-cell leukaemia: a clinicopathological study of five cases. *Blood*, **62**, 758–766.

179. Yetgin S & Ozsoylu S (1982) Myeloid metaplasia in Vitamin D deficiency rickets. *Scandinavian Journal of Haematology*, **28**, 180–185.

180. Yoo D, Pierce LE & Lessin LS (1983) Acquired pure red cell aplasia associated with chronic lymphocytic leukaemia. *Cancer*, **51**, 844–850.

181. You W & Weisbrot IM (1979) Chronic neutrophilic leukaemia, report of two cases and review of the literature. *American Journal of Clinical Pathology*, **72**, 233–242.

9. Interpretation – red cells and platelets

HYPOCHROMIC AND MICROCYTIC RED CELLS

THE DIFFERENTIAL DIAGNOSIS OF IRON DEFICIENCY, THALASSAEMIA TRAIT AND THE ANAEMIA OF CHRONIC DISEASE

Cells which are microcytic are usually also hypochromic. Other types of red cell of reduced size (such as irregularly contracted cells, fragments or microspherocytes) have a different significance and will be discussed separately. If a blood film appears hypochromic and microcytic it is first necessary to note whether it is from a child or an adult since cells which would be considered hypochromic and microcytic in an adult may be normal in a child; only if the red cell size and degree of haemoglobinization fall below what would be expected at a given age should the cells be considered as hypochromic and microcytic. The ethnic origin should also be noted since some of the causes of microcytosis are much commoner in some ethnic groups than in others.

If a film is assessed as hypochromic and/or microcytic the differential diagnosis usually lies between iron deficiency, the anaemia of chronic disease and α -or β-thalassaemia trait. Other causes of hypochromia and microcytosis are much less common (see Fig. 3.73). It is necessary not only to assess the red cell morphology but also to consider the relationship between the haemoglobin concentration and the red cell indices. A correct interpretation often also requires a knowledge of the medical history. For example, the haemoglobin and red cell indices in a patient who has had repeated venesec-

tion for the treatment of polycythaemia rubra vera are often very similar to those found in thalassaemia trait. Similarly, a dimorphic film may give a clue to a diagnosis of sideroblastic anaemia, but if the patient is known to be receiving iron therapy a response to the medication is a more likely explanation.

The correct diagnosis of this group of conditions is of some importance. Many patients with sideroblastic anaemia or thalassaemia trait have been mistakenly prescribed iron, sometimes for years. Some patients with thalassaemia trait have developed serious iron overload as a result. Patients with thalassaemia trait or the anaemia of chronic disorders have also been subjected to extensive investigations for suspected gastrointestinal blood loss because of a mistaken assumption that their microcytosis is due to iron deficiency. The laboratory detection of β-thalassaemia trait is of particular importance in patients in the reproductive age range since, although the condition is of little significance in itself, a quarter of the offspring of two affected subjects will, on average, have thalassaemia major.

Iron deficiency

In iron deficiency a normocytic, normochromic anaemia with anisocytosis precedes the development of anisochromasia, hypochromia and microcytosis. Morphological changes are not usually marked until the Hb falls below 10–11 g/dl when the blood film shows anisocytosis, poikilocytosis, hypochromia,

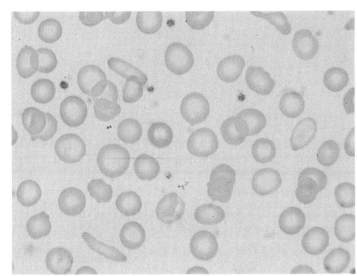

Fig. 9.1 *The blood film of a patient with iron deficiency showing anisocytosis, poikilocytosis (including elliptocytes[(1)]), hypochromia and microcytosis . The automated blood count (Coulter S Plus IV) was: RBC 4.22 × 10⁹/l, Hb 7 g/dl, PCV 0.29, MCV 67 fl, MCH 16.6 pg, MCHC 24.5 g/dl.*

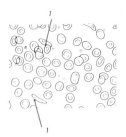

and microcytosis (Fig. 9.1). Poikilocytes include elliptocytes, particularly very thin elliptocytes which are often described as pencil cells. Occasional target cells can be present but they are not numerous. Basophilic stippling is infrequent. The presence of anisochromasia is a useful sign, since it is usually absent in thalassaemia trait. Polychromasia is sometimes present.

The earliest blood count evidence of iron deficiency is usually an increase in the RDW (red cell distribution width). This parameter, which measures anisocytosis, becomes abnormal before anaemia develops.[10] The next change observed is a fall of the Hb, RBC and PCV followed by a fall in the MCV and MCH. A low MCHC is a sensitive indicator of iron deficiency when it is calculated from a microhaematocrit or when it is measured on a Technicon H.1 automated counter. When it is measured on Coulter or Ortho instruments or on one of the earlier models of Technicon instruments, it is insensitive falling only when the anaemia is fairly marked. A low MCHC on a Coulter instrument is, however, relatively specific for iron deficiency since it is almost normal in thalassaemia trait and in the anaemia of chronic disease. The reticulocyte percentage may be normal or elevated, while the absolute reticulocyte count is normal or reduced.

Patients with iron deficiency not infrequently have an elevated platelet count, which may be consequent on the iron deficiency itself or on blood loss or underlying malignant disease. In severe iron deficiency the platelet count may be low. Leucopenia and granulocytopenia

occur in up to 10 percent of patients. Hypersegmented neutrophils are sometimes present and are not necessarily indicative of coexisting vitamin B_{12} or folic acid deficiency. In geographic areas where hookworm infestation occurs the observation of eosinophilia may suggest that this is the cause of the iron deficiency.

Certain supplementary laboratory tests are useful in confirming the diagnosis of iron deficiency. In the uncomplicated case the serum iron and the serum ferritin are low and the serum transferrin or total iron-binding capacity is elevated (Fig. 9.2). The definitive test is the demonstration of absence of bone marrow iron.

β-thalassaemia trait

β-thalassaemia trait refers to heterozygosity for β-thalassaemia. The majority of such subjects are not anaemic and have no abnormal clinical features. The clinical diagnosis of β-thalassaemia minor in general corresponds to heterozygous β-thalassaemia.

β-thalassaemia trait is common in Italy and in Greece; in some regions of these two countries the prevalence is 15–20 percent. A similar prevalence is observed in Cyprus, among both Greek and Turkish Cypriots. The prevalence in some parts of India and in Thailand and other parts of South-east Asia reaches 5–10 percent. In American Blacks the prevalence is about 1 percent and in West Indians it is about 0.5 percent. β-thalassaemia trait occurs in virtually all ethnic groups although in Caucasians of Northern European origin it is very infrequent.

The majority of subjects with β-thalassaemia trait have a normal Hb; a minority are mildly anaemic. Anaemia is commoner among Greeks and Italians than among Blacks. Despite the usual lack of anaemia microcytosis is characteristically marked (Fig. 9.3 and see also Fig. 3.71). The blood film may or may not show hypochromia. The haemoglobin content of the red cells appears fairly uniform, in contrast to the anisochromasia which is usually seen in a patient who is developing iron deficiency. Poikilocytosis varies from trivial to marked. Target cells may be prominent but in some patients they are infrequent or absent (Fig. 9.3b). A few irregularly contracted cells are seen in some patients (Fig. 9.3a). Occasional patients have marked elliptocytosis but in general elliptocytes are not a feature. Basophilic stippling is quite common in Mediterranean subjects with β-thalassaemia trait but is much less often seen when the condition occurs in Black or Oriental subjects. The reticulocyte percentage and absolute count are often somewhat elevated.[63] In a patient with uncomplicated thalassaemia trait the white cells and platelets are normal. In distinguishing between β-thalassaemia trait and iron-deficiency polycythaemia rubra vera, which may have very similar red cell indices, useful features are the anisochromasia, leucocytosis and thrombocytosis which can occur in the latter conditon.

SOME SUPPLEMENTARY TESTS USEFUL IN DISTINGUISHING BETWEEN IRON DEFICIENCY AND OTHER CAUSES OF HYPOCHROMIA OR MICROCYTOSIS				
test	iron deficiency	anaemia of chronic disease	iron deficiency plus the anaemia of chronic disease	thalassaemia trait
serum iron	low	low	low	normal
transferrin or TIBC (total iron-binding capacity)	increased	normal or decreased	normal or decreased	normal
serum ferritin	decreased	normal or increased	low in the normal range	normal
RDW	usually increased	usually normal	usually increased	usually normal
free erythrocyte protoporphyrin*	increased	increased	increased	normal

* Also elevated in sideroblastic anaemia and lead poisoning.

Fig. 9.2 Some supplementary tests which are useful in distinguishing between iron deficiency and some of the other causes of hypochromia or microcytosis.

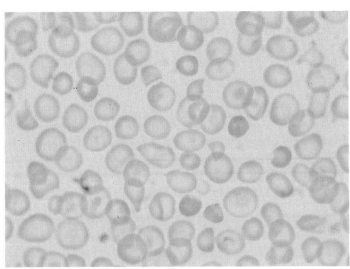

Fig. 9.3 The blood films of three healthy subjects with β-thalassaemia trait showing the range of morphological features which may be observed:

(a) a blood film showing anisocytosis, poikilocytosis, hypochromia, microcytosis, occasional target cells[1] and several irregularly contracted cells[2];

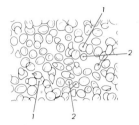

(b) a blood film showing only microcytosis and slight poikilocytosis; the diagnosis could easily have been missed in this subject if the red cell indices (see Fig. 9.4b) had not been available;

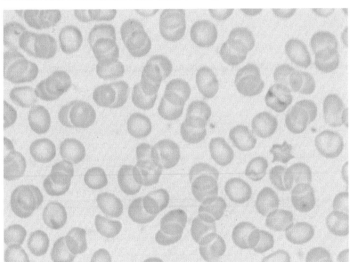

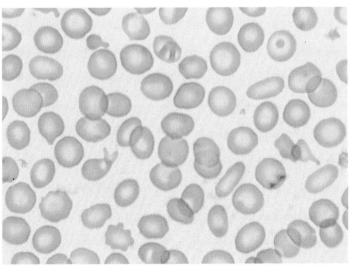

(c) a blood film showing anisocytosis, poikilocytosis (including target cells[1] and elliptocytes[2]) and microcytosis; this patient was shown by family studies to have β⁰-thalassaemia trait.

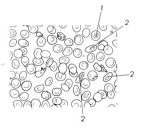

The automated blood counts corresponding to **(a)** and **(b)** are shown in Fig. 9.4a, b.

The red cell indices of β-thalassaemia trait are very characteristic (Fig. 9.4a,b,c) and it is often easier to make a correct provisional diagnosis from the indices than from the blood film. The Hb and PVC are normal or close to normal with the MCV usually being markedly reduced. The MCH is reduced proportionately to the MCV. The MCHC is usually normal. It has been reported that, in contrast to the findings in iron deficiency, the RDW is usually normal.[10] However, when a patient with β-thalassaemia trait is anaemic the RDW tends to rise[10] so that this parameter is least useful when most needed, and other observers have found it commonly elevated, even in non-anaemic cases.[61]

Various formulae have been devised in an attempt to separate iron deficiency and β-thalassaemia trait on the basis of the relationship between the various red cell indices (Fig. 9.5). Although these formulae may identify the majority of uncomplicated cases they do not work well in childhood, during pregnancy or when there are complicating factors.

β-thalassaemia trait is a heterogeneous disorder. In some cases the abnormal gene leads to no β chain production (β⁰-thalassaemia) whereas in others the abnormal gene permits β chain synthesis at a reduced rate (β⁺-thalassaemia). The haematological features of individuals who are heterozygous for B⁰ thalassaemia and

β⁺ thalassaemia respectively cannot be distinguished, although there are some slight differences between groups of patients.

Specific tests required for the definitive diagnosis of β-thalassaemia trait are haemoglobin electrophoresis and the measurement of the percentage of haemoglobin A_2 in the red cells. In β-thalassaemia trait the haemoglobin A_2 percentage is almost always elevated. The haemoglobin F level is also elevated in a third to a half of cases. In subjects with δβ- rather than β-thalassaemia trait the haemoglobin A_2 level is normal or low but the haemoglobin F percentage is elevated. It should be noted that in a small percentage of subjects the β-thalassaemia gene is silent, that is, there is no apparent haematological defect (in the heterozygote): such cases cannot, by definition, be diagnosed from the haematological features. In occasional patients with the blood count and film features of thalassaemia trait an abnormal haemoglobin is present which is synthesized at a reduced rate and thus produces a thalassaemic disorder. The commonest such β chain abnormality is that which gives rise to haemoglobin Lepore; this abnormality is readily detected on haemoglobin electrophoresis.

The diagnosis of β-thalassaemia trait during pregnancy is clinically important because of the possibility of β-thalassaemia major in the infant if the father is also

TYPICAL AUTOMATED BLOOD COUNTS IN THREE HEALTHY SUBJECTS WITH β-THALASSAEMIA TRAIT				
	a	b	c	d
Case	male, aged 16	male, aged 40	pregnant female aged 30	
			24 weeks gestation	33 weeks gestation
Instrument	Coulter S	Coulter S	S Plus IV	
RBC ($\times 10^{12}$/l)	5.78	7.3	4.17	3.5
Hb (g/dl)	10.5	14.3	10	8.9
PCV	0.32	0.43	0.31	0.28
MCV (fl)	56	59	74	80
MCH (pg)	18.2	19.7	23.6	25.5
MCHC (g/dl)	32.3	32.8	32	32

Fig. 9.4 Typical red cell indices of three healthy subjects with β-thalassaemia trait.

affected. Many women with β-thalassaemia trait enter pregnancy without this diagnosis having been made; since antenatal diagnosis of thalassaemia major is now possible it is important that the laboratory should detect possible cases of thalassaemia trait and should initiate confirmatory tests as early in pregnancy as possible. If the haematologist does not suggest the diagnosis and initiate diagnostic tests many cases go undiagnosed with the low MCV either going unnoticed or being assumed to be due to iron deficiency. The detection of thalassaemia trait during pregnancy can be difficult, for several reasons. Firstly, the red cell indices are less characteristic since haemodilution, which is a physiological effect of pregnancy, lowers the Hb, RBC and PCV; the Hb may fall as low as 5–6 g/dl.[112] The rise of the MCV which occurs in pregnancy also contributes to the red cell indices being less characteristic than in a non-pregnant subject (Fig. 9.4d). The majority of the formulae which have been recommended for the diagnosis of thalassaemia trait become quite unreliable in pregnancy.[4] Secondly, iron deficiency has an increased incidence during pregnancy and when the two conditions coexist diagnosis is complicated. Not only is the relationship between the Hb and the red cell indices no longer characteristic but the haemoglobin A_2 percen-

tage is lowered by iron deficiency, sometimes to a level which is no longer diagnostic of thalassaemia trait. In the non-pregnant patient the correct diagnosis is usually made when the microcytosis fails to correct following adequate iron therapy. In the pregnant patient, since it is important that no cases should go undiagnosed it is necessary to investigate all women with a low MCV or MCH regardless of whether the indices are characteristic of thalassaemia trait, and regardless of the degree of anaemia.[4]. β-thalassaemia trait should be particularly suspected in high incidence groups such as Greeks, Turks, Cypriots, Italians and to a lesser extent subjects from the Indian subcontinent. However it can occur in subjects of any ethnic origin, including Caucasians of northern European origin.

α-thalassaemia trait

Haematologically normal subjects have four α genes. α-thalassaemia trait may be due to lack of two of the four genes (or a functionally equivalent disorder) in which case it is designated α-thalassaemia-1 trait, or may be due to a lack of one of the four α genes (or a functionally equivalent disorder) in which case it is designated α-thalassaemia-2 trait.

SOME FORMULAE WHICH HAVE BEEN RECOMMENDED FOR DISTINGUISHING BETWEEN β-THALASSAEMIA TRAIT AND IRON DEFICIENCY			
Formula	β-thalassaemia trait	iron deficiency	reference
$\dfrac{MCV}{RBC}$	<13	>13.3	66
MCV – RBC – (Hb × 5) – constant*	<0	>0	35,36
$\dfrac{MCH}{RBC}$	<3.8	>3.8	102
$\dfrac{MCV^2 \times MCH}{100}$	<1530	>1530	101
RDW (Coulter S Plus IV)	<14.6	>14.6	10

* The constant is 3.4 with a plasma trapping correction in the MCV[35] and 8.4 with no plasma trapping correction.[36]

Fig. 9.5 Various formulae which have been recommended to aid in the distinction between β-thalassaemia trait and iron deficiency.

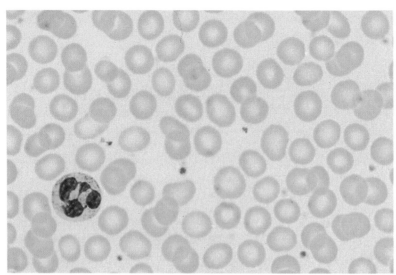

Fig. 9.6 The blood film of a healthy subject with α_1-thalassaemia trait showing microcytosis and mild hypochromia. The automated blood count (Coulter S) was RBC 6.24 × 10⁹/l, Hb 14.1 g/dl, PCV 0.45, MCV 72 fl, MCH 23 pg, MCHC 31.3 g/dl.

α-thalassaemia is common in many ethnic groups. A high incidence is found among various South-east Asian ethnic groups, particularly among Thais and Chinese. Among American Blacks α-thalassaemia-2 trait occurs in about 25–30 percent of subjects and α-thalassaemia-1 trait in about 1–2 percent.[32] In Jamaicans the prevalence is approximately 30 percent and 3 percent respectively.[98] In Nigerians the prevalence is even higher with 33 percent having α-thalassaemia-2 trait and 8 percent α-thalassaemia-1 trait.[38] α-thalassaemia-2 trait occurs in about 7 percent of Greeks[109] and is also common in some regions of Italy. In some parts of the tropics the prevalence of α-thalassaemia trait is as high as 85 percent.

α-thalassaemia-1 trait produces haematological features very similar to those of β-thalassaemia trait (Fig. 9.6); basophilic stippling may occur but target cells are not very prominent. α-thalassaemia-2 trait produces a lesser abnormality which has red cell indices overlapping with both those of normal subjects and those of subjects with α-1- or β-thalassaemia trait. α-thalassaemia trait should be suspected when a subject has persistent microcytosis without biochemical evidence of iron deficiency, elevation of the haemoglobin A₂ percentage, or the presence of an abnormal haemoglobin. There is no simple test to confirm the diagnosis. The likelihood of α-thalassaemia trait is increased if the microcytosis is shown to be familial. It is supported if a small percentage of cells (about one per thousand) are found to form haemoglobin H inclusions (see Fig. 7.8a) but inclusions are not demonstrable in all cases. The most definitive tests for α-thalassaemia trait are expensive and time-consuming. The relative rates of synthesis of α and β chains can be studied in reticulocytes; a reduced rate of synthesis of α chains supports the diagnosis of α-thalassaemia trait but there is some overlap of test results with those of normal subjects. The most definitive test is DNA analysis demonstrating the absence of one or both α genes.

A condition resembling α-thalassaemia trait is also produced by the presence of haemoglobin Constant Spring which has an abnormal α chain and is synthesized at a reduced rate. It is not uncommon in South-east asia and occurs to a lesser extent in the Caribbean area, around the Mediterranean, in the Middle East and in the Indian subcontinent. It is detected by haemoglobin electrophoresis, though sometimes with difficulty since it constitutes a low percentage of the haemoglobin.

In ethnic groups where α-thalassaemia-1 trait is due to absence of both the α genes from a single chromosome there is a risk of offspring totally lacking α globin genes; this causes haemoglobin Bart's hydrops fetalis, a condition incompatible with fetal survival and sometimes also associated with obstetric complications in the mother. In these ethnic groups (Oriental) the diagnosis of α-thalassaemia trait is important. In other ethnic groups where, in general, only a single α gene is missing from any one chromosome the risk of this condition is very low and diagnosis is only important to prevent inadvertent iron therapy.

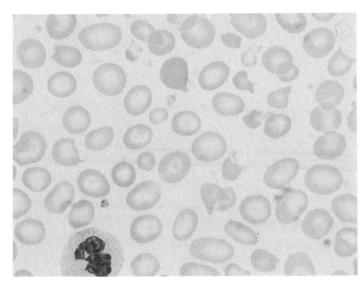

Fig. 9.7 *The blood film of a patient with haemoglobin H disease showing anisocytosis, marked poikilocytosis, hypochromia and microcytosis; the corresponding red cell indices are shown in Fig. 9.8a and the haemoglobin H preparation in Fig. 7.8a.*

Haemoglobin H disease

The lack of three of the four α chain genes (or a functionally equivalent disorder)[112] produces haemoglobin H disease. Haemoglobin H disease is most often seen in subjects of South-east Asian origin including Thais, Chinese and Indonesians, and is also seen in Greeks and Cypriots and less often in a variety of other ethnic groups. Clinical features are a chronic haemolytic anaemia with hepatomegaly and splenomegaly.

Haemoglobin H disease can usually be suspected from the blood film and the red cell indices. There is an anaemia of moderate degree; the Hb concentration is typically 6–10 g/dl, but is lower during pregnancy, during infections and after exposure to oxidant drugs. The blood film shows marked hypochromia, microcytosis and poikilocytosis, often including target cells (Fig. 9.7); all these abnormalities are more marked than in α- or β-thalassaemia trait. Basophilic stippling is seen. Polychromasia is present and the reticulocyte percentage and absolute count are elevated.

The red cell indices show the MCV and the MCH to be generally lower than in β-thalassaemia trait, and unlike β-thalassaemia trait the MCHC is often reduced and the RDW is increased (Fig. 9.8).

The condition is confirmed by the demonstration of haemoglobin H inclusions in red cells (see Fig. 7.8) and by electrophoresis which shows 2–40 percent of haemoglobin H.

Haemoglobin H disease occurs rarely as a feature of myelodysplasia.

TYPICAL AUTOMATED BLOOD COUNTS IN TWO PATIENTS WITH HAEMOGLOBIN H DISEASE		
Case	**male, aged 40**	**male, aged 13**
Instrument	Coulter S Plus IV	Coulter S
RBC ($\times 10^{12}$/l)	4.95	6.06
Hb (g/dl)	9.6	10
PCV	0.299	0.34
MCV (fl)	60.5	56
MCH (pg)	19.4	16.5
MCHC (g/dl)	32.1	29.6
RDW	25.7	–
Reticulocyte count ($\times 10^9$/l)	237	963

Fig. 9.8 *Typical red cell indices in two patients with haemoglobin H disease.*

Other conditions with red cell indices similar to those of thalassaemia trait

Red cell indices similar to those of thalassaemia trait also occur in subjects with certain abnormal haemoglobins. Haemoglobin Constant Spring not only produces a condition similar to α-thalassaemia trait but can also interact with α-thalassaemia genes to cause haemoglobin H disease. A number of other haemoglobins with an abnormal α chain are synthesized at a reduced rate and thus simulate α-thalassaemia trait.[112] The same is true with certain rare, highly unstable α chains which are largely degraded before haemoglobin can be formed.

Haemoglobin Lepore is an abnormal β-δ fusion chain which is synthesized at a slow rate and produces a blood film and indices identical to that of β-thalassaemia trait. It is detectable on haemoglobin electrophoresis; haemoglobin A_2 is lowered rather than elevated. Several rare unstable β chain variants with a decreased rate of synthesis can also produce haematological features which simulate β-thalassaemia trait, including in this case an elevated haemoglobin A_2 level. The same haematological features can be produced when a highly unstable β chain is synthesized at a normal rate.

Red cell indices suggestive of thalassaemia trait are usual in haemoglobin E disease and common in haemoglobin E trait, the β^E chain being synthesized at a slower rate than the β^A chain (see below). Thalassaemic indices are also seen not infrequently in association with sickle cell trait, haemoglobin C trait and haemoglobin C disease (see below).

β-thalassaemia major

Thalassaemia major which is consequent on homozygosity or double heterozygosity for β-thalassaemia genes produces a severe anaemia due to ineffective erythropoiesis. Clinical features include splenomegaly and bone deformity due to expansion of the marrow cavity.

Although there is marked hypochromia and microcytosis the laboratory features are not likely to be confused with iron deficiency or thalassaemia trait. Anaemia is severe with the Hb sometimes being as low as 2–3 g/dl. Anisocytosis and poikilocytosis are also very marked, with the poikilocytes including target cells, tear-drop cells, elliptocytes, fragments and many cells of bizarre shape (Fig. 9.9). Both basophilic stippling and Pappenheimer bodies are present. NRBC are frequent; the circulating erythroblasts are micronormoblastic and show dyserythropoietic features, defective haemoglobinization and the presence of Pappenheimer bodies. The total nucleated cell count as measured on automated counters is markedly increased because of the presence of NRBC, but there is often also a true leucocytosis; in children the absolute lymphocyte count may be increased and in older subjects the neutrophil count. The platelet count may be normal or

Fig. 9.9 The blood film of a patient with β-thalassaemia major who has been splenectomized and is receiving intermittent blood transfusions. The blood film is dimorphic with about two-thirds of the cells being donor cells. The patient's own red cells show marked anisocytosis, poikilocytosis and hypochromia; target cells[1], Pappenheimer bodies[2] and three NRBC[3] are present; there are inclusions[4] which represent precipitated α chains in one of the very hypochromic erythrocytes and in one of the NRBC.

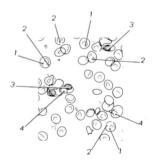

increased; in advanced disease with marked spleno-megaly the platelet count falls. Heinz body preparations show inclusions in a small percentage of cells. Following splenectomy the WBC and the platelet count rise: the blood film is even more strikingly abnormal with an increase of target cells, relatively large hypochromic cells, Pappenheimer bodies and NRBC and the appearance of many Howell–Jolly bodies. Post-splenectomy, Heinz body preparations show ragged inclusions in 10–20 pecent of red cells; these inclusions, which are composed of precipitated α chains, differ from the Heinz bodies consequent on oxidant stress in that they are not attached to the red cell membrane, and are present in NRBC as well as in mature erythrocytes.[80]

In thalassaemia major there is a reduction of the MCV, MCH and MCHC with a marked increase in the RDW.

The diagnosis of thalassaemia major is confirmed by haemoglobin electrophoresis which shows haemoglobin F to be the major haemoglobin with haemoglobin A being either absent or markedly reduced.

Thalassaemia intermedia

Thalassaemia intermedia is the name given to a genetically heterogeneous group of conditions of a clinical severity intermediate between that of thalassaemia major and that of thalassaemia minor; the haematological features are also intermediate.

The anaemia of chronic disease

'The anaemia of chronic disease' is a term used to describe the anaemia which is consequent on chronic infection of inflammation or, less often, malignant disease, which is characterized by a low serum iron and defective incorporation of iron into haemoglobin despite adequate iron in reticuloendothelial stores.

The anaemia of chronic disease, when mild, is normocytic and normochromic, but as it becomes more severe hypochromia and microcytosis develop (Fig. 9.10). In severe chronic inflammation the degree of microcytosis may be just as marked as in iron deficiency. The RDW has been reported to be normal in the anaemia of chronic disease[10] but this has not been a consistent observation.[61] Associated features may be useful in the differential diagnosis. There may be neutrophilia, increased rouleaux formation, increased background staining and an elevated ESR, all consequent on the inflammatory or malignant condition which is causing the anaemia.

The supplementary tests which are useful in distinguishing the anaemia of chronic disease from other common causes of hypochromia and microcytosis are shown in Fig. 9.2 Diagnosis is most difficult when a patient with an anaemia of chronic disease due to malignancy or inflammation develops iron deficiency. In this circumstance the transferrin and iron binding capacity commonly fail to rise and although the serum ferritin falls it may not fall to the levels usually associated with iron deficiency. It may be impossible to diagnose such a complex situation from the peripheral blood features and biochemical tests. A bone marrow aspiration showing whether or not storage iron is present will allow a correct appraisal.

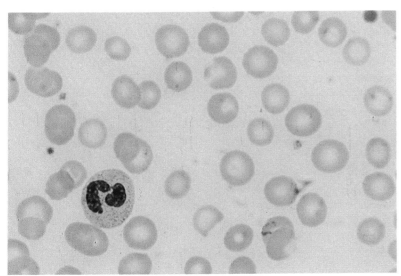

Fig. 9.10 The blood film of a patient with the anaemia of chronic disease consequent on a lymphoma, showing mild anisocytosis, poikilocytosis and hypochromia. The automated blood count (Coulter S) was RBC 3.10 × 10⁹/l, Hb 7.4 g/dl, PCV 0.23, MCV 75.6 fl, MCH 23.8 pg, MCHC 31.5 g/dl.

Sideroblastic anaemia

Congenital sideroblastic anaemia (Fig. 9.11) is a rare condition which is easily confused with iron deficiency since the dominant features are hypochromia and microcytosis.

Haemoglobin levels range from 3–4 g/dl up to almost normal levels. The blood film may be dimorphic or may show uniform hypochromia and microcytosis. Occasionally target cells and basophilic stippling are present. Poikilocytosis is sometimes marked and Pappenheimer bodies may be detectable. In older subjects hypersplenism due to iron overload can cause mild leucopenia and thrombocytopenia.

MCV and MCH are reduced and MCHC is sometimes reduced. Histograms of red cell size may show two populations of cells.

Congenital sideroblastic anaemia is observed predominantly in males, but female cases also occur.[93] Female carriers who are not anaemic may have a small percentage of hypochromic, microcytic cells.

In sideroblastic anaemia induced by drugs marked microcytosis can occur, together with a dimorphic blood film.

In idiopathic acquired sideroblastic anaemia (also designated refractory anaemia with ringed sideroblasts) (see page 218) the dominant population is usually either macrocytic or normocytic and normochromic with only a small population of hypochromic microcytes (see Figs 3.76 and 8.32b). In a minority of patients the blood film is dimorphic but the major population is also hypochromic and microcytic. Only this latter group is likely to be confused with other causes of hypochromic and microcytic anaemia. The observation of a dimorphic blood film together with other features of myelodysplasia suggests the correct diagnosis.

The definitive diagnosis of sideroblastic anaemia requires a bone marrow aspiration to demonstrate the high percentage of ring sideroblasts. However, the diagnosis can often be predicted from the peripheral blood finding when a dimorphic blood film is associated with Pappenheimer bodies and with ring sideroblasts demonstrable by an iron stain of a buffy coat preparation (see Fig. 7.10b).

The diagnosis of sideroblastic anaemia is important both because treatment is possible in some patients and in order to avoid iatrogenic iron overload if a patient is mistakenly assumed to be iron deficient. Patients may become iron overloaded even in the absence of exogenous iron or blood transfusion.[77] The correct diagnosis of patients with a mild congenital sideroblastic anaemia can be important since some of them will respond to pyridoxine therapy and some can tolerate regular venesection which will alleviate iron overload.

Other causes of hypochromic, microcytic anaemia

Lead poisoning may produce either a normochromic, normocytic anaemia or a hypochromic, microcytic anaemia. In the latter case the MCV, MCH and MCHC are reduced. Pappenheimer bodies may be detected, since lead causes sideroblastic erythropoiesis. Basophilic stippling is often a prominent feature which may suggest the diagnosis. The reticulocyte percentage is sometimes elevated.

Other causes of hypochromic, microcytic blood films (see Fig. 3.73) are rare.

MACROCYTIC RED CELLS AND THE DIFFERENTIAL DIAGNOSIS OF MEGALOBLASTIC ANAEMIA

MEGALOBLASTIC ANAEMIA

The haematological features due to a deficiency of vitamin B_{12} or a deficiency of folic acid are indistinguishable from each other. The diagnosis of megaloblastic anaemia can generally be made only by examination of a bone marrow aspirate, although it can be strongly suspected from the peripheral blood findings. Characteristic features are anaemia, macrocytosis, anisocytosis, poikilocytosis (including the presence of oval macrocytes) and neutrophil hypersegmentation (Fig. 9.12a). Macropolycytes (see page 47) may be seen as well as hypersegmented neutrophils (see page 38 and Fig. 3.14). Oval macrocytes are important in the diagnosis since they are not usually seen when macrocytosis is associated with macronormoblastic erythropoiesis; they are not, however, specific — being seen also in South-east Asian ovalocytosis and in myelofibrosis and myelodysplastic states. Tear-drop poikilocytes are also common, and basophilic stippling may be seen. Because of the increased thickness of the red cells central pallor is reduced or absent. As anaemia becomes more severe poikilocytosis and fragmentation become increasingly marked to the extent that the measured MCV may fall despite the presence of numerous macrocytes. When megaloblastic anaemia is very severe thrombocytopenia and leucopenia develop. Occasional circulating megaloblasts can be present (Fig. 9.12b), particularly when anaemia is severe.

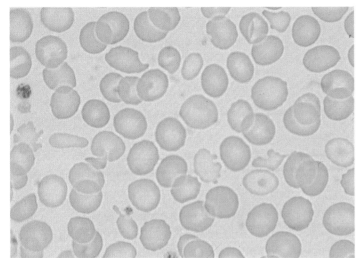

Fig. 9.11 *A dimorphic blood film from a patient with congenital sideroblastic anaemia. There is a minor population of cells which are hypochromic and microcytic and tend to form target cells; there is also poikilocytosis. The patient had previously responded to pyridoxine with a rise of Hb and was taking pyridoxine when this blood specimen was obtained.*

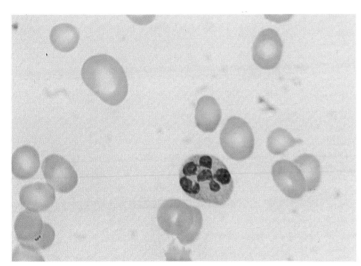

Fig. 9.12 *The blood films of two patients with megaloblastic anaemia:*
(a) from an elderly woman with both malabsorption of vitamin B_{12} and dietary deficiency of folic acid showing marked anisocytosis, macrocytosis, several oval macrocytes[1], a tear-drop poikilocyte[2] and a hypersegmented neutrophil. The automated blood count (Coulter S Plus IV) was WBC 4.2 × 10⁹/l, RBC 0.76 × 10⁹/l, Hb 4.2 g/dl, PCV 0.10, MCV 133 fl, MCH 47.4 pg, MCHC 35.7 g/dl and platelet count 50 × 10⁹/l;

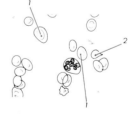

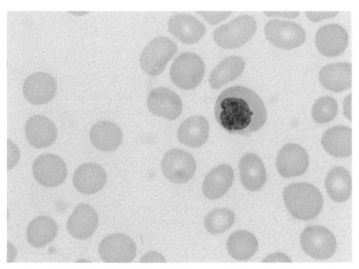

(b) from a patient with pernicious anaemia showing macrocytosis and a circulating megaloblast.

In megaloblastic anaemia the red cell indices show a reduction of the Hb, PCV and RBC and an elevation of the MCV and MCH. The percent and absolute reticulocyte count is reduced. The RDW tends to be increased, whereas in macrocytosis associated with macronormoblastic erythropoiesis it is more likely to be normal.[10] When the platelet count is reduced the electronically measured mean platelet volume remains relatively low in contrast to the high mean platelet volume which is observed when thrombocytopenia is due to decreased platelet life span.[9]

In patients presenting with neurological manifestations of pernicious anaemia haematological abnormalities may be very minor. The Hb and the MCV may both be normal and the blood film may show only an occasional macrocyte or hypersegmented neutrophil.

Folic acid antagonists produce haematological abnormalities which are indistinguishable from those of folic acid or vitamin B_{12} deficiency but when megaloblastic anaemia is due to other drugs interfering more directly with DNA synthesis hypersegmentation of neutrophils is not a feature.

When there is a double deficiency of iron and either vitamin B_{12} or folic acid the film may show hypochromic microcytes in addition to macrocytes, or the features of iron deficiency may dominate with only the presence of hypersegmented neutrophils suggesting the possibility of a double deficiency. Hypersegmented neutrophils may, however, be seen in uncomplicated iron deficiency. Iron deficiency is sometimes unmasked when vitamin B_{12} or folic acid therapy is given to a patient with inadequate iron stores; following an initial satisfactory rise of Hb and the production of well haemoglobinized cells iron stores are exhausted, hypochromic microcytes are produced and the blood film becomes dimorphic. Thalassaemia trait, like iron deficiency, can prevent the development of macrocytosis when a patient develops a megaloblastic anaemia; the MCV rises into the normal range rather than above it.

The diagnosis of megaloblastosis which develops very rapidly causing acute pancytopenia has been discussed in Chapter 8 (see page 247).

Megaloblastosis can be unsuspected and therefore difficult to diagnose when it is superimposed on a condition which itself causes major morphological abnormalities. Such can be the case with myelofibrosis or thalassaemia major; there may be little more than a fall in the haemoglobin concentration and the appearance of hypersegmented neutrophils to suggest it.

If megaloblastosis occurs in a hyposplenic or asplenic subject then morphological changes are very striking (Fig. 9.13). Numerous large Howell–Jolly bodies are seen and Pappenheimer bodies may be present. The combination of hyposplenism and megaloblastic erythropoiesis is most often seen in patients with coeliac disease in whom splenic atrophy and folic acid deficiency are both common, in patients who have had a

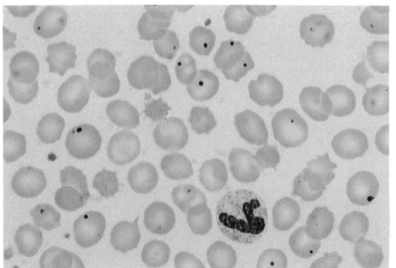

Fig. 9.13 The blood film of a splenectomized post renal transplant patient with megaloblastic anaemia due to azathioprine therapy; Howell–Jolly bodies are particularly prominent because more are formed when erythropoiesis is megaloblastic and in the absence of a spleen they cannot be pitted from the circulating cells.

total gastrectomy and splenectomy but have not been given replacement vitamin B_{12}, and in splenectomized renal transplant patients who are receiving azathioprine therapy.

When effective treatment is given to a patient with megaloblastic anaemia there is a lag phase of a few days and then a rise of the WBC and platelet count occurs followed by the production of polychromatic macrocytes and a rise of the Hb. If the patient has been pancytopenic there may be a rebound thrombocytosis and leucocytosis, often associated with a left shift or a leucoerythroblastic blood film. Hypersegmented neutrophils persist in the blood for 5–7 days or even longer following treatment and in those who were initially pancytopenic they may actually increase.

The diagnosis of megaloblastic anaemia generally requires a bone marrow examination but if for any reason this is not possible, examination of a buffy coat preparation may show sufficient megaloblasts for a confident diagnosis to be made.

OTHER CAUSES OF MACROCYTOSIS
Alcohol intake and liver disease

Excess alcohol intake can cause a megaloblastic anaemia consequent on associated folic acid deficiency of interference with folic acid metabolism. Both liver disease and alcohol abuse can also cause a macrocytic anaemia which is independent of any deficiency on vitamin B_{12} or folic acid and is associated with macronormoblastic erythropoiesis. Although a bone marrow examination is required for differentiation between megaloblastic and macronormoblastic erythropoiesis certain peripheral blood features are helpful. When macrocytosis is due to liver disease and/or alcohol abuse the amount of anisocytosis and poikilocytosis is usually less than in a megaloblastic anaemia with a similar MCV. Oval macrocytes and hypersegmented neutrophils are absent whereas target cells and stomatocytes can be present. Thrombocytopenia and leucopenia can occur in both conditions. The RDW may be helpful, being more likely to be abnormal in a megaloblastic anaemia and normal in a macronormoblastic anaemia.[10]

Sideroblastic anaemia

When macrocytosis is due to primary acquired sideroblastic anaemia the diagnosis can usually be suspected from the peripheral blood examination because of the presence of a small percentage of hypochromic microcytes (see Fig. 8.32b), often in association with other features of myelodysplasia such as hypogranular neutrophils or monocytosis. Pappenheimer bodies are usually detectable. Hypersegmented neutrophils are absent.

Refractory anaemia

Refractory anaemia as part of a myelodysplasia may be macrocytic. This diagnosis is suspected when the other features of myelodysplasia (see page 214) are noted. The association of a macrocytic anaemia and thrombocytosis raised the possibility of the 5q– syndrome.

Haemolytic anaemia and blood loss

A striking degree of macrocytosis (for example an MCV of 115–120 fl) can be seen in chronic haemolytic anaemia. This is due not only to increased numbers of reticulocytes but also to the fact that 'stress reticulocytes' (see page 70), which are larger than normal reticulocytes, mature into macrocytes rather than normocytes. A lesser degree of macrocytosis occurs when the bone marrow is responding to recent blood loss. The presence of polychromasia together with an increased reticulocyte count suggests that a macrocytosis is due to either haemolysis or recent blood loss.

Macrocytosis is a feature of some of the congenital dyserythropoietic anaemias (see page 292). Further causes of macrocytosis are shown in Fig. 3.74.

TARGET CELLS AND THE HAEMATOLOGICAL FEATURES OF HAEMOGLOBINOPATHIES

TARGET CELLS

If target cells are present in a blood film it is useful to consider the size and degree of haemoglobinization of the cells and also whether there are any associated diagnostic features such as the presence of other changes of hyposplenism or of sickle cells. Some of the causes of target cell formation are shown in Fig. 3.90 and the mechanism of their formation is discussed on page 78. If target cells are associated with hypochromic, microcytic red cells then the differential diagnosis lies between iron deficiency, a haemoglobinopathy and a thalassaemic condition. If target cells are associated with macrocytosis then liver disease or obstructive jaundice is suggested. If target cell formation is associated with normocytic, normochromic red cells then the differential diagnosis includes hyposplenism, a haemoglobinopathy, obstructive jaundice and liver disease.

THE HAEMATOLOGICAL FEATURES OF HAEMOGLOBINOPATHIES

Sickle cell anaemia

The term sickle cell anaemia refers to the homozygous state for the sickle cell gene. The term sickle cell disease may be used synonymously or may be used to refer more widely to all haemoglobinopathies characterized by sickling which include, for example, double heterozygosity for haemoglobin S and either β-thalassaemia or an abnormal haemoglobin such as haemoglobin C, haemoglobin E, haemoglobin O^{Arab}, haemoglobin $D^{Los Angeles}$ (also called haemoglobin D^{Punjab}) or haemoglobin Lepore. The sickle cell gene and therefore sickle cell anaemia have the greatest frequency in Blacks but they are seen also in Indians, Greeks, Italians, Turks, Cypriots, Spaniards, Arabs, North Africans and subjects from Central and South America.

Clinical features of sickle cell anaemia are splenomegaly during childhood, chronic anaemia, and painful crises due to tissue infarction following vascular obstruction by sickled cells.

In sickle cell anaemia[95] the haemoglobin concentration is usually of the order of 7–8 g/dl, but with a range of 4–11 g/dl or even greater. Higher Hb levels are characteristic of Arabs with sickle cell anaemia. A typical blood film (Fig. 9.14) shows sickle cells which are characteristically crescent or sickle shaped, boat-shaped cells, target cells, polychromasia, macrocytosis, basophilic stippling, NRBC and the features of hyposplenism.

The hyposplenic features are consequent initially on reduction of function and subsequently on progressive infarction of the spleen. The reticulocyte count is usually 10–20 percent. The MCV is not elevated to a degree commensurate with the increase of the reticulocyte count;[43] this may be regarded as a relative microcytosis. The RDW is increased. The Technicon H.1 automated counter may show a population of cells with an increased MCHC in patients with sickle cell anaemia; these are probably irreversibly sickled cells.

At birth, when only a small percentage of haemoglobin S is present, the haemoglobin concentration, red cell indices and blood film are normal. Haematological abnormalities appear during the first year of life.[25,97] The Hb falls below the normal range at 1–6 months of age. A few sickle cells and other features of sickle cell anaemia begin to appear at 4–6 months of age; features of hyposplenism usually appear at 9–12 months of age but sometimes as early as 6 months. In early infancy hyposplenism is reversible by blood transfusion but later it is not. The features of hyposplenism appear at about the time that splenomegaly is detected. NRBC only become common after 12 months of age.

Sometime subjects, although homozygous for the sickle cell gene, have a normal or near normal Hb and very few signs or symptoms of sickle cell anaemia; they are mainly Arabs with an unusually high percentage of haemoglobin F which is ameliorating the condition. In such subjects the morphological abnormalities may also be slight.

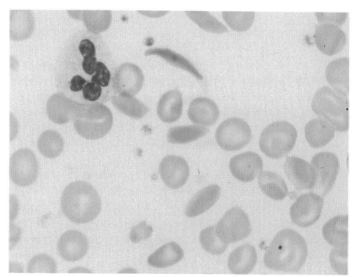

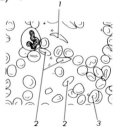

Fig. 9.14 The blood film of a patient with sickle cell anaemia showing one sickle cell[(1)] and several boat-shaped cells[(2)]; the latter are also consequent on polymerization of haemoglobin S, but are not diagnostic since poikilocytes of similar shape are sometimes seen in other conditions. One cell contains a Howell–Jolly body[(3)].

Sickle cells are not seen in the blood films of subjects with sickle cell trait. They may, however, be seen in subjects with the double heterozygous states which clinically are characterized by sickling episodes, and in heterozygotes for haemoglobin S[Antilles], an abnormal haemoglobin which is even more prone to cause sickling than is haemoglobin S itself.[69]

During a sickle cell crisis typical changes are leucocytosis (with the WBC sometimes as high as 40–50 × 10^9/l), neutrophilia, increasing polychromasia, the appearance of NRBC and an increase in the reticulocyte count. The neutrophil alkaline phosphatase score is not elevated when neutrophilia is due to sickle cell crisis alone without underlying infection. During a crisis the number of sickle cells increases but as recognition of this requires a knowledge of the usual findings in the individual patient this is not diagnostically very useful.

The laboratory should be alert to a sudden fall of the Hb in patients with sickle cell anaemia. This may be due to: acute sequestration of red cells in the spleen or less often the liver in young subjects; red cell aplasia, usually due to a parvovirus infection; megaloblastic erythropoiesis consequent on the increased need for folic acid which is a feature of any haemolytic anaemia; suppression of erythropoiesis due to infection; or bone marrow infarction. Peripheral blood features which are useful in the differential diagnosis of a falling haemoglobin concentration are: a fall of the platelet count and an increase in the reticulocyte percentage and the number of NRBC in acute sequestration, macrocytosis and hypersegmented neutrophils in megaloblastosis; a disappearance of polychromasia and of reticulocytes and sometimes associated thrombocytopenia in parvovirus-induced red cell aplasia; and marked leucoerythroblastic features and sometimes circulating megakaryocytes in bone marrow infarction.

When α-thalassaemia trait coexists with sickle cell anaemia there are subtle differences in the red cell indices, but only when groups of patients are considered. Individuals cannot be distinguished on haematological grounds. In a group with coexisting α-thalassaemia trait the Hb and RBC are higher, whereas the MCV, MCH, MCHC, reticulocyte count and degree of polychromasia are lower.

The diagnosis of sickle cell anaemia requires demonstration that only haemoglobins S, F and A_2 are present; in some patients who are microcytic family studies are also required to distinguish between sickle cell anaemia and the compound heterozygous state for sickle cell anaemia and β^0-thalassaemia

Sickle cell trait

Some patients with sickle cell trait have small numbers of target cells. Others, however, have no morphological abnormality so that the blood film cannot be relied on for diagnosis. A sickle cell solubility test must be performed whenever it is necessary to diagnose or exclude sickle cell trait; a positive test must be followed by confirmatory haemoglobin electrophoresis to show that both haemoglobin A and haemoglobin S are present, with the percentage of haemoglobin A being higher than the percentage of haemoglobin S. Subjects with sickle cell trait have normal haemoglobin levels; they are more often microcytic than are other Blacks.[99] Although the microcytosis may be partly due to a slightly higher incidence of α-thalassaemia trait in patients with sickle cell trait,[65] this does not appear sufficient to explain the frequency of microcytosis; it appears that the β^S gene must also make a contribution to the microcytosis.

Compound heterozygosity for haemoglobin S and β-thalassaemia

Subjects who are heterozygous for both haemoglobin S and either β^0-thalassaemia or β^+-thalassaemia cannot generally be distinguished from sickle cell anaemia on the basis of their clinical features, blood films (Fig. 9.15) or blood counts although as a group some differences do exist. In the compound heterozygotes the disease may be milder and splenomegaly is much more likely to persist beyond early childhood. The Hb, RBC and PCV are generally higher and the MCV, MCH, MCHC, reticulocyte percentage and reticulocyte absolute count are usually lower;[94,96] target cells are numerous but sickle cells are less frequent than in sickle cell anaemia. Cytopenias due to hypersplenism can occur as a consequence of the persisting splenomegaly.

Because there is considerable overlap between the features of the three groups a reliable distinction cannot be made on the basis of the blood film and count. The β^+-thalassaemia/haemoglobin S compound heterozygote has red cell indices which differ more from sickle cell anaemia than do those of the/β^0-haemoglobin S compound heterozygote. β^+-thalassaemia/ haemoglobin S can be distinguished from sickle cell anaemia by haemoglobin electrophoresis which shows some haemoglobin A, but with the percentage of haemoglobin S being higher than the percentage of haemoglobin A. β^0/haemoglobin S has no haemoglobin A and can be distinguished from sickle cell anaemia only by family studies.

Compound heterozygosity for haemoglobin S and pancellular hereditary persistence of fetal haemoglobin (HPFH)

Compound heterozygosity for haemoglobin S and pancellular hereditary persistence of fetal haemoglobin (HPFH) have a mild clinical condition with a lesser degree of anaemia than is usual in sickle cell anaemia; the blood film usually lacks the features of hyposplenism and shows only small numbers of sickle cells. Haemoglobin electrophoresis shows haemoglobins S and F but no haemoglobin A. This compound heterozygous state is distinguished from compound heterozygosity for haemoglobin S and β^0-thalassaemia by the much milder clinical and haematological abnormalities, and by the higher percentage of haemoglobin F — 20–30 percent rather than the level of 0.5–15 percent which is usual in sickle cell anaemia. An intermediate level of haemoglobin F is seen in subjects with sickle cell anaemia and either heterocellular HPFH or an inherited ability to increase the percentage of haemoglobin F in response to anemia.

Compound heterozygosity for haemoglobin S and haemoglobin C (SC disease)

Compound heterozygosity for haemoglobins S and C causes a sickling disorder of very variable severity, ranging from virtually asymptomatic to a severity comparable with that of sickle cell anaemia. Splenomegaly is present in childhood and may persist into adult life.

In SC disease the Hb is higher than in sickle cell anaemia with little overlap, levels of 8–14 g/dl being seen in women and 8–17 g/dl in men.[94] SC disease can usually be distinguished from sickle cell anaemia on the basis of the peripheral blood film (Fig. 9.16a) and count, although haemoglobin electrophoresis showing the presence of the two haemoglobins is needed for confirmation. The blood film shows more target cells than in sickle cell anaemia but fewer NRBC, less polychromasia and very few sickle cells. Some irregularly contracted cells are present. Howell–Jolly bodies and Pappenheimer bodies consequent on hyposplenism are less common and develop much later in life. Deformed cells containing both haemoglobin S and haemoglobin C can be distinguished from sickle cells by their having some straight edges or by being angulated or branched; such cells are detectable in the majority of patients with sickle cell/haemoglobin C disease[28] (Fig. 9.16b), but in my experience only a few patients have numerous cells of this type. Occasional cells may be seen with crystals of the same form as haemoglobin C crystals. The RBC on average is higher than in sickle cell anaemia and the MCV and reticulocyte count are lower, the latter averaging 3 percent rather than 10 percent.[94] The MCV can be below the normal range, even in those who do not have coexisting α-thalassaemia trait.[5] The MCHC is higher than in sickle cell disease, often falling above the normal range.

A sudden fall of the Hb may be due to superimposed megaloblastosis, and macrocytes and hypersegmented

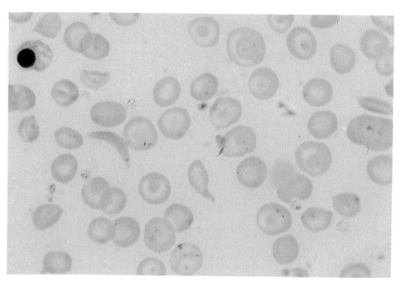

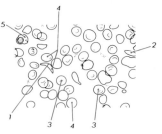

Fig. 9.15 *The blood film of a patient with sickle cell/β^0-thalassaemia showing one sickle cell[1], one boat-shaped cell[2], target cells[3], numerous Pappenheimer bodies[4] and one NRBC[5].*

neutrophils should be sought; this complication is particularly likely during pregnancy. Bone marrow necrosis also has an increased frequency during pregnancy. Aplastic crises can occur and are likely to be viral in origin.

Haemoglobin C disease (Haemoglobin C homozygosity)

The only major incidence of haemoglobin C is in Blacks originating from West Africa, west of the Niger river; there is a much lower rate of occurrence in North Africa, Sicily, other parts of Italy and Spain. Haemoglobin C disease causes chronic haemolysis and usually a haemolytic anaemia. The spleen is enlarged and the incidence of gallstones is increased.

The blood film is characterized by large numbers of target cells and large numbers of irregularly contracted cells (Fig. 9.17 and see also Fig. 3.92). Some cells appear spherocytic but close inspection shows that the majority are, in fact, irregular in shape. Polychromasia and some NRBC may be noted. Haemoglobin C crystals (Fig. 9.18) are uncommon but when present are sufficiently distinctive to confirm the presence of this haemoglobin.

There is usually a mild to moderate anaemia with the reticulocyte percentage and absolute count being somewhat increased. A markedly reduced MCV and MCH is common, with the MCHC being increased.[5] The low MCV and MCH occur even in the absence of coexisting α-thalassaemia trait. Diagnosis requires haemoglobin electrophoresis which shows predominantly haemoglobin C with some haemoglobin F and a total absence of haemoglobin A. A definite distinction between haemoglobin C disease and a compound heterozygous state for haemoglobin C and β^0-thalassaemia (Fig. 9.18) requires family studies.

Haemoglobin C trait

Haemoglobin C trait is an asymptomatic abnormality of no significance apart from the possibility of a more severe condition in offspring. The haemoglobin concentration is normal. The blood film commonly shows some target cells (Fig. 9.19), varying from occasional to frequent, and red cells are often hypochromic and microcytic,[5] even in the absence of coexisting α-thalassaemia trait. Some patients have occasional irregularly contracted cells. The reticulocyte count is

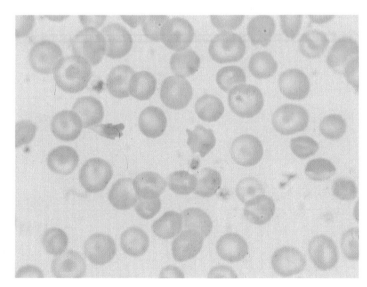

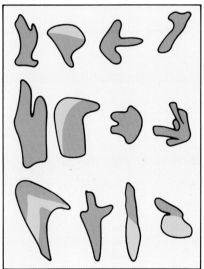

Fig. 9.16 (a) *The blood film of a patient with sickle cell/haemoglobin C disease showing target cells and one cell of bizarre shape (centre) characteristic of this compound heterozygous condition. The automated blood count (Coulter S Plus IV) was RBC 3.8 × 10⁹/l, Hb 12.2 g/dl, PCV 0.35, MCV 93 fl, MCH 32.1 pg, MCHC 34.5 g/dl; the reticulocyte count was 243 × 10⁹/l.*

(b) *Drawing of the characteristic misshapen cells which are seen in sickle cell/haemoglobin C disease.*

normal. Some subjects have a normal blood film and indices so that, although this trait can often be suspected from the blood film, haemoglobin electrophoresis is required to confirm or exclude the diagnosis, this is necessary, for example, if genetic counselling is to be carried out.

Haemoglobin E disease

Haemoglobin E occurs frequently in Thailand, Burma, Cambodia, Laos, Vietnam and Malaya and to a lesser extent in other countries in South-east Asia stretching from Indonesia to Nepal. It has a very low frequency in Blacks and Caucasians.

Haemoglobin E disease (homozygosity for haemoglobin E)[57] is an asymptomatic condition; there is a mild anaemia or even a normal haemoglobin concentration. The spleen is usually not enlarged.

The blood film shows target cells (ranging from few to very numerous), irregularly contracted cells, hypochromia, microcytosis and often bizarre poikilocytes (Fig. 9.20). Red cell indices are usually similar to those of thalassaemia trait with an elevated RBC, a reduced MCV and MCH and a normal MCHC. The reticulocyte count is usually normal. Diagnosis requires haemoglobin electrophoresis which shows the presence of haemoglobin E and 5–10 percent of haemoglobin F

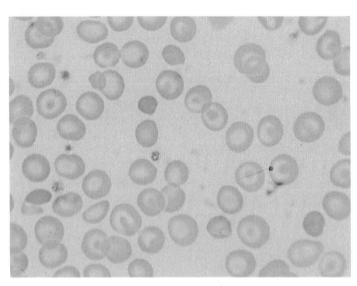

Fig. 9.17 *The blood film of a patient with haemoglobin C disease showing a mixture of target cells and irregularly contracted cells.*

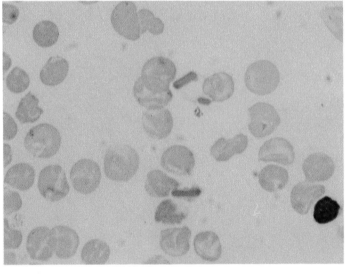

Fig. 9.18 *The blood film of a patient who was a compound heterozygote for haemoglobin C and β^0-thalassaemia showing crystals of haemoglobin C, contained within cells which otherwise appear empty of haemoglobin[1]; one cell contains two crystals.*

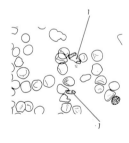

with a total absence of haemoglobin A. There are some haematological and electrophoretic differences between groups of patients with haemoglobin E disease and the compound heterozygous state for haemoglobin E and β^0-thalassaemia respectively (see below) but individuals cannot always be distinguished with certainty and family studies may be needed for definite diagnosis.

Haemoglobin E trait

Haemoglobin E trait (heterozygosity for haemoglobin E) is a completely asymptomatic condition. The Hb is almost always normal. The blood film (Fig. 9.21) usually shows a few target cells, often hypochromia and microcytosis and sometimes a few irregularly contracted cells. The red cell indices are often similar to those of thalassaemia trait. Confirmation of diagnosis is by haemoglobin electrophoresis which shows haemoglobins A and E, but with the amount of E often being considerably less than the amount of A since the abnormal β chain is synthesized at a slower rate.

Compound heterozygosity for haemoglobin E and β-thalassaemia

The compound heterozygous state for haemoglobin E and β-thalassaemia in general is more severe than haemoglobin E disease. Anaemia, hepatomegaly and

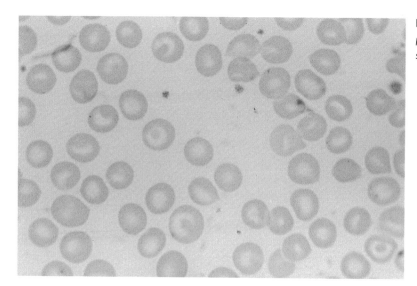

Fig. 9.19 *The blood film of a patient with haemoglobin C trait showing several target cells.*

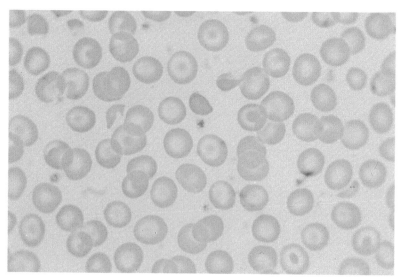

Fig. 9.20 *The blood film of a patient with haemoglobin E disease showing hypochromia, microcytosis, target cells and occasional poikilocytes and irregularly contracted cells. The automated blood count (Coulter S) was RBC 6.84 × 10⁹/l, Hb 11.9 g/dl, PCV 0.37, MCV 54 fl, MCH 17.4 pg, MCHC 26.7 g/dl.*

splenomegaly are usual. Some cases require blood transfusion. The degree of severity may resemble that of thalassaemia major or thalassaemia intermedia. In South-east Asia most cases are β^0-thalassaemia/haemoglobin E but in India β^+-thalassaemia/haemoglobin E occurs and can also be quite severe.

The anaemia is usually moderate, typical Hb levels being 7–9 g/dl, but ranging from 2–13 g/dl.[18]

Marked hypochromia and microcytosis are usual blood film features, together with basophilic stippling (some cases), anisocytosis and poikilocytosis — with the poikilocytes including target cells, keratocytes, tear drop cells, fragments and irregularly contracted cells. The reticulocyte percentage is increased and some NRBC may be present. The MCV and MCH are reduced and, in contrast to haemoglobin E disease and E trait the MCHC can be reduced. Haemoglobin electrophoresis shows haemoglobin E and haemoglobin F, with F levels varying from less than 10 percent to well over 50 percent. In β^+-thalassaemia/haemoglobin E disease haemoglobin A will also be present with the level being about 30 percent.

Complicating conditions which have been reported in β-thalassaemia/haemoglobin E include aplastic crises, megaloblastic anaemia and hypersplenism.

Homozygosity for Haemoglobin D^Los Angeles

Haemoglobin D^Los Angeles (previously also known as haemoglobin D^Punjab) is found in North-west India, Pakistan, Afghanistan and Iran and less commonly in Blacks and in a varity of other ethnic groups. Homozygotes for haemoglobin D are clinically well and have either a mild anaemia or a normal Hb.

The blood film shows target cells and some irregularly contracted cells. Diagnosis is by haemoglobin electrophoresis. Haemoglobin D moves with haemoglobin S at alkaline pH but it does not sickle and at acid pH it moves with haemoglobin A rather than with haemoglobin S. Although haemoglobin D disease is very mild and of little importance to the individual the correct diagnosis is important since the compound heterozygous state with haemoglobin S produces a sickling disorder.

Haemoglobin D^Los Angeles trait

Subjects with haemoglobin D trait may have a normal blood film or the film may show a small number of target cells. The Hb and MCV are normal. The trait is of no consequence except for the possible interaction with haemoglobin S.

Haemoglobin O^Arab

Haemoglobin O^Arab has been found in Arabs, North Africans, Blacks and in subjects from Eastern Europe. Homozygotes have a moderately severe haemolytic anaemia with target cells in the blood film. Compound heterozygotes with β^0-thalassaemia/haemoglobin O^Arab have a thalassaemic disorder of moderate severity.

Unstable haemoglobins

Unstable haemoglobins may produce mild, moderate or severe haemolytic anaemia, depending on the severity of the molecular defect. Some unstable haemoglobins also have a high oxygen affinity and are therefore associated with polycythaemia. Haemolysis is sometimes precipitated by infection or exposure to oxidant drugs. Splenomegaly can occur and patients sometimes complain of passage of dark urine after intravascular haemolysis.

The blood film findings are very variable. Sometimes the blood film is normal or shows only macrocytosis associated with an elevated reticulocyte count. In other patients there may be anisocytosis, poikilocytosis, hypochromia, irregularly contracted cells, 'bite cells' (that is, cells which appear to have had a bite taken out of them, probably resulting from removal of Heinz bodies by the spleen), basophilic stippling, and polychromasia (Fig. 9.22). Non-splenectomized subjects may be thrombocytopenic, consequent on hypersplenism. Heinz body preparations are positive following splenectomy and during haemolytic crises in some non-splenectomized subjects. A haemolytic crisis can also cause the appearance of other signs of hyposplenism, such as Howell–Jolly bodies and target cells.

The automated blood count may show an elevated MCV or a reduction of the MCH and MCHC (Fig. 9.22) attributable to removal of haemoglobin as Heinz bodies by the spleen. In some cases a discrepancy has been noted between a low MCH and MCHC and a lack of hypochromia on the blood film. This has been attributed to the fact that the unstable haemoglobin may lose some of its haem groups; the staining of the red cells is dependent on their globin content whereas the accurate measurement of the haemoglobin concentration requires the presence of the haem group.[83]

Confirmation of the diagnosis is by haemoglobin electrophoresis and a test for an unstable haemoglobin such as a heat or isopropanol instability test.

Very unstable haemoglobins can also produce a disorder similar to thalassaemia consequent on very rapid breakdown of the abnormal chain.

High oxygen affinity haemoglobins

High oxygen affinity haemoglobins cause polycythaemia. They should be suspected when polycythaemia occurs with no signs of a myeloproliferative disorder, particularly if the subject is young or there is a family history of a high Hb. The blood film is 'packed' but shows no other abnormality. Confirmation of diagnosis is by haemoglobin electrophoresis and measurement of oxygen affinity.

POIKILOCYTOSIS

A striking degree of poikilocytosis with red cells of a variety of abnormal shapes is seen in: idiopathic myelofibrosis and infiltrative disease of the bone marrow (see page 220); severe megaloblastic anaemia (see page 264); thalassaemia major and haemoglobin H disease (see pages 262 and 261); congenital and acquired dyserythropoietic anaemias (see page 292) and certain haemolytic anaemias (see microangiopathic haemolytic

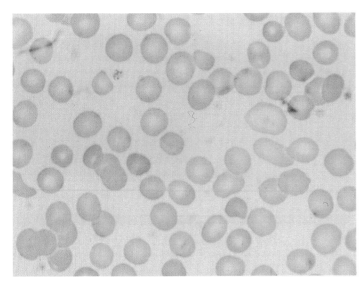

Fig. 9.21 *The blood film of a patient with haemoglobin E trait showing hypochromia, microcytosis and occasional irregularly contracted cells. The automated blood count (Coulter S Plus IV) was RBC 4.39 × 10⁹/l, Hb 11 g/dl, PCV 0.32, MCV 74 fl, MCH 25.1 pg, MCHC 33.2 g/dl.*

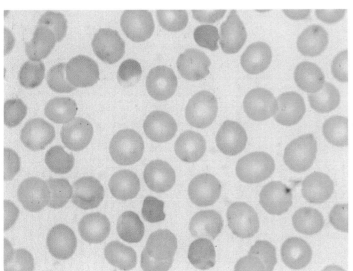

Fig. 9.22 *The blood film of a patient who was heterozygous for haemoglobin Köln showing several irregularly contracted cells including one in which the haemoglobin has retracted from the cell margin[1]. The automated blood count (Coulter S Plus IV) was RBC 4.04 × 10⁹/l, Hb 11.9 g/dl, PCV 0.40, MCV 100 fl, MCH 29.5 pg, MCHC 29.4 g/dl.*

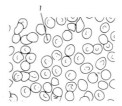

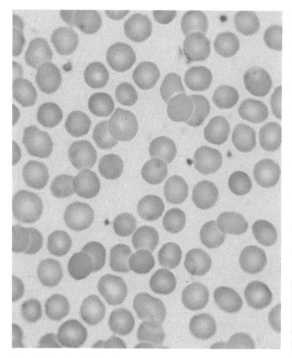 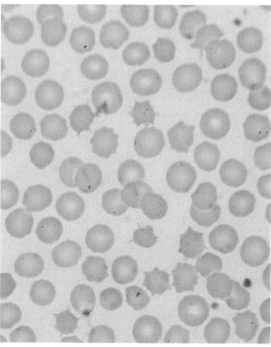

Fig. 9.23 *Blood films from patients with hereditary spherocytosis:* **(a)** *a patient with mild chronic haemolysis without anaemia;*

(b) *a patient who has had a splenectomy; this patient was the father of the first patient;*

anaemia and congenital pyropoikilocytosis, pages 284 and 283). In other conditions one specific type of poikilocyte, for example the spherocyte or the elliptocyte, predominates.

SPHEROCYTOSIS

Some of the causes of spherocytosis are shown in Fig. 3.81. When the major feature of a blood film is spherocytosis the differential diagnosis usually lies between hereditary spherocytosis and warm autoimmune haemolytic anaemia (AIHA). The blood films of these two conditions are often indistinguishable.

Hereditary spherocytosis

Hereditary spherocytosis (Fig. 9.23) is an inherited condition in which a reduction or abnormality of spectrin in the red cell membrane leads to chronic haemolysis. Depending on the severity of the haemolysis, there may or may not be chronic anaemia. Inheritance is

usually autosomal dominant but in some families is autosomal recessive.

The blood film shows spherocytosis, and in the more severe cases anaemia and polychromasia. Ultrastructural studies have shown that in hereditary spherocytosis only a minority of the red cells are actually microspherocytes or spherocytes; the majority of the cells are discocytes, stomatocytes or stomatospherocytes[105] (see Fig. 3.80). In mild cases of hereditary spherocytosis it is sometimes very difficult to be certain whether or not spherocytes are present and an osmotic fragility test is needed for confirmation; this is not a specific test for the inherited condition but merely confirms the presence of osmotically fragile spherocytes, irrespective of the mechanism of their formation. In other patients the spherocytosis is obvious with there being marked polychromasia and numerous polychromatic macrocytes. In severe cases of hereditary spherocytosis other poikilocytes may also be present.

Automated blood counts may show the MCHC to be elevated and with counts performed on the Technicon

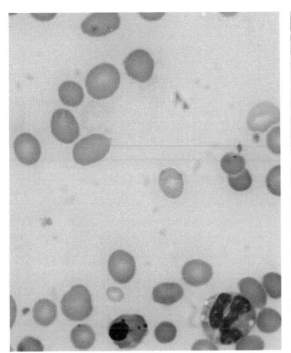

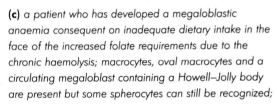

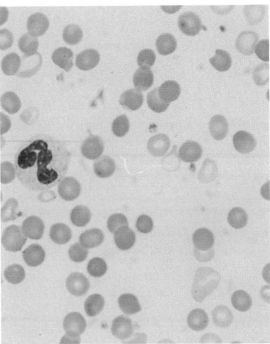

(c) *a patient who has developed a megaloblastic anaemia consequent on inadequate dietary intake in the face of the increased folate requirements due to the chronic haemolysis; macrocytes, oval macrocytes and a circulating megaloblast containing a Howell–Jolly body are present but some spherocytes can still be recognized;*

(d) *a patient who has developed a superimposed anaemia of chronic disease due to an intercurrent infection; some cells have developed central pallor and have become hypochromic and microcytic; this is the same patient as shown in* **(c)**.

H.1 a minor population of cells with increased haemoglobin concentration may be identifiable on the histogram.

Since the blood films of hereditary spherocytosis and autoimmune haemolytic anaemia can be identical the differential diagnosis requires personal and family history and a direct antiglobulin test (DAGT, Coombs' test) to exclude autoimmune haemolytic anaemia.

Complications of hereditary spherocytosis which may be suspected from examining the blood film include megaloblastic anaemia due to folic acid deficiency (Fig. 9.23c), and pure red cell aplasia, usually consequent on parvovirus infection. A worsening of the anaemia should therefore lead to the blood film being examined for macrocytes — particularly oval macrocytes — for hypersegmented neutrophils, and for a lack of the polychromasia which would be appropriate to the degree of anaemia. Reticulocytopenia is seen in red cell aplasia, and leukopenia and thrombocytopenia sometimes also occur. Previously undiagnosed cases of hereditary spherocytosis may be unmasked by the occurrence of parvovirus-induced red cell aplasia, and also by the development of infectious mononucleosis — in which case the mechanism is a worsening of the haemolysis. Haemolytic episodes can also be precipitated by pregnancy[48] or induced by exercise. In the neonatal period symptomatic ABO haemolytic disease of the newborn is a great deal more common in babies which are subsequently found to have hereditary spherocytosis.

As for any chronic haemolytic anaemia, patients with this condition are predisposed to gallstones as a consequence of the increased haemoglobin breakdown. If they develop obstructive jaundice the spherocytosis lessens as more lipid is taken up into the red cell membrane, and the osmotic fragility becomes more normal. The development of iron deficiency anaemia or the anaemia of chronic disease also leads to a lessening of the degree of spherocytosis and the blood film may become dimorphic (Fig. 9.23d).

When a patient with hereditary spherocytosis has a splenectomy the cells remain spherocytic, although osmotic fragility tests may show that a small population of very fragile cells which was previously present has disappeared; it is likely that this population was composed of abnormal cells which, rather than being removed by the spleen, were being further damaged by it. Ultrastructural study shows that postsplenectomy the minor population of microspherocytes has largely disappeared.[105] The usual features of a postsplenectomy blood film are modified by spherocytosis; target cells are not usual, and spheroacanthocytes are formed (Fig. 9.23b)

Warm autoimmune haemolytic anaemia

Warm autoimmune haemolytic anaemia is an acquired haemolytic anaemia in which red cell membranes are damaged by an antibody and whole red cells and parts of their membranes are removed by phagocytic cells in the spleen, and to a lesser extent the liver.

As with hereditary spherocytosis, the blood film shows spherocytosis and sometimes also polychromasia and polychromatic macrocytes (Fig. 9.24a); the MCHC may be increased. In severe autoimmune haemolytic anaemia white cell precursors and NRBC can be present. In occasional patients tear-drop poikilocytes have been prominent and have disappeared following splenectomy.[40] Associated features which may be seen in autoimmune haemolytic anaemia and which suggest this diagnosis rather than hereditary spherocytosis are red cell agglutination, occasional erythrophagocytosis by monocytes (Fig. 9.24b), and thrombocytopenia — which also has an immune basis. The combination of autoimmune haemolytic anaemia and autoimmune thrombocytopenia is referred to as Evans' syndrome. A rare phenomenon is the rosetting of red cells around neutrophils.[78] Confirmation of the diagnosis of autoimmune haemolytic anaemia requires a direct antiglobulin test to detect immunoglobulin or complement on the surface of the red cells. In rare cases with a negative antiglobulin test diagnosis rests on even more sensitive tests for antibody on red cells or on the response to immunosuppressive therapy.

When warm autoimmune haemolytic anaemia occurs as a complication of chronic lymphocytic leukaemia, lymphoma or angioimmunoblastic lymphadenopathy the features of the primary disease will be seen in the blood film.

The autoimmune haemolytic anaemia which follows therapy with α-methyldopa and, less often, a small number of other drugs is indistinguishable both morphologically and serologically from idiopathic autoimmune haemolytic anaemia.

Other causes of spherocytosis

Large numbers of spherocytes are also present in several conditions where the nature of the condition is readily deduced from the clinical history. These include some drug-induced immune haemolytic anaemias (innocent-bystander mechanism), *Clostridium welchii* sepsis, Zieve's syndrome and severe burns. In *Clostridium welchii* sepsis the spherocytes may be so fragile that lysis occurs in the blood specimen causing an artefactual elevation of the MCH and MCHC (page 132). Zieve's syndrome is a spherocytic haemolytic anaemia in a patient with severe alcoholic liver disease; there is associated hypercholesterolaemia. In severe burns striking spherocytosis occurs with quite distinctive morphological features (Fig. 9.25a), minute microspherocytes or microvesicles containing haemoglobin being present, and sometimes also dumb-bell-shaped red cells.

In a delayed transfusion reaction spherocytosis is also marked but as only the donor cells are affected the film is dimorphic (see Fig. 3.79). The direct antiglobulin test is positive. When blood group O plasma containing anti-A antibodies in high titre is transfused into a group A subject spherocytosis is generalized and may persist for weeks.[37] Marked spherocytosis has also been reported in hypophosphataemia due to severe diabetic ketoacidosis;[100] as the mechanism is likely to be ATP depletion it is likely that the cells are actually spheroechinocytes rather than spherocytes.

Normal neonates have moderate numbers of spherocytes but when large numbers are present a diagnosis of ABO haemolytic diseases of the newborn is suggested (Fig. 9.25b), a diagnosis which is confirmed by a positive direct antiglobulin test and the finding of a high titre IgG anti-A, or less often anti-B, in the maternal serum. Erythrophagocytosis of the antibody-coated cells is common. The degree of spherocytosis in Rhesus haemolytic disease of the newborn (Fig. 9.25c) is less; this diagnosis is confirmed by a positive direct antiglobulin test and by the finding of anti-D or another Rhesus antibody in the maternal serum which reacts with an antigen on the neonatal cells. Spherocytosis in the neonate may also be due to heredity spherocytosis, homozygous hereditary elliptocytosis or congenital pyropoikilocytosis (see page 283).

Small numbers of spherocytes are seen in many conditions (see Fig. 3.81). In hyposplenism and microangiopathic haemolytic anaemia detection of the associated features indicates the aetiology. In an immediate transfusion reaction most of the incompatible cells are destroyed rapidly so that, in contrast to a delayed transfusion reaction, only small numbers of spherocytes are seen. Diagnosis is apparent from the clinical setting and is confirmed by failure of the Hb to rise appropriately, and serological demonstration of incompatibility. During attacks of paroxysmal cold haemoglobinuria some

erythrophagocytosis may be present in addition to small numbers of spherocytes; associated haematological features are leucopenia due to neutropenia, eosinopenia and monocytopenia together with a lesser degree of lymphopenia.[52] Diagnosis is confirmed by demonstration of the Donath–Landsteiner antibody, which causes haemolysis on rewarming a previously chilled specimen. In chronic cold haemagglutinin disease and acute cold haemolytic anaemia due to a cold agglutinin small numbers of spherocytes may be present (Fig. 9.25d); these diagnoses are usually readily

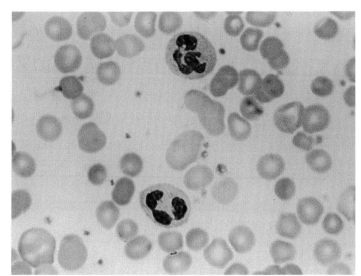

Fig. 9.24
(a) The blood film of a patient with autoimmune haemolytic anaemia showing spherocytes[1] and polychromatic macrocytes[2].

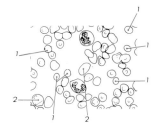

(b) A blood film taken during haemodialysis from a patient with chronic renal failure who had a positive antiglobulin test but no overt haemolysis; it shows erythrophagocytosis by monocytes.

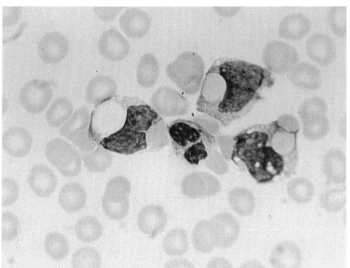

apparent because of the artefactual macrocytosis on automated blood counts (page 132) and the agglutination of red cells which is present unless the film is made from warm blood (Fig. 9.25e, and see also Fig. 3.7); confirmation is by demonstrating the presence of complement on the red cells and a cold antibody in high titre or with a high thermal amplitude in the serum.

ELLIPTOCYTOSIS, OVALOCYTOSIS AND PYROPOIKILOCYTOSIS

The presence of more than 25 percent of elliptocytes or ovalocytes has been suggested as a diagnostic criterion for the diagnosis of elliptocytosis or ovalocytosis; as discussed on page 72 the terms elliptocyte and ovalocyte have been used inconsistently in the haematological literature. When a high percentage of cells are elliptical or oval the diagnosis of hereditary elliptocytosis is very probable. Rare patients with developing myelofibrosis have had similar numbers of elliptocytes.[30] Confirmation is by demonstrating the familial nature of the condition or, in the research laboratory, by biochemical investigation of the red cell membrane.

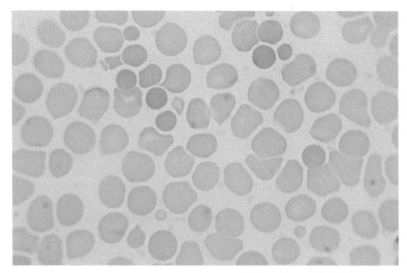

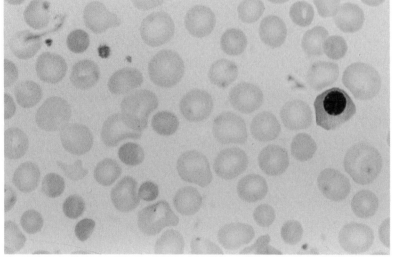

Fig. 9.25 Blood films showing other causes of spherocytosis: **(a)** spherocytosis due to severe burns; microspherocytes, some of which are minute, are present;

(b) blood film of a baby with ABO haemolytic disease of the newborn showing marked spherocytosis and an NRBC;

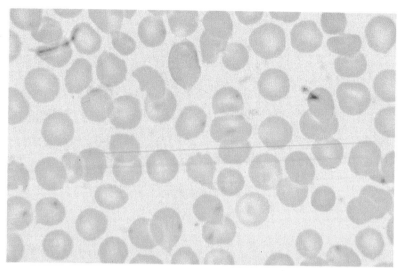

(c) *blood film of a baby with Rhesus haemolytic disease of the newborn showing that the degree of spherocytosis is much less than that which is seen in ABO haemolytic disease of the newborn;*

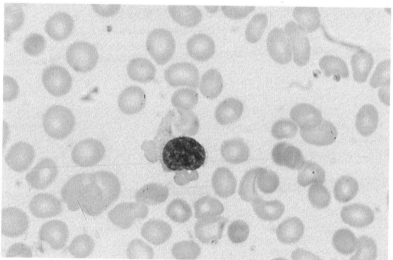

(d) *blood film of a patient with infectious mononucleosis who had acute haemolytic anaemia due to an anti-i cold antibody; the film shows spherocytes, an atypical lymphocyte and a very small red cell agglutinate;*

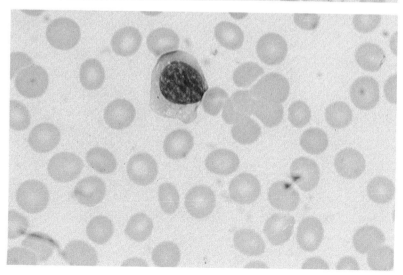

(e) *another area of the same film a shown in (d) showing an atypical lymphocyte and a larger red cell agglutinate.*

Hereditary elliptocytosis (and ovalocytosis)

A variety of genetic and biochemical abnormalities underlie hereditary elliptocytosis (Fig. 9.26). Inheritance is usually autosomal dominant with severe disease occurring in the occasional homozygotes. The biochemical defect resides either in the red cell membrane protein 4.1 or in the α or the β chain of the spectrin molecule.

The characteristic cell shape varies between kindreds, and to a very considerable extent within kindreds. Within a kindred there is a correlation between the degree of abnormality of cell shape and the severity of haemolysis. There is considerably less correlation between these two factors if different kindreds are considered. Some kindreds with primarily ovalocytes have overt haemolysis while others with marked elliptocytosis do not. However the presence of other poikilocytes including some spherocytes and fragments does correlate with the severity of haemolysis. Within the one kindred the degree of morphological abnormality and the severity of the haemolysis correlate but the same qualitative biochemical defect (for example a specific abnormality of the α chain of spectrin) may be found in an asymptomatic carrier with less than 2 percent elliptocytes, in a subject with hereditary elliptocytosis with or without haemolysis, and in a subject with hereditary pyropoikilocytosis (see below).[21] Similarly heterozygotes for a lack of the red cell membrane protein 4.1 may have morphologically normal red cells or few or numerous elliptocytes.[70,106]

Hereditary elliptocytosis therefore manifests itself either as a morphological abnormality without haemolysis or as elliptocytosis with haemolysis which is either minimal and compensated, more severe but intermittent, or chronic and severe. In the majority of cases there is either mild, well-compensated haemolysis or no shortening of red cell life span so that elliptocytosis is the only feature observed. In a small minority there is polychromasia or even anaemia.

The rare homozygotes for hereditary elliptocytosis are likely to have marked morphological abnormality and overt haemolysis; the blood film may show spherocytes, fragments, microelliptocytes, and irregularly contracted cells in addition to elliptocytes.[21,81,106] They are usually transfusion dependent.

In general, subjects with hereditary elliptocytosis have very few elliptocytes at birth. However some who, in later life, appear to have typical hereditary elliptocytosis with only mild haemolysis may, in the neonatal period, have severe haemolysis and a blood film showing not only some elliptocytes but also fragments, irregularly contracted cells and microcytes.[3,21] Some cases with haemolysis in the neonatal period have, at that stage, morphological features very similar to those of hereditary pyropoikilocytes (see below).

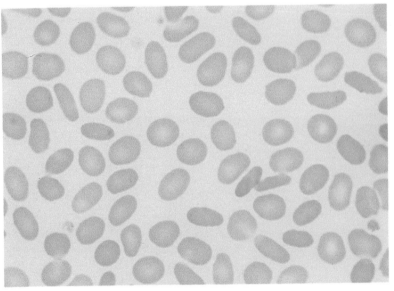

Fig. 9.26 *The blood film of a patient with hereditary elliptocytosis showing elliptocytes and ovalocytes; the patient had a normal haemoglobin concentration and reticulocyte count.*

Patients with hereditary elliptocytosis who require splenectomy may thereafter have marked poikilocytosis, in addition to the usual postsplenectomy features; the poikilocytes include prominent spherocytes, microelliptocytes and fragments.

Hereditary pyropoikilocytosis

Hereditary pyropoikilocytosis is a congenital haemolytic anaemia with autosomal recessive inheritance which is characterized by a bizarre blood film with gross anisocytosis and poikilocytosis including microspherocytes, micropoikilocytes and cells with bud-like projections;[116] there are few elliptocytes. The condition is defined by fragmentation of red cells on *in vitro* heating which occurs at a lower than normal temperature. This feature is indicated in the name 'pyropoikilocytosis'. Hereditary elliptocytosis manifests a similar but lesser abnormality on *in vitro* heating. Hereditary pyropoikilocytosis, like hereditary elliptocytosis, can be due to a defect in the association of spectrin dimers to form spectrin tetramers. It has been found that at least in some cases one parent of an affected case has typical hereditary elliptocytosis with an abnormal spectrin molecule while the other has morphologically normal red cells. It seems that, in these families, hereditary pyropoikilocytosis is due to double heterozygosity for an α spectrin mutant and another abnormality which is silent in the simple heterozygotes.[21,67] In other families neither parent has had elliptocytosis; these cases may be due to homozygosity or double heterozygosity for recessive genes.

South-east Asian ovalocytosis

South-east Asian ovalocytosis is a distinct form of inherited ovalocytic disorder which has also been designated hereditary ovalocytosis of Melanesians and stomatocytic elliptocytosis. It has been described in Melanesia, Papua and New Guinea, Indonesia, the Philippines and in Malaysian aboriginals. Inheritance is autosomal recessive. In some of the affected ethnic groups as many as 20–30 percent of the population are homozygotes.

The morphological features observed in the peripheral blood film are pathognomonic (Fig. 9.27). Red cells are oval rather than elliptical. A small number of macro-ovalocytes, approximately twice the size of normal red cells, are present. Stomatocytes are seen, but in addition to typical stomatocytes there are ovalocytes with a longitudinal stoma and cells with two areas of central pallor, or with a Y-shaped or V-shaped area of central pallor. In contrast to hereditary elliptocytosis, the condition is readily detectable at birth. Subjects with South-east Asian ovalocytosis usually have no anaemia or polychromasia. The blood film is so distinctive that nothing beyond its examination is required for confirmation of the diagnosis. Subjects with this condition have reduced expression of many red cell antigens.

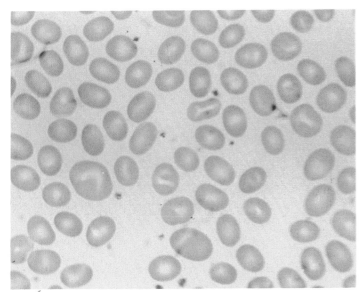

Fig. 9.27 *The blood film of a patient with South-east Asian ovalocytosis showing several macro-ovalocytes one of which has a Y-shaped stoma[1] and the other an eccentric transverse stoma[2]; many of the smaller cells are either stomatocytes[3], ovalocytes[4] or stomato-ovalocytes[5].*

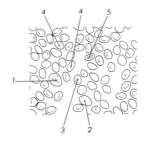

SPICULATED CELLS

The terminology applied to spiculated cells is discussed on page 73. Schistocytes and keratocytes have only a few spicules and are of distinctive appearance. Both are formed as a result of mechanical damage to cells and their significance is similar. They are discussed below. Echinocytes and acanthocytes have more numerous spicules. They may resemble each other but are readily distinguished from fragments and keratocytes.

Echinocytes and acanthocytes

When a film shows spiculated cells other than fragments and keratocytes it is first necessary to determine whether they are echinocytes or acanthocytes since the possible aetiologies differ. By far the commonest cause of spiculated cells is an echinocytic change due to ageing of the blood sample, often referred to as red cell crenation. The blood film should therefore be examined for other abnormalities suggesting prolonged storage (see page 86). It is preferable that the presence of spiculated cells be confirmed on a blood film prepared from a freshly drawn non-anticoagulated blood specimen.

The medical history may suggest the reason for the presence of spiculated cells, as when echinocytes occur following blood transfusion (see Fig. 3.84) or when acanthocytes occur in association with abetalipoproteinaemia, degenerative neurological disease, liver disease (Fig. 9.28a), hypothyroidism, anorexia nervosa (see Fig. 3.85) or hyposplenism. The blood film should be examined for abnormal features which may suggest any of these diagnoses, for example the macrocytosis which can occur in hypothyroidism or the mild pancytopenia of anorexia nervosa. Hyposplenism may sometimes cause acanthocytosis as the dominant feature (Fig. 9.28b) so the other features of hyposplenism should be carefully sought. Acanthocytes were a feature of one family with a variant of hereditary spherocytosis.[6] If the cause of acanthocytosis is not apparent thyroid function tests and studies of serum lipids can be helpful.

Schistocytes and microangiopathic haemolytic anaemia

Schistocytes or fragments are produced when cells are torn in pieces by mechanical damage or by contact with fibrin strands, tumour cells, an abnormal blood vessel wall or a foreign surface. Schistocytes take a variety of forms including small, angular fragments and microspherocytes (see page 76); keratocytes, which are larger with paired spicules, have a similar significance to schistocytes. When appreciable numbers of fragments occur in association with anaemia, reticulocytosis and signs of haemolysis in the term microangiopathic haemolytic anaemia (Fig. 9.29a) may be used. Similar pathological changes in the red cells can occur when cells are damaged by turbulent flow around defective prosthetic valves (mechanical haemolytic anaemia) (Fig. 9.29b, c) or can be consequent on lesions in large vessels. Some of the causes of red cell fragmentation are shown in Fig. 9.30. Patients with fragments commonly also have some degree of thrombocytopenia, due to consumption of platelets, consequent on the same pathological process. Platelets tend to be large. If there is marked thrombocytopenia the diagnosis of thrombotic thrombocytopenic purpura should be considered. It is important for the laboratory to appreciate that an anaemia is microangiopathic in nature so that a correct diagnosis can be made and appropriate treatment can be given for those conditions where treatment is available (for example thrombotic thrombocytopenic purpura). Correct diagnosis also allows the avoidance of platelet transfusion which may be harmful in patients with thrombotic thrombocytopenic purpura.[44]

The blood film does not usually give any indication of the nature of the underlying disease but the differential diagnosis can be narrowed if other clinical features are considered together with the peripheral blood findings. Many of the conditions listed in Fig. 9.30 cause both microangiopathic haemolytic anaemia and renal failure. This combination constitutes the haemolytic–uraemic syndrome, a syndrome with multiple causes but which, in its most characteristic form, follows infection by either *Shigella dysenteriae* or verotoxin-secreting strains of *Escherichia coli*.[56] In thrombotic thrombocytopenic purpura, renal failure is a less consistent feature, but thrombocytopenia is present together with signs or symptoms suggestive of thrombotic lesions in other tissues, as well as in the kidneys; confirmation of the diagnosis requires histological demonstration of thrombi in small vessels. Thrombotic thrombocytopenic purpura is also a syndrome with multiple causes, and there is some overlap between this condition and haemolytic uraemic syndrome. When microangiopathic haemolytic anaemia occurs without renal failure and in the presence of normal blood pressure metastatic malignant disease is very likely; anaemia of this type is sometimes the presenting feature of metastatic malignancy and in this circumstance leucoerythroblastic features can also be present.

When there is chronic intravascular haemolysis due to red cell fragmentation, haptoglobin becomes saturated by the haemoglobin which is released from the red cells and free haemoglobin (containing iron) is then lost in the urine; iron deficiency may be the consequence (Fig. 9.29c). The iron deficiency then worsens the anaemia which in turn leads to a hyperdynamic circulation; in conditions such as defective prosthetic valves this causes further aggravation of the anaemia. It is therefore important to note the additional blood film features suggesting iron deficiency.

Fragments may also be seen as one feature of an abnormal blood film in patients with intrinsically defective red cells as in: pyropoikilocytosis; homozygotes for heredity elliptocytosis or other hereditary elliptocytosis with overt haemolysis; haemolytic anaemia due to reduction of high-affinity binding sites for ankyrin;[2] thalassaemia major; haemoglobin H disease and various dyserythropoietic anaemias. In some of these patients the abnormal red cells may be damaged and undergo fragmentation as they are squeezed through the sinusoids of the spleen.

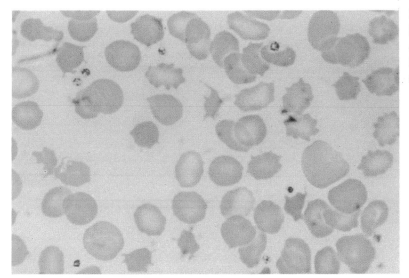

Fig. 9.28
(a) A blood film showing acanthocytosis due to fulminant hepatic failure of unknown aetiology.

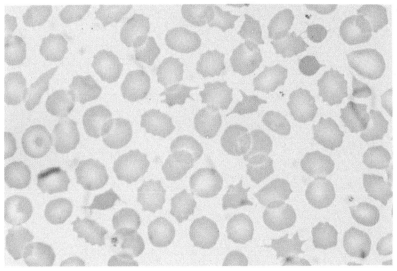

(b) The blood film of a subject who was previously haematologically normal but who has had a splenectomy, showing unusually numerous acanthocytes. There are also crenated cells, fragments and one target cell.

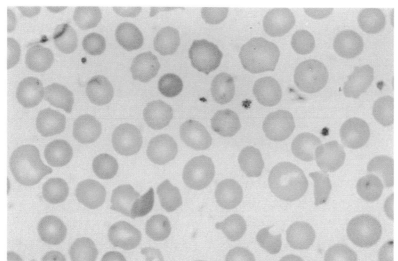

Fig. 9.29
(a) The blood film from an adult with the haemolytic uraemic syndrome showing fragments, several spherocytes and several polychromatic macrocytes.

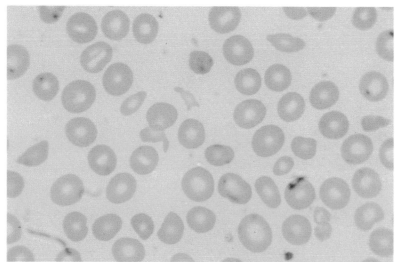

(b) The blood film of a patient with mechanical haemolytic anaemia due to a defective prosthetic mitral valve showing numerous fragments.

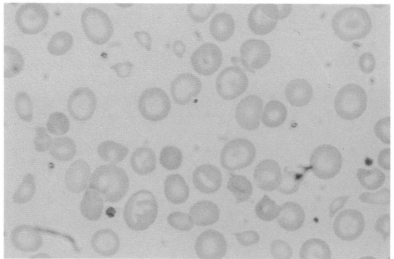

(c) The blood film of a patient with iron deficiency due to mechanical haemolysis from d defective prosthetic valve showing hypochromia and microcytosis in addition to fragments; the patient also had haemoglobin C trait and one target cell is shown.

SOME CAUSES OF RED CELL FRAGMENTATION

Microangiopathic haemolytic anaemia

epidemic or sporadic haemolytic uraemic syndrome (may follow infection by *Shigella* or toxin-producing *E. coli*)

thrombotic thrombocytopenic purpura

haemolytic uraemic syndrome or thrombocytopenic purpura-like illnesses following vaccination (influenza, polio, measles, smallpox, triple antigen or TAB vaccination)[15] or bacterial, viral, rickettsial or fungal infection[56,73,85,108]

familial haemolytic uraemic syndrome

pregnancy-associated thrombotic thrombocytopenic purpura and haemolytic uraemic syndrome associated with pregnancy, oral contraceptive intake or the post-partum state

other pathological processes involving the kidney (with or without other vascular disease)

    pregnancy associated hypertension (toxaemia of pregnancy)
    malignant hypertension
    renal cortical necrosis
    microscopic polyarteritis nodosa
    acute glomerulonephritis
    systemic lupus erythematosus with renal involvement
    systemic sclerosis (scleroderma) involving the kidney[89]
    Wegener's granulomatosis
    irradiation of the kidney
    rejection of a transplanted kidney

diabetic angiopathy[16]

systemic amyloidosis

toxicity of mitomycin C, bleomycin, other chemotherapeutic agents, cyclosporin A, penicillin and penicillamine[56]

disseminated intravascular coagulation (including DIC associated with malignant disease, aortic aneurysm and renal vein thrombosis)

therapeutic defibrination with Arvin (occasionally)

disseminated carcinoma (particularly mucin-secreting adenocarcinoma, particularly carcinoma of the stomach)

congenital microangiopathic haemolytic anaemia with thrombocytopenia[92,110]

thymoma (1 case)[82]

bee sting[56]

thrombotic microangiopathy following bone marrow transplantation

thrombotic microangiopathy following arteriography[39]

associated with vascular malformations or other vascular lesions

haemangioma

haemangioendothelioma of the liver

haemangioendotheliosarcoma

plexiform lesions of pulmonary hypertension

plexiform pulmonary lesions in cirrhosis[76]

giant cell arteritis[117]

mechanical fragmentation

prosthetic aortic valves (aortic more than mitral, much more common when there is regurgitation around a valve)

prosthetic patches

homograft valves (less likely than with prosthetic valves)

fascia lata autograft valves (less likely than with prosthetic valves)

xenograft valves (porcine) (less likely than with prosthetic valves)

severe aortic stenosis (very uncommon)

severe mitral valve disease and following valvuloplasty for mitral valve disease (rare)

aortic coarctation (rare)

Fig. 9.30 *Some of the causes of red cell fragmentation.*

STOMATOCYTOSIS

Occasional stomatocytes are seen in the blood films of healthy subjects. Stomatocytosis (see Fig. 3.91) refers to an increase in the number of stomatocytic cells. The only common cause of stomatocytosis is alcohol excess and alcoholic liver disease. The frequent coexistence of macrocytosis is helpful in suggesting this diagnosis. Triconcave cells can also be present, particularly in those with very advanced liver disease.[114]

Stomatocytes have been associated with a great variety of clinical conditions[24,68] but an aetiological connection has not been established. Phenothiazines can cause a stomatocytic change *in vitro*; it appears likely that their administration to patients can also cause stomatocytosis since an association has been observed.[24]

Hereditary stomatocytosis, the condition in which stomatocytes were first described,[60] is one of the less common causes of this morphological abnormality. The term hereditary stomatocytosis covers a heterogeneous group of conditions in which the morphological abnormality is associated with a chronic haemolytic state of variable severity. The inheritance is usually autosomal dominant. The haemolysis may be compensated or there may be an anaemia which is mild, moderate or severe. The majority of such patients have an abnormality of cation flux and an increase of intracellular sodium. They have been divided into two main groups. In the overhydrated variety the MCV is increased and the MCHC is decreased; the osmotic fragility is increased.[115] In the dehydrated variety[68] the MCV is decreased and the MCHC is increased; the osmotic fragility is decreased, although there may be a fragile tail of cells. In the latter variety the stained blood film usually shows target cells and occasional irregularly contracted cells, echinocytes, and cells with haemoglobin concentrated to the periphery or to one or two edges of the cell. Stomatocytes are infrequent; more numerous stomatocytes are seen on a wet preparation. Because of the paucity of stomatocytes in the stained blood film in the dehydrated variant of 'hereditary stomatocytosis' alternative designations of 'hereditary xerocytosis' and 'dessicytosis' have been suggested, together with 'hydrocytosis' for the overhydrated variant. In addition to these two groups Rhesus null cells are stomatocytic. Two patients have also been described in whom haemolytic anaemia and stomatocytosis were associated with mild thrombocytopenia; in one of these cases the platelets were noted to be large and investigation of the red cells did not disclose any abnormality of membrane lipids or cation flux.[104] A quite frequent occurrence of stomatocytosis in association with large platelets has been described in subjects of Mediterranean (Greek and Italian) origin in Australia;[50] strangely, stomatocytosis does not appear at all common in subjects of similar ethnic origin in the UK.

Stomatocytosis occurs in South-east Asian ovalocytosis; the other distinctive morphological features (see page 283) make this an easy diagnosis to make from the blood film.

The occurrence of stomatocytosis may be a useful indication of alcohol excess or liver disease. If this possibility has been excluded it is usually only useful to investigate stomatocytosis if there is a likelihood of haemolysis as evidenced by reticulocytosis with or without anaemia and splenomegaly. Investigations then indicated are Rhesus typing and studies of osmotic fragility and red cell cation content and flux.

IRREGULARLY CONTRACTED CELLS AND G6PD DEFICIENCY

Irregularly contracted cells (see page 79) occur in several unrelated conditions. The commonest causes are administration of oxidant drugs, haemolytic episodes in glucose-6-phosphate dehydrogenase (G6PD) deficiency and haemoglobin C disease. The morphological features of haemoglobin C disease, with coexistence of target cells and irregularly contracted cells, are distinctive and are described above (see page 271)

Exposure to oxidant drugs and chemicals

When oxidant drugs are administered in sufficient dosage to subjects who were previously haematologically normal, chronic haemolysis occurs and some patients become anaemic. The blood film shows macrocytosis, polychromasia and irregularly contracted cells (Fig. 9.31a). Occasional 'bite cells' (see below) and cells with retracted haemoglobin are seen. A Heinz body preparation may show occasional Heinz bodies, but if the spleen is functioning normally they are often not found. Haemolysis of this type was previously common with phenacetin but the drugs now most often incriminated are dapsone and sulphasalazine. A similar type of haemolysis can occur with abuse of volatile nitrites.[12]

With a very severe oxidant stress, for example exposure to poisons such as lysol, acute haemolysis can occur even in those whose red cells are metabolically normal. The morphological features are the same as those seen in acute episodes of haemolysis in patients with G6PD deficiency. The term 'Heinz body haemolytic anaemia' has been used.

G6PD deficiency

In subjects who are deficient in G6PD acute haemolysis can follow infection or exposure to fava beans, naphthalene or oxidant drugs. Because the haemolysis is acute, polychromasia and macrocytosis are not initally seen. Irregularly contracted cells are seen together with cells in which the haemoglobin has retracted away from the edge of the cell (see Fig. 9.31b, c). Sometimes half of the cell appears empty; these cells have been called hemi-ghosts (Fig. 9.31b). Rarely a few complete ghosts are detectable (Fig. 9.31b) 'Bite cells' may also be noted; these are cells from which a 'bite' appears to have been taken (Fig. 9.31c); they are thought to be formed when the spleen removes a Heinz body from a cell. In patients with very acute haemolysis not all Heinz bodies are removed so that a Heinz body preparation is positive and in the Romanowsky-stained blood film a protrusion may be seen at the margin of the cell (Fig. 9.31b). Features of hyposplenism can appear at the height of the

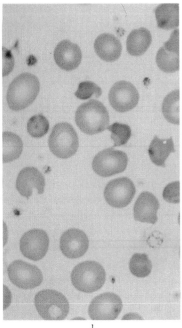

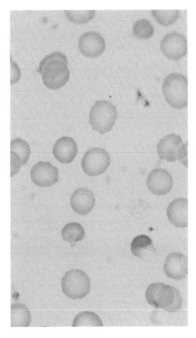

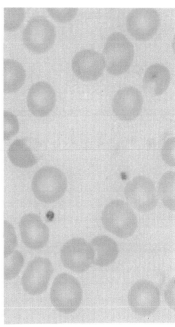

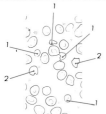

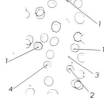

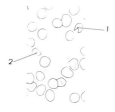

Fig. 9.31 (a) *The blood film of a patient taking dapsone for a skin condition showing macrocytosis, irregularly contracted cells[1] and several bite cells[2].*

(b) *The blood film of a Black child with deficiency of G6PD who had suffered an episode of acute haemolysis. The film shows anaemia, irregularly contracted cells[1], a hemighost[2], a complete ghost[3] and a cell with a protrusion attributable to a Heinz body[4]; the Heinz body preparation was positive.*

(c) *The blood film of a patient with acute haemolysis associated with G6PD deficiency showing a bite cell[1], and a cell with haemoglobin retracted from the cell margin[2].*

haemolytic episode as a consequence of reticulo-endothelial overload.

Some variants of G6PD are associated with a chronic haemolytic anaemia with nonspecific morphological features such as anisocytosis, poikilocytosis, macrocytosis and basophilic stippling; G6PD deficiency therefore enters into the differential diagnosis of congenital nonspherocytic haemolytic anaemia (see below) as well as the differential diagnosis of irregularly contracted cells.

Other causes of irregularly contracted cells

Other less common causes of appreciable numbers of irregularly contracted cells are other defects of the red cell pentose phosphate shunt and unstable haemoglobins. Other defects of the pentose phosphate shunt will produce the same blood film findings as are seen in G6PD deficiency. Unstable haemoglobins may be associated either with episodic haemolysis following infection or oxidant drug exposure, in which case irregularly contracted cells are the major feature, or with chronic haemolysis in which some irregularly contracted cells are seen together with macrocytosis and polychromasia (see Fig 9.22).

Some but not all patients with acute haemolysis in association with Wilson's disease (see page 292) have shown irregularly contracted cells, possibly attributable to an oxidant action of free copper.[47]

Small numbers of irregularly contracted cells are sometimes seen in β-thalassaemia trait, haemoglobin E disease and trait, haemoglobin H disease, the dehydrated variant of hereditary stomatocytosis and congenital dyserythropoietic anaemia.

OTHER HAEMOLYTIC ANAEMIAS
Other congenital haemolytic anaemias

I have already discussed the morphological features of hereditary spherocytosis (page 276), hereditary elliptocytosis (page 282), hereditary pyropoikilocytosis (page 283) hereditary stomatocytosis (page 288) and glucose-6-phosphate deficiency and other defects of the red cell pentose shunt pathway (page 289). Several other congenital haemolytic anaemias have morphology which is sufficiently distinctive that the diagnosis can be suspected from the blood film. This is so for some cases of pyrimidine 5' nucleotidase deficiency in which basophilic stippling is very prominent and for the very rare congenital haemolytic anaemia consequent on reduction of high-affinity binding sites for ankyrin which has microcytosis and red cell fragmentation in addition

to marked anisocytosis and poikilocytosis.[2] The basophilic stippling of pyrimidine 5' nucleotidase deficiency is best seen in blood films made from heparinized or native blood rather than EDTA-anticoagulated blood.[7]

Other congenital haemolytic anaemias have less distinctive morphological features. They have been grouped together under the general heading of congenital, nonspherocytic haemolytic anaemias, the majority being due to a deficiency of one of the enzymes of the glycolytic pathway. The commonest is pyruvate kinase deficiency. They have in common macrocytosis, polychromasia, and an elevated reticulocyte count; if haemolysis is severe there may be NRBC (Fig. 9.32). Minor morphological abnormalities such as anisocytosis, poikilocytosis and some basophilic stippling are not uncommon. A small number of dense spiculated cells may be present; it has been postulated that these are cells which have become depleted of ATP and are at the end of their lifespan. Spiculated cells which most closely resemble abnormal echinocytes have been noted to be very frequent postsplenectomy in some cases of pyruvate kinase deficiency[59] (Fig. 9.32b), but this finding has not been consistent. In pyruvate kinase deficiency there may be improvement of the haemolysis after splenectomy but with the reticulocyte percentage being paradoxically higher; the probable explanation is that prior to splenectomy some highly defective newly produced cells were removed rapidly by the spleen but in its absence are surviving. Patients with congenital nonspherocytic haemolytic anaemia sometimes have leucopenia, probably as a consequence of hypersplenism. Occasional cases of congenital haemolytic anaemia due to abnormality of the glycolytic pathway have had more marked morphological abnormality. For example, one family with hexokinase deficiency showed spherocytes, ovalocytes, cells resembling sickle cells, and cells with a polar haemoglobin distribution.[72]

Certain uncommon variants of glucose-6-phosphate dehydrogenase have the clinical picture of congenital nonspherocytic haemolytic anaemia, rather than the more usual episodic haemolysis in association with infection or oxidant drugs.

Congenital erythropoietic porphyria also causes chronic haemolysis with or without a haemolytic anaemia, with there being no specific morphological features on a Romanowsky-stained blood film. When this diagnosis is suspected from the striking clinical features it can be confirmed by examination of the peripheral blood under ultraviolet light; a proportion of the erythrocytes and the nuclei of circulating erythroblasts[47] exhibit fluorescence.

Congenital haemolytic anaemia should be suspected, and relevant investigations should be performed, not only when there is a marked morphological abnormality but also when there is anaemia with macrocytosis and a high reticulocyte count, particularly when these features are detected early in life.

Other acquired haemolytic anaemias

I have already discussed chronic cold haemagglutinin disease (page 242), warm autoimmune haemolytic anaemia and other acquired causes of spherocytosis (page 278), oxidant damage to red cells (page 288) and microangiopathic haemolytic anaemia and other fragmentation syndromes (page 284). In other acquired haemolytic anaemias the morphology is less distinctive. In acute haemolytic anaemias mediated by a cold agglutinin, such as that occurring during *Mycoplasma* infection or less often during infectious mononucleosis, the blood film is likely to show red cell agglutinates and a few spherocytes with subsequently the development of polychromasia. Erythrophagocytosis may be observed. The presence of atypical lympocytes and a cold agglutinin mediated haemolytic anaemia is very likely to be due to infectious mononucleosis (see Fig. 9.25d, e).

In paroxysmal cold haemoglobinuria, which now most often is transient and follows measles and other viral infections, small numbers of spherocytes may be seen during the acute attack and erythrophagocytosis may occur.

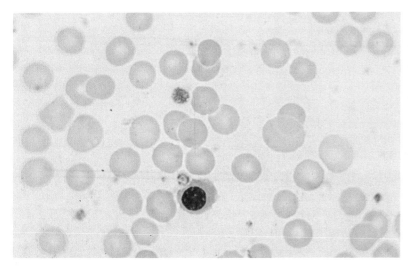

Fig. 9.32

(a) *The blood film of a patient with pyruvate kinase deficiency showing anisocytosis, macrocytosis, polychromasia and an NRBC.*

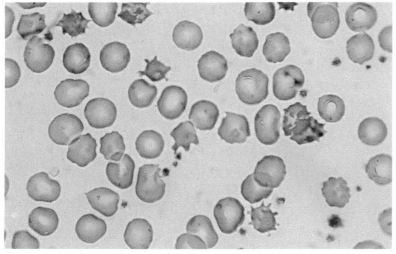

(b) *The blood film of a patient with pyruvate kinase deficiency who has been splenectomized, showing macrocytosis and abnormal spiculated cells.*

In acute immune haemolytic anaemia induced by drugs small numbers of spherocytes are seen. Rarely agglutinates are seen.

Haemolysis induced by industrial exposure to arsine gas is characterized by prominent red cell ghosts.

Certain acquired haemolytic anaemias produce no distinctive morphological abnormality. This is often so of the acute haemolytic anaemia due to Wilson's disease. This is an important diagnosis to make since haemolysis may be the presenting feature of this disease which is fatal if left untreated; Wilson's disease can be readily diagnosed by clinical features and biochemical tests as long as the diagnosis is considered. The condition should therefore always be considered when there is acute unexplained haemolysis in a young person.

There are also rarely any specific features in those with chronic or intermittent haemolysis due to severe exercise or physical trauma ('march haemoglobinuria' or haemolysis due to jogging on hard surfaces or karate or drumming with the hands). These conditions should be sought for by specific interrogation when there is mild intravascular haemolysis in an apparently fit, usually young, person.

Paroxysmal nocturnal haemoglobinuria may have associated leucopenia or thrombocytopenia but has no characteristic red cell features; specific investigations for this condition should be carried out when there is an acquired haemolytic anaemia for which no cause is readily apparent.

CONGENITAL DYSERYTHROPOIETIC ANAEMIA

Congenital dyserythropoietic anaemias characteristically cause a mild to moderate anaemia with marked poikilocytosis and a normal absolute reticulocyte count. In a minority of cases the anaemia is severe. Three types of congenital dyserythropoietic anaemia (CDA) have been well characterized (Fig. 9.33). Diagnosis requires examination of the bone marrow and, in the case of type II CDA, the demonstration of a positive acidified-serum lysis test; the diagnosis can, however, be suspected from the peripheral blood features (Figs 9.33 and 9.34).

Fig. 9.33 *The peripheral blood features of the congenital dyserythropoietic anaemias.*

INHERITANCE PATTERN AND MORPHOLOGICAL FEATURES IN THE CONGENITAL DYSERYTHROPOIETIC ANAEMIAS			
Type	Inheritance	Red cell size	Other morphological features
type I	autosomal recessive	macrocytic	oval macrocytes, marked anisocytosis, marked poikilocytosis, basophilic stippling, irregularly contracted cells, polychromasia
type II (Hempas)*	autosomal recessive	normocytic	moderate anisocytosis, moderate poikilocytosis including 'pincer cells'[64] and irregularly contracted cells, some NRBC polychromasia
type III	autosomal dominant	normocytic or slightly macrocytic	marked anisocytosis, marked poikilocytosis including fragments and irregularly contracted cells, basophilic stippling, polychromasia

*Hempas = hereditary erythroid multinuclearity with positive acidified-serum lysis test.

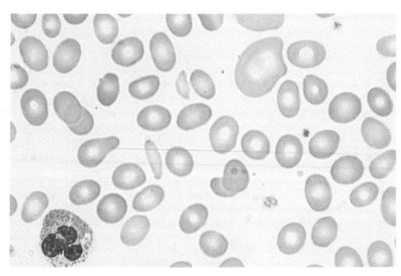

Fig. 9.34 *Blood films of patients with congenital dyserythropoietic anaemias:*
(a) *CDA type I showing anisocytosis, macrocytosis, and poikilocytosis, with the poikilocytes including fragments and tear drop cells;*

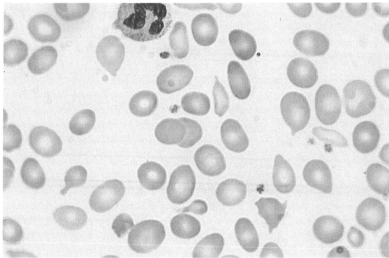

(b, c) *CDA type III showing anisocytes and poikilocytosis.*

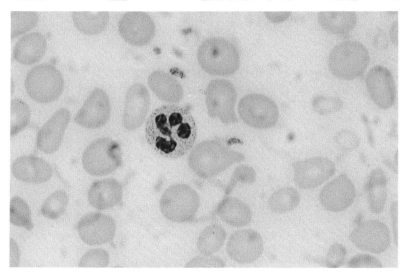

A number of cases have been reported which do not appear to belong to the three well recognized categories. In one family the condition resembled CDA type I but the inheritance appeared to be autosomal dominant rather than autosomal recessive.[90] Another family had marked microcysosis (due to sideroblastic erythropoiesis) together with marked anisocytosis and poikilocytosis.[14] Some cases have had circulating NRBC which have become very numerous after splenectomy.[11]

HYPOSPLENISM

Hyposplenism means that splenic function is absent or reduced. The haematological features which allow this diagnosis to be made are discussed on page 84. The most reliable blood film indication of reduced spleen function is the presence of Howell–Jolly bodies; target cells, acanthocytes and thrombocytosis have multiple causes but Howell–Jolly bodies are very rarely seen except in hyposplenic subjects. The detection of hyposplenism by the laboratory is of considerable importance. Firstly, it may be of diagnostic importance. In coeliac disease or amyloidosis, for example, this may be the finding which first raises suspicion of the correct diagnosis. In one series of patients six cases of coeliac disease were diagnosed as a result of investigating 13 patients who were noted to be hyposplenic.[17] Secondly, the finding is of therapeutic importance, since subjects with reduced splenic function are at risk of infection; when a patient is found to be hyposplenic there is an indication for prophylactic penicillin if a child and for vaccination with pneumococcal antigens if an adult. Quite often patients are noted to be hyposplenic when neither they nor their medical attendants were aware that the spleen had been removed during prior surgery. Thirdly, the appreciation of the cause of the haematological abnormalities may save needless investigation, for example in those patients where the most striking abnormality is the presence of a lymphocytosis or of target cells or acanthocytes. Some of the causes of hyposplenism are shown in Fig. 9.35.

Occasionally the blood film may provide evidence of the cause of the hyposplenism. This is so in sickle cell disease, sickle cell/haemoglobin C disease, essential thrombocythaemia (when the elevation of the platelet count is much more than in hyposplenism from other causes), and in some patients in whom the spleen is infiltrated by leukaemic cells or by lymphoma. If the distinctive features suggesting the coexistence of megaloblastic anaemia and hyposplenism (see Fig. 9.13) are

seen the diagnosis of coeliac disease with secondary folic acid deficiency is among the conditions which should be suspected (see page 266). When the patient has had a splenectomy for a haematological disease the underlying disease may also be revealed by the blood film. For example, a patient with autoimmune thrombocytopenic purpura may have persisting thrombocytopenia or the platelets may be larger than those usually seen postsplenectomy, indicating that platelet turnover is increased. A patient who has been splenectomized for hereditary spherocytosis will have large numbers of spheroacanthocytes and will lack the usual target cells, whereas some patients who have been splenectomized for pyruvate kinase deficiency have prominent spiculated cells.

In febrile hyposplenic subjects it is useful to examine the blood film specifically for malarial parasites and for *Babesiae* (in the relevant geographic areas) and for bacteria within white blood cells (see pages 46 and 191).

The failure to detect the features of hyposplenism may be significant in a patient who is known to have had a splenectomy. Small fragments of spleen may have been seeded within the peritoneal cavity and may have undergone hyperplasia, or a splenunculus may have enlarged. If a patient who has had a splenectomy for autoimmune thrombocytopenic purpura has had regrowth of splenic tissue the disease may relapse and may respond again if the residual tissue is removed. In a relapsed patient the absence of the expected morphological features is an indication to investigate for residual splenic tissue. However the demonstration of the blood film features of hyposplenism, although making it less likely that there is appreciable residual functioning spleen, does not exclude this possibility since quite a small amount of splenic tissue may be sufficient to cause disease relapse.

ANAEMIA WITH NORMOCYTIC NORMOCHROMIC RED CELLS

Normocytic normochromic anaemia can occur as part of a pancytopenia (see Fig. 8.62). Other conditions which can cause a normocytic, normochromic anaemia as the predominant or only haematological abnormality are shown in Fig. 9.36, together with associated features which, if present, may help in the differential diagnosis.

The commonest cause of a normocytic, normochromic anaemia is the anaemia of chronic disease, associated with infection, inflammation or malignancy (see page 263).

If the cause of a normocytic, normochromic anaemia is not apparent, investigations which may be helpful include serum iron and transferrin levels, serum ferritin level, red cell folate and serum vitamin B_{12} assays and tests of hepatic, renal and thyroid function. In some patients a bone marrow aspiration and trephine biopsy may be necessary for diagnosis.

POLYCYTHAEMIA RUBRA VERA AND OTHER CAUSES OF POLYCYTHAEMIA

Polycythaemia means the presence of increased numbers of red cells. Conventionally the term is applied to patients who have a high haemoglobin concentration and a high PCV in addition to a high RBC. In true polycythaemia the total volume of red cells in the circulation is increased above what would be expected in a healthy person of the same age, sex, height and weight, whereas in relative or pseudopolycythaemia the total red cell volume is normal but the plasma volume is reduced. The two conditions cannot be distinguished on a blood film which in both cases shows a 'packed' film (Fig. 9.37) since the increased viscosity prevents the spreading of a thin film of blood. To determine whether a polycythaemia is true or relative requires measurement of total red cell and plasma volumes by isotopic dilution studies.

A high haemoglobin should be verified on a further blood specimen, preferably obtained without use of a tourniquet, to exclude dehydration during an acute illness or haemoconcentration during venesection.

Some of the causes of a true polycythaemia are shown in Fig. 9.38. True polycythaemia is further divided into polycythaemia rubra vera (also designated primary proliferative polycythaemia) which is a myeloproliferative disorder, and secondary polycythaemia, in which the bone marrow is responding to a physiological stimulus or to a non-haemopoietic disorder.

POLYCYTHAEMIA RUBRA VERA

Polycythaemia rubra vera (PRV) is a myeloproliferative disorder in which there is increased production of erythrocytes and often also of granulocytes and platelets. It is largely a disease of the middle-aged and elderly, although occasional cases are seen in younger adults and very rare cases in children. Common clinical features are those resulting from the hyperviscosity of the polycythaemic blood such as cerebrovascular accidents and peripheral gangrene, together with those indicative of the myeloproliferative disorder such as hepatomegaly, splenomegaly and itch. The designation idiopathic erythrocytosis has been used for patients who do not have any clear evidence of a myeloproliferative disorder but in whom no primary disease responsible for the polycythaemia can be found. It appears that some but probably not all of these patients actually do have early polycythaemia rubra vera.

SOME CAUSES OF HYPOSPLENISM

Physiological

neonatal period (particularly in premature babies), old age

Pathological

congenital absence or hypoplasia (can be associated with situs invertus and cardiac anomalies; can be hereditary;[53] has followed maternal coumarin intake, occurs in reticular agenesis)

congenital polysplenism[86]

splenectomy

splenic infarction (sickle cell anaemia, sickle cell/haemoglobin C disease and other sickling disorders; essential thrombocythaemia; polycythaemia;[58] following splenic torsion)

splenic atrophy (associated with coeliac disease, dermatitis herpetiformis, ulcerative colitis,[88] Crohn's disease,[88] tropical sprue,[22] autoimmune thyroid disease, systemic lupus erythematosus;[29] other autoimmune splenic atrophy;[111] graft-versus-host disease;[26] Fanconi's anaemia; following splenic irradiation[23] or Thorotrast administration[8])

splenic infiltration or replacement (amyloidosis,[42] sarcoidosis, leukaemia and lymphoma (occasionally), carcinoma[55] and sarcoma[103] (rarely),

reticuloendothelial overload (severe haemolytic anaemia or immune-complex diseases)

Fig. 9.35 *Some of the causes of hyposplenism.*

SOME CAUSES OF A NORMOCYTIC NORMOCHROMIC ANAEMIA	
Causative condition	**Morphological and other peripheral blood features which may sometimes be present and which may help in the differential diagnosis**
early iron deficiency*	a few hypochromic or microcytic cells may be present; RDW elevated
anaemia of chronic disease*	increased rouleaux, less often increased white cell count or platelet count, RDW often normal, elevated ESR
lead poisoning*	basophilic stippling, polychromasia
double deficiency of iron and either vitamin B_{12} or folic acid	hypersegmented neutrophils, increased RDW
bone marrow infiltration	may be leucoerythroblastic but this is not necessarily so, poikilocytosis, ESR often elevated
multiple myeloma	increased rouleaux, increased background staining, circulating plasma cells, elevated ESR
primary acquired*† sideroblastic anaemia	dimorphic, Pappenheimer bodies, other features of myelodysplasia (see below)
other myelodysplastic syndromes†	other cytopenias, hypogranular and pseudo-Pelger neutrophils, immature myeloid cells
paroxysmal nocturnal haemoglobinuria	other cytopenias — particularly neutropenia, low neutrophil alkaline phosphatase score
blood loss†	polychromasia subsequently develops, reticulocyte count becomes elevated, leucoerythroblastosis occurs only if the blood loss is acute and severe
renal failure	keratocytes, schistocytes
liver failure†	target cells, stomatocytes, other cytopenias
hypothyroidism†	acanthocytes
Addison's disease	neutropenia, monocytopenia, lymphocytosis, eosinophilia
hypopituitarism	as for Addison's disease
hyperparathyroidism[13]	nil
anorexia nervosa	acanthocytes, other cytopenias, poikilocytosis, basophilic stippling
pure red cell aplasia† (PRCA)	lack of polychromasia, reticulocytes infrequent or absent; in constitutional PRCA (Diamond–Blackfan syndrome) there is often a mild macrocytosis and the platelet count may be elevated at the onset; chronic acquired PRCA may be associated with chronic lymphocytic leukaemia (T or B cell) of a proliferation of large granular lymphocytes in which case a lymphocytosis will be present

* Anaemia may also be microcytic.
† Anaemia may also be macrocytic.

Fig. 9.36 *Some causes of a normocytic normochromic anaemia.*

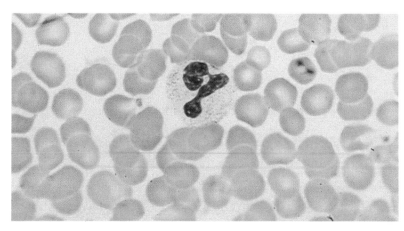

Fig. 9.37 A 'packed film' consequent on post-transplant polycythaemia. The haemoglobin was 20 g/dl and the PCV 0.59. The MCV was increased to 114 fl as a consequence of azathioprine therapy.

SOME CAUSES OF TRUE POLYCYTHAEMIA	
Primary	**Secondary**
polycythaemia rubra vera (primary proliferative polycythaemia) essential erythrocytosis	**increased oxygen affinity of haemoglobin** high affinity haemoglobins including some methaemoglobins and some cases of hereditary persistence of fetal haemoglobin deficiency of diphosphoglycerate mutase with consequent very low levels of 2,3 DPG (2,3 diphosphoglycerate) increasing the oxygen affinity of haemoglobin[87]
Secondary	
secondary to hypoxia residence at high altitude smoking chronic obstructive airways disease and other hypoxic lung diseases cyanotic heart disease hepatic cirrhosis (consequent on pulmonary arteriovenous shunting)[49] sleep apnoea and other hypoventilation syndromes including morbid obesity (Pickwickian syndrome) **secondary to inadequate oxygen-carrying capacity** chronic carbon monoxide poisoning chronic methaemoglobinaemia and sulphaemoglobinaemia (exogenous causes) congenital deficiency of NAD-linked or NADH-linked methaemoglobin reductase with consequent methaemoglobinaemia	**increased secretion of erythropoietin (proven or presumptive) other than due to hypoxia[45]** **renal lesions** renal carcinoma (hypernephroma), Wilms' tumour, renal adenoma, renal haemangioma, renal sarcoma, renal cysts including polycystic disease of the kidney, renal artery stenosis, post-transplant polycythaemia, hydronephrosis, horseshoe kidney,[20] nephrocalcinosis[41] cerebellar haemangioblastoma uterine fibroids hepatoma tumours of the adrenal gland, ovary, lung and thymus **familial erythrocytosis of either autosomal dominant[46] or autosomal recessive inheritance[1]** **androgen administration or androgen-secreting tumours in women, Cushing's syndrome, primary aldosteronism**

Fig. 9.38 Some of the causes of polycythaemia.

Certain features on the blood film are helpful in making a diagnosis of polycythaemia rubra vera. The total white cell count, neutrophil count and basophil count are elevated in the majority of cases; an elevation of the eosinophil and monocyte counts is less common. The elevated basophil count, when present, is of particular diagnostic importance since this is not associated with other causes of polycythaemia. The platelet count is elevated in the majority and platelet size may be increased; the red cells are often hypochromic and microcytic as the hyperplastic erythropoiesis has led to exhaustion of the iron stores. The neutrophil alkaline phosphatase score can be useful since it is usually elevated in polycythaemia rubra vera and is usually normal in secondary polycythaemia. A bone marrow aspiration and trephine biopsy is indicated when PRV is suspected; there is erythroid and usually megakaryocytic and granulocytic hyperplasia.

DIFFERENTIATION OF PRV FROM OTHER CAUSES OF POLYCYTHAEMIA

The blood film in patients with secondary polycythaemia sometimes shows features which are also seen in PRV but may show other features which are useful in the differential diagnosis. One of the commonest causes of a high haemoglobin concentration is heavy smoking, which can cause both a true polycythaemia and a reduction of plasma volume. Heavy smokers may have macrocytosis, neutrophilia, monocytosis and lymphocytosis; they do not have the marked basophilia and the thrombocytosis which can be features of polycythaemia rubra vera. Patients with chronic obstructive airways disease may have macrocytic red cells whereas in PRV red cells are normocytic or microcytic. A patient with polycythaemia apparently caused by heavy alcohol intake also had macrocytic red cells.[74] Thrombocytosis can occur in malignant disease including carcinoma of the kidney but in this case the platelets are small or normal in size as opposed to the large platelets which can be seen in PRV.

COMPLICATING FACTORS IN POLYCYTHAEMIA RUBRA VERA

Some patients with PRV present with anaemia due to complicating deficiency of vitamin B_{12} or folic acid. They are only diagnosed when replacement therapy is followed by a rise of the haemoglobin above the normal range. More commonly PRV presents with complicating iron deficiency causing the Hb and PCV to remain within normal limits (Fig. 9.39). The RBC is usually markedly elevated. The red cell indices may be very similar to those of thalassaemia trait except that the MCHC is likely to be low and the RDW to be elevated; thrombocytosis, neutrophilia and basophilia may also suggest that thalassaemia trait is not the correct diagnosis. It is important that the correct diagnosis should be made in such patients; they should not be given iron therapy which will render them overtly polycythaemic.

PRV may transform into myelofibrosis. A fall of the haemoglobin level and the development of

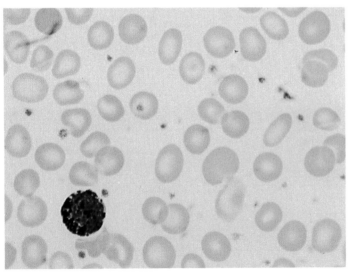

Fig. 9.39 The blood film of a patient with polycythaemia rubra vera complicated by iron deficiency, showing anaemia and thrombocytosis and some hypochromic and microcytic cells. The white cell is a basophil. The automated blood count (Coulter S Plus IV) was WBC 6.7 × 10⁹/l, RBC 4.38 × 10⁹/l, Hb 10.6 g/dl, PCV 0.328, MCV 75 fl, MCH 24.2 pg, MCHC 32.3 g/dl, RDW 24.9, platelet count 1056 × 10⁹/l.

leucoerythroblastic features and marked anisocytosis and poikilocytosis suggest that this complication is occurring. PRV may terminate in acute myeloblastic leukaemia with or without preceding myelofibrosis or myelodysplasia. In some cases the terminal acute leukaemia has been erythroleukaemia. The likelihood of acute leukaemia supervening is mugh higher in those who develop myelofibrosis.[34]

POLYCYTHAEMIA IN NEONATES
The healthy neonate has a much higher haemoglobin concentration than is found at any other period of life but neonates can also have polycythaemia with a number of aetiologies which are unique to this period of life. They include twin-to-twin transfusion, maternofetal transfusion and intrauterine hypoxia and growth retardation.

THROMBOCYTOSIS
Thrombocytosis refers to an increase in the platelet count above that expected in a healthy subject of the same age and sex. The term thrombocythaemia is usually restricted to a thrombocytosis which represents a myeloproliferative disorder; alternative designations are essential thrombocythaemia and essential thrombocytosis. Some of the causes of thrombocytosis are shown in Fig. 9.40.

ESSENTIAL THROMBOCYTHAEMIA
Thrombocythaemia is a myeloproliferative disorder consequent on a clonal proliferation of a multipotent stem cell but mainly manifest in the platelet lineage. Clinical features are mainly due to impaired flow in the microcirculation as a direct consequence of the thrombocytosis. Other clinical features, due to the myeloproliferation, are itch, splenomegaly and hepatomegaly. Splenomegaly is present in less than half and hepatomegaly in fewer still.[71]

The blood film shows thrombocytosis with giant platelets (Fig. 9.41). Some of the platelets can be hypogranular. Neutrophilia is present in about a third. The basophil count may be slightly elevated but is characteristically less than 3 percent.[71] Occasional nucleated red cells and occasional immature granulocytes can be present. The features of iron deficiency are quite common, usually indicating prior occult haemorrhage, but it should be noted that iron deficiency itself can cause thrombocytosis. The blood film features of hyposplenism are sometimes present and are indicative of prior

---

SOME CAUSES OF THROMBOCYTOSIS

Primary

essential thrombocythaemia (idiopathic or essential thrombocytosis)

chronic granulocytic leukaemia

myelofibrosis (early in the disease course)

polycythaemia rubra vera

myelodysplasia, particularly in the 5q− chromosome syndrome and in association with sideroblastic anaemia

acute megakaryoblastic leukaemia (some cases)[19]

myeloproliferative disorder associated with Down's syndrome

Secondary

response to infection

response to inflammation

response to haemorrhage

response to surgery and trauma

malignant disease

iron deficiency

rebound after alcohol withdrawal

rebound following treatment of megaloblastic anaemia

severe haemolytic anaemia (particularly after unsuccessful splenectomy)

adrenaline administration

vinca alkaloid administration

associated with vitamin E deficiency in premature infants[84]

associated with infantile cortical hyperostosis[79]

Redistributional

splenectomy and hyposplenism

Unknown mechanism

tidal platelet dysgenesis

Fig. 9.40 *Some of the causes of thrombocytosis.*

splenic infarction as a consequence of microvascular obstruction. The neutrophil alkaline phosphatase score is low in a small minority of patients; it is elevated in some patients and normal in the majority.[71]

Automated full blood counters show an increased mean platelet volume and platelet distribution width.

As with other myeloproliferative disorders essential thrombocythaemia may terminate in acute myeloid leukaemia, but this is quite uncommon. It may also terminate in myelofibrosis.

Other causes of thrombocytosis and their distinction from essential thrombocythaemia

Thrombocythaemia can usually be readily distinguished from chronic granulocytic leukaemia because of the characteristic features of the latter condition. However a small number of patients in whom the major disease manifestation is thrombocytosis are found to have the Ph' chromosome. Their prognosis is much worse than that of patients without the Ph' chromosome, with a high rate of development of acute myeloid leukaemia or overt chronic granulocytic leukaemia. They are therefore better regarded as a variant of chronic granulocytic leukaemia rather than as essential thrombocythaemia. A basophil count of 3 percent or higher has been found helpful in identifying these patients, but the neutrophil alkaline phosphatase score was not found to be useful since it was often not reduced.[71]

It can be difficult to distinguish between polycythaemia rubra vera which is complicated by iron deficiency to the extent of having a low or normal haemoglobin concentration (see Fig. 9.39) and thrombocythaemia with iron deficiency. Platelet size can be increased in both conditions but giant platelets are much commoner in thrombocythaemia. The estimation of total red cell volume following iron repletion will make the distinction, but this will complicate the management. It may well be possible to treat the patient effectively without distinguishing between these two diagnostic possibilities. The distinction between iron deficiency anaemia with thrombocytosis and essential thrombocythaemia is more straightforward. In the former condition platelet size is reduced rather than increased and there is no neutrophilia or basophilia. The platelet count returns to normal following iron therapy.

Myelodysplasia rather than thrombocythaemia is suggested by the coexistence, with the thrombocytosis, of other more common features of myelodysplasia; macrocytosis and thrombocytosis together suggest specifically the 5q− syndrome, the other characteristic feature of which is the presence of non-lobulated megakaryocytes in the bone marrow. The 5q− acquired chromosomal abnormality can also be associated with isolated thrombocytois.

Marked thrombocytosis can occur in idiopathic myelofibrosis but this condition is usually easily distinguished from essential thrombocythaemia on the basis on the more marked splenomegaly and the leucoerythroblastic blood film. Extreme thrombocytosis with counts as high as $3500–10\,000 \times 10^9/l$ has been

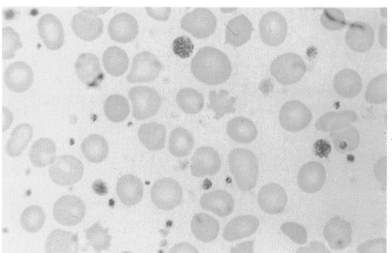

Fig. 9.41 The blood film of a patient with essential thrombocythaemia showing thrombocytosis with giant platelets; there is also red cell anisocytosis and poikilocytosis.

reported when idiopathic myelofibrosis terminates in a megakaryocytic leukaemia.[33]

Most patients with acute megakaryoblastic leukaemia have generalized pancytopenia. A minority have thrombocytosis with counts as high as 1000–1500 × 10^9/l.[19] This condition can be distinguished from thrombocythaemia by the presence of features of acute leukaemia such as anaemia or neutropenia or the presence of at least a small number of blasts in the peripheral blood. If there is any difficulty in the differential diagnosis a bone marrow aspirate and/or biopsy will allow the distinction.

The distinction between essential thrombocythaemia with prior splenic infarction, and thrombocytosis as a feature of hyposplenism is made mainly on the degree of elevation of the count. In hyposplenism *per se* the platelet count is usually of the order of 400–600 × 10^9/l, unless there is in addition a stimulus to increased platelet production, whereas in essential thrombocythaemia with complicating splenic infarction and atrophy the platelet count is likely to be well over 1000 × 10^9/l. In both these conditions platelet size is increased.

In most patients with reactive thrombocytosis the clinical features suggest the correct diagnosis, since most conditions capable of causing a significant thrombocytosis are readily apparent. When the differential diagnosis lies between thrombocythaemia and a reaction to malignancy or occult infection or inflammation the most helpful laboratory features are the degree of elevation of the platelet count and the size and morphology of the platelets. Counts of over 1500 × 10^9/l are rarely seen in reactive conditions. Counts over 1000 × 10^9/l for which there is no obvious explanation are also quite likely to be due to a myeloproliferative disorder; platelet counts of this level can occur in reactive conditions, for example, shortly after splenectomy or when there is very severe infection or inflammation, but in these patients the likely cause is usually readily apparent; this is not necessarily so when thrombocytosis is reactive to nonhaemopoietic malignancy. Occult malignancy can produce a very high platelet count, for example between 1000 and 1500 × 10^9/l.

The conditions found responsible for platelet counts of more then 900 × 10^9/l[51] and more than 1000 × 10^9/l[91] respectively in two studies have been tabulated in Fig. 9.42. It will be seen that haematological disorders, cancer, splenectomy and fever/inflammation were each responsible for between a fifth and a quarter

THE LIKELY CAUSES OF MARKEDLY ELEVATED PLATELET COUNTS		
	platelet count greater than 900 × 10^9/l[51]	platelet count greater than 1000 × 10^9/l[91]*
total number of patients	526	102
myeloproliferative or other haematological disorder	26%	28%
cancer	27%	24%
splenectomy	20%	40%
fever or inflammation	19%	30%
connective tissue disorder	9%	2%
lymphoma	–	21%
iron deficiency	–	4%
* In this series patients who had more than one possible cause of thrombocytosis have been tabulated under both possible causes.		

Fig. 9.42 *The likely causes of an elevated platelet count.*

SOME CAUSES OF THROMBOCYTOPENIA
(excluding conditions which usually cause pancytopenia)

FAILURE OF PLATELET PRODUCTION

Congenital
May-Hegglin anomaly
Bernard–Soulier syndrome
Epstein's syndrome (thrombocytopenia with deafness and renal disease)
other inherited thrombocytopenias, some with large platelets and some with platelets of normal size
megakaryocytic hypoplasia, inherited or due to intrauterine events
Fanconi's anaemia

Acquired
following marrow damage by some of the drugs which can cause aplastic anaemia or as the first manifestation of aplastic anaemia
myelodysplasia
severe iron deficiency
parvovirus infection (rarely)
thiazide administration
interferon therapy
paroxysmal nocturnal haemoglobinuria
acquired amegakaryocytic thrombocytopenia

INCREASED PLATELET DESTRUCTION OR CONSUMPTION

Immune mechanisms
Congenital
alloimmune thrombocytopenia in the newborn
immune thrombocytopenia in the newborn due to passively acquired maternal autoantibody
maternal drug hypersensitivity

Acquired
destruction of platelets by autoantibody
   primary: autoimmune thrombocytopenic purpura
   secondary: (associated with systemic lupus erythematosus,
      rheumatoid arthritis, chronic lymphocytic leukaemia, Hodgkin's disease, non-Hodgkin's lymphoma, sarcoidosis,[27]
      angioimmunoblastic lymphadenopathy)
drug-induced immune thrombocytopenia
postinfection thrombocytopenia, particularly after rubella, but also after other viral infections and vaccinations
immune thrombocytopenia associated with human immunodeficiency virus infection
post-transfusion purpura
anaphylaxis

Non-immune mechanisms

Congenital
The Schulman–Upshaw syndrome[92,110]

Acquired
disseminated intravascular coagulation
associated with microangiopathic haemolytic anaemia (including thrombotic thrombocytopenia purpura)
viral haemorrhagic fevers
Brazilian haemorrhagic fever (*Haemophilus aegyptis* infection)
other bacterial, viral and protozoan diseases
extracorporeal circulation and massive transfusion
Kaposi's sarcoma[107]
DDAVP therapy in type IIB Von Willebrand's disease[31]

REDISTRIBUTION OF PLATELETS

Congenital
hypersplenism

Acquired
hypersplenism (including acute sequestration in sickle cell disease)
hypothermia[75]

UNCERTAIN OR COMPLEX MECHANISMS

Congenital
congenital infections (toxoplasmosis, cytomegalovirus infection, rubella, syphilis, listeriosis, Coxsackie B infection, herpes virus infection)
associated with severe Rhesus haemolytic disease of the newborn
idiopathic hyperglycinaemia[113]
methylmalonic acidaemia[113]
isovaleric acidaemia[113]
Wiskott–Aldrich syndrome
the grey platelet syndrome
Chédiak–Higashi anomaly
cyclical thrombocytopenia and tidal platelet dysgenesis
Mediterranean macrothrombocytosis[50]
some cases of type IIB Von Willebrand's disease[31]

Acquired
neonatal herpes simplex infection
phototherapy[62]
alcohol-induced thrombocytopenia
heparin-induced thrombocytopenia
associated with cyanotic congenital heart disease
Graves' disease[54]

Fig. 9.43 *Some of the causes of thrombocytopenia.*

of counts showing thrombocytosis. When the platelet count exceeded 2000 × 10⁹/l the likelihood of a myeloproliferative disorder was very high: of 12 such cases two had essential thrombocythaemia and another nine other myeloproliferative disorders; three of the latter group had also been splenectomized.[91]

The platelet size is useful in the differential diagnosis of thrombocytosis since large platelets are observed in myeloproliferative disorders and in hyposplenic subjects, whereas patients with reactive thrombocytosis have small platelets. Measurements of platelet volume on automated instruments similarly demonstrate that in reactive conditions the mean platelet volume (MPV) falls as the platelet count rises so that the normal relationship is preserved; in myeloproliferative disorders the normal relationship between the MPV and platelet count is disturbed.[9] Observation of platelet morphology is likewise of use. The presence of hypogranular or agranular platelets, platelets of bizarre shape, or micromegakaryocytes suggests a myeloid stem cell disorder not a reactive condition. Basophilia is not seen in reactive thrombocytosis.

When the cause of thrombocytosis cannot be determined from the clinical history and examination of the blood film a bone marrow examination is indicated. Definitive diagnosis of essential thrombocythaemia requires not only examination of the bone marrow but also cytogenetic studies and, if the haemoglobin concentration is not unequivocally normal, estimation of total red cell volume.

THROMBOCYTOPENIA

Thrombocytopenia is a reduction of the platelet count below the level expected in a healthy subject of the same age and sex. It is possible that the normal range should also be adjusted for ethnic origin but it is not yet clear whether the lower levels observed in Blacks in comparison with Caucasians represent an ethnic variation or the presence of occult disease.

Thrombocytopenia may be congenital or acquired and may be due to reduced production, redistribution between the spleen and the circulating blood, or increased destruction, consumption or extravascular loss. Some of the causes of thrombocytopenia are shown in Fig. 9.43.

Congenital thrombocytopenia may represent an inherited condition or may be consequent on an infective agent or a toxin operating during intrauterine life. Congenital megakaryocytic hypoplasia is a very heterogeneous group of conditions. Some cases are inherited

and some are due to events during pregnancy such as rubella infection or exposure to thiazides or related drugs. Some cases are associated with chromosome defects, specifically with trisomy 13 and trisomy 18. Megakaryocytic hypoplasia can occur as an isolated anomaly or in association with absent radii (a relatively common association designated the TAR or thrombocytopenia with absent radii syndrome), absent ulnars and radii, absence of all long bones, anomalies of the digits, dyskeratosis congenita, congenital heart disease, microcephaly, micrognathia and renal defects. The very rare condition previously thought to result from defective platelet production and attributed to a deficiency of thrombopoietin is now thought to be due to diminished platelet survival.[92,110] Thrombocytopenia may be the first manifestation of Fanconi's anaemia; this disorder has been tabulated with the congenital conditions since the disease, although not the thrombocytopenia, is present at birth.

Acquired thrombocytopenia may similarly be due to failure of production, increased destruction or redistribution.

All unexpectedly low platelet counts should be verified on a blood film in order to exclude pseudothrombocytopenia due to platelet aggregation or satellitism. Having confirmed the thrombocytopenia consideration can be given to determining the cause of thrombocytopenia. The platelet size should first be assessed. Thrombocytopenia of many, but not all, aetiologies is associated with an increase in platelet size (Figs 9.44 and 9.45) as is shown in Fig. 3.62. Conversely, small platelets are seen in association with thrombocytopenia in the Wiskott–Aldrich syndrome (Fig. 9.46) and in bone marrow failure.

Measurements of platelet size on automated instruments have also been applied in the differential diagnosis of thrombocytopenia. It has been demonstrated that when the mechanism of thrombocytopenia is increased platelet destruction, as in autoimmune thrombocytopenic purpura, the electronically determined platelet size increases as the platelet count falls.[9] When thrombocytopenia is due to megaloblastic anaemia or bone marrow failure the platelet size is reduced so that the normal relationship between count and size is disturbed. The usefulness of automated measurements of platelet size is reduced by the fact that in many patients with severe thrombocytopenia the platelet sizes do not conform to a logarithmic distribution and the data is therefore rejected for computation of mean platelet volume.

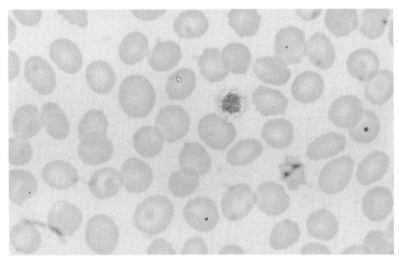

Fig. 9.44 The blood film of a patient with autoimmune thrombocytopenic purpura who has been splenectomized, showing postsplenectomy features and a single giant platelet.

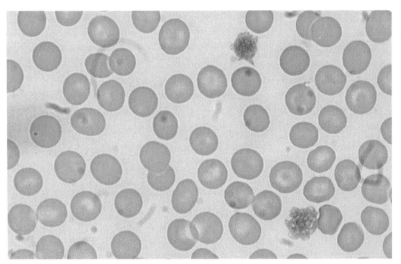

Fig. 9.45 The blood film of a patient with Bernard–Soulier syndrome showing two giant platelets.

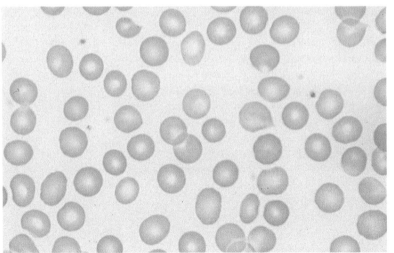

Fig. 9.46 The blood film of a patient with Wiskott–Aldrich syndrome showing thrombocytopenia and four quite small platelets.

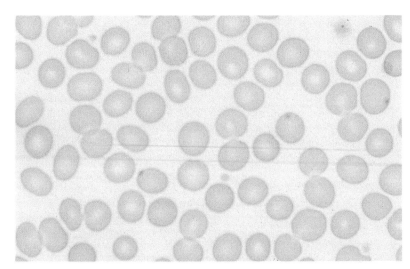

Fig. 9.47 The blood film of a patient with the grey platelet syndrome showing three agranular platelets[1]

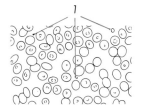

Platelet morphology has a limited application in the differential diagnosis of thrombocytopenia. In the grey platelet syndrome (Fig. 9.47), which sometimes is associated with thrombocytopenia, the platelets are agranular and therefore stain a pale blue or grey. Similarly agranular platelets are sometimes seen in hairy cell leukaemia and in myelodysplastic disorders.

Associated features can be important in suggesting the cause of thrombocytopenia. The presence of microangiopathic features suggests a certain range of diagnostic possibilities (see Fig. 9.30). The May–Hegglin anomaly can be diagnosed from the association between large platelets and the characteristic white cell inclusions (see Fig. 3.26). Myelodysplasia will usually have other features in the blood film. The presence of spherocytes suggests autoimmune thrombocytopenic purpura plus autoimmune haemolytic anaemia. The presence of lymphoma cells or the lymphocytes of chronic lymphocytic leukaemia with a thrombocytopenia disproportionate to the reduction of other cells suggests autoimmune destruction of platelets.

References

1. Adamson JW, Stamatoyannopoulos G, Kontras S, Lascari A & Detter J (1973) Recessive familial erythrocytosis. *Blood*, **41**, 641–652.
2. Agre P, Orringer EP, Chui DH & Bennett V (1981) A molecular defect in two families with hemolytic poikilocytic anaemia: reduction of high affinity membrane binding sites for ankyrin. *Journal of Clinical Investigation*, **68**, 1566–1576.
3. Austrin RF & Desforges JF (1969) Hereditary elliptocytosis: an unusual presentation of hemolysis in the new born associated with transient morphologic abnormalities. *Pediatrics*, **44**, 196–200.
4. Bain BJ (1988) Screening antenatal patients in a multiethnic community for β-thalassaemia trait. *Journal of Clinical Pathology*, **41**, 481–485.
5. Ballas SK, Larner J, Smith ED, Surrey S, Schwartz E & Rappaport EF (1987) The xerocytosis of SC disease. *Blood*, **69**, 124–128.
6. Becker PS & Lux SE (1985) Hereditary spherocytosis and related disorders. *Clinics in Hematology*, **14**, 15–44.
7. Ben-Bassat I, Brok-Simoni F, Kende G, Holtzmann F & Ramot B (1976) A family with red cell pyrimidine 5′-nucleotidase deficiency. *Blood*, **47**, 919–922.
8. Bensinger TA, Keller AR, Merrell LF & O'Leary DS (1971) Thorotrast-induced reticuloendothelial blockade. *American Journal of Medicine*, **51**, 663–668.
9. Bessman JD, Williams LJ & Gilmer PR (1982) Platelet size in health and disease. *American Journal of Clinical Pathology*, **78**, 150–153.

10. Bessman JD, Gilmer PR & Gardner FH (1983) Improved classification of the anemias by MCV and RDW. *American Journal of Clinical Pathology*, **80**, 322–326.

11. Bethlenfalvay NC, Hadnagy Cs & Heimpel H (1985) Unclassified type of congenital dyserythropoietic anaemia (CDA) with prominent peripheral erythroblastosis. *British Journal of Haematology*, **60**, 541–550.

12. Bogart L, Bonsignore J & Carvalho A (1986) Massive hemolysis following inhalation of volatile nitrites. *American Journal of Hematology*, **22**, 327–329.

13. Boxer M, Ellman L, Gillis R & Wang C-A (1977) Anemia in primary hyperparathyroidism. *Archives of Internal Medicine*, **137**, 588–590.

14. Brien WF, Mant MJ & Etches WS (1985) Variant congenital dyserythropoietic anaemia with ringed sideroblasts. *Clinical and Laboratory Haematology*, **7**, 231–237.

15. Brown RC, Blecher TE, French EA & Toghill PJ (1973) Thrombotic thrombocytopenic purpura and influenza vaccination. *British Medical Journal*, **2**, 303 (letter).

16. Brunning RD, Jacob HS, Brenckman WD, Jimenez-Pasquau F & Goetz FC (1976) Fragmentation haemolysis in patients with severe diabetic angiopathy. *British Journal of Haematology*, **34**, 283–289.

17. Bullen AW, Hall R, Gowland G, Rajah S & Losowsky MS (1981) Hyposplenism, adult coeliac disease and autoimmunity. *Gut*, **22**, 28–33.

18. Bunyaratvej A, Sahaphong S, Bhamarapravati N & Wasi P (1985) Quantitative changes in red blood cell shapes in relation to clinical features in β-thalassemia/hemoglobin E disease. *American Journal of Clinical Pathology*, **83**, 555–559.

19. Chan BWB, Flemans RJ & Sbinden G (1971) Acute leukemia with megakaryocytic predominance. *Cancer*, **28**, 1343–1349.

20. Clinicopathologic conference (1978) Erythrocytosis. *American Journal of Medicine*, **65**, 1007–1014.

21. Coetzer T, Lawler J, Prchal JT & Palek J (1987) Molecular determinants of clinical expression of hereditary elliptocytosis and pyropoikilocytosis. *Blood*, **70**, 766–772.

22. Corazzo GR & Gasbarrini G (1983) Defective splenic function and its relation to bowel disease. *Clinics in Gastroenterology*, **12**, 651–669.

23. Dailey MO, Coleman CN & Fajardo LF (1981) Splenic injury caused by therapeutic irradiation. *American Journal of Surgical Pathology*, **5**, 325–331.

24. Davidson RJ, How J & Lessels S (1977) Acquired stomatocytosis: its prevalence and significance in routine haematology. *Scandinavian Journal of Haematology*, **19**, 47–53.

25. Davis LR (1976) Changing blood picture in sickle-cell anaemia from shortly after birth to adolescence. *Journal of Clinical Pathology*, **29**, 898–901.

26. Demetrakopoulos GE, Tsokos GC & Levine AS (1982) Recovery of splenic function after GVHD-associated functional asplenia. *American Journal of Hematology*, **12**, 77–80.

27. Dickerman JD, Holbrook PR & Zinkham WH (1972) Etiology and therapy of thrombocytopenia associated with sarcoidosis. *Journal of Pediatrics*, **81**, 758–764.

28. Diggs LW & Bell A (1965) Intraerythrocytic hemoglobin crystals in sickle-cell hemoglobin C disease. *Blood*, **25**, 218–223.

29. Dillon AM, Stein HB & English RA (1982) Splenic atrophy in systemic lupus erythematosus. *Annals of Internal Medicine*, **96**, 40–43.

30. Djaldetti M, Cohen A & Hart J (1984) Elliptocytosis preceding myelofibrosis in a patient with polycythemia vera. *Acta Haematologica*, **72**, 26–28.

31. Donnér M, Holmberg L & Nilsson IM (1987) Type IIB Von Willebrand's disease with probable autosomal recessive inheritance and presenting as thrombocytopenia in infancy. *British Journal of Haematology*, **66**, 349–354.

32. Dozy AM, Kan YW, Embury SH, Mentzer WC, Wang WC, Lubin B, Davis JR & Koenig HM (1979) α-globin gene organization in blacks precludes the severe form of α-thalassaemia. *Nature*, **280**, 605–607.

33. Egner JR, Aabo D & Dimitrov NV (1982) Megakaryocytic leukaemia as a phase of myeloproliferative disorders. *Scandinavian Journal of Haematology*, **28**, 186–191.

34. Ellis JT, Peterson P, Geller SA & Rappaport H (1986) Studies of the bone marrow in polycythemia vera and the evolution of myelofibrosis and second hematologic malignancies. *Seminars in Hematology*, **23**, 144–155.

35. England JM & Fraser PM (1973) Differentiation of iron deficiency from thalassaemia trait by routine blood count. *Lancet*, **i**, 449–452.

36. England JM, Bain BJ & Fraser PM (1973) Differentiation of iron deficiency from thalassaemia trait *Lancet*, **i**, 1514 (letter).

37. Ervin DM, Christian RM & Young LE (1950) Dangerous universal donors. *Blood*, **5**, 553–567.

38. Falusi AG, Esan GJF, Ayyub H & Higgs DR (1987) Alpha-thalassaemia in Nigeria: its interaction with sickle-cell disease. *European Journal of Haematology*, **38**, 370–375.

39. Fairley S & Ihle BU (1986) Thrombotic microangiopathy and acute renal failure associated with arteriography. *British Medical Journal*, **293**, 922–933.

40. Farolino DL, Rustagi PK, Currie MS, Doeblin TD & Logue GL (1986) Teardrop-shaped red cells in autoimmune hemolytic anemia. *American Journal of Hematology*, **21**, 415–418.

41. Feest TG, Proctor S, Brown R & Wrong ON (1978) Nephrocalcinosis: another cause for renal erythrocytosis. *British Medical Journal*, **ii**, 605.

42. Gertz MA, Kyle RA & Greipp PR (1983) Hyposplenism in primary systemic amyloidosis. *Annals of Internal Medicine*, **98**, 475–477.

43. Glader BE, Propper RD & Buchanan GR (1979) Microcytosis associated with sickle cell anaemia. *American Journal of Clinical Pathology*, **72**, 63–64.

44. Gordon LI, Kwaan HC & Rossi EC (1987) Deleterious effects of platelet transfusions and recovery thrombocytosis in patients with thrombotic microangiopathy. *Seminars in Hematology*, **24**, 194–201.

45. Hammond D & Winnick S (1974) Paraneoplastic erythrocytosis and ectopic erythropoietins. *Annals of the New York Academy of Science*, **230**, 219–227.

46. Hellmann A, Rotoli B, Cotes PM & Luzzatto L (1983) Familial erythrocytosis with overproduction of erythropoietin. *Clinical and Laboratory Haematology*, **5**, 335–342.

47. Hoffbrand AV & Pettit JE (1987) *Clinical Haematology Illustrated.* Edinburgh: Churchill Livingstone; London: Gower Medical Publishing.

48. Ho-Yen DO (1984) Hereditary spherocytosis presenting in pregnancy. *Acta Haematologica*, **72**, 29–33.

49. Hutchinson DCS, Sapru RP, Sumerling MD, Donaldson GWK & Richmond J (1968) Cirrhosis, cyanosis and polycythemia: multiple pulmonary arteriovenous anastomoses. *American Journal of Medicine*, **45**, 139–151.

50. Jackson JM, Stanley ML, Crawford IG, Barr AL & Hilton HB (1978) The problem of Mediterranean stomatocytosis. *Australian and New Zealand Journal of Medicine*, **8**, 216–217 (Abstr).

51. Jones MJ & Pierre RV (1981) The causes of extreme thrombocytosis. *American Journal of Clinical Pathology*, **76**, 349 (Abstract).

52. Jordan WS, Prouty RL, Heinle RW & Dingle JH (1952) The mechanism of hemolysis in paroxysmal cold hemoglobinuria. *Blood*, **7**, 387–403.

53. Kevy SV, Tefft M, Vawter GF & Rosen FS (1968) Hereditary splenic hypoplasia. *Pediatrics*, **42**, 752–757.

54. Kurata Y, Nishiõeda Y, Tadahiro T & Kitani T (1980) Thrombocytopenia in Graves' disease: effect of T_3 on platelet kinetics. *Acta Haematologica*, **63**, 185–190.

55. Kurth D, Deiss A & Cartwright GE (1969) Circulating siderocytes in human subjects. *Blood*, **34**, 754–764.

56. Kwaan HC (1987) Miscellaneous secondary thrombotic microangiopathy. *Seminars in Hematology*, **24**, 141–147.

57. Lachant NA (1987) Hemoglobin E: an emerging hemoglobinopathy in the United States. *American Journal of Hematology*, **25**, 449–462.

58. Larrimer JH, Mendelson DS & Metz EN (1975) Howell–Jolly bodies. A clue to splenic infarction. *Archives of Internal Medicine*, **135**, 857–858.

59. Leblond PF, Lyonnais J & Delage J-M (1978) Erythrocyte populations in pyruvate kinase deficiency anaemia following splenectomy. *British Journal of Haematology*, **39**, 55–61.

60. Lock SP, Smith RS & Hardisty RM (1961) Stomatocytosis: a hereditary red cell anomaly associated with haemolytic anemia. *British Journal of Haematology*, **7**, 303–314.

61. Marsh WL, Bishop JW & Darcy TP (1987) Evaluation of red cell volume distribution width (RDW). *Hematologic Pathology*, **1**, 117–123.

62. Maurer HM, Fratkin M, McWilliams NB, Kirkpatrick D, Draper D, Haggins JC & Hunter CR (1976) Effects of phototherapy on platelet counts in low-birthweight infants and on platelet production and life span in rabbits. *Pediatrics*, **57**, 506–512.

63. Mazza V, Saglio G, Cappio FC, Camaschella C, Neretto G & Gallo E (1976) Clinical and haematological data in 254 cases of beta-thalassaemia trait in Italy. *British Journal of Haematology*, **33**, 91–99.

64. McCann SR, Firth R, Murray N & Temperley IJ (1980) Congenital dyserythropoietic anaemia type II (HEMPAS): a family study. *Journal of Clinical Pathology*, **33**, 1197–1201.

65. Mears JG, Lachman HM, Labie D & Nagel RL (1983) Alpha-thalassaemia trait is related to prolonged survival in sickle cell anaemia. *Blood*, **62**, 286–290.

66. Mentzer WC (1973) Differentiation of iron deficiency from thalassaemia trait. *Lancet*, **i**, 882 (letter).

67. Mentzer WC, Turetsky T, Mohandas N, Schrier S, Wu C-Sc & Koenig H (1984) Identification of the hereditary pyropoikilocytosis carrier state. *Blood*, **63**, 1439–1446.

68. Miller DR, Rickles FR, Lichtman MA, La Celle PL, Bates J & Weed RI (1971) A new variant of hereditary hemolytic anemia with stomatocytosis and erythrocyte cation abnormality. *Blood*, **38**, 184–204.

69. Monplaisir N, Merault G, Poyart C, Rhoda MD, Craescu CT, Vidaud M, Galacteros Y, Blouquit Y & Rosa J (1987) Hb S-Antilles ($\alpha_2\beta_2$Glu→Val, 23Val→Ile): a new variant with lower solubility than Hb S and producing sickle cell disease in heterozygotes. *Acta Haematologica*, **78**, 222 (Abstr).

70. Morlé L, Garbarz M, Alloisio N, Girot R, Chaveroche I, Boivin P & Delaunay J (1985) The characterization of protein 4.1 Presles, a shortened variant of RBC membrane protein 4.1 *Blood*, **65**, 1511–1517.

71. Murphy S, Iland H, Rosenthal D & Laszlo J (1986) Essential thrombocythemia: an interim report from the Polycythemia Vera Study Group. *Seminars in Hematology*, **23**, 177–182.

72. Newman P, Muir A & Parker AC (1980) Non-spherocytic haemolytic anaemia in mother and son associated with hexokinase deficiency. *British Journal of Haematology*, **46**, 537–547.

73. Nishiura T, Miyazaki Y, Oritani K, Tominaga N, Tomiyama Y, Katagiri S, Kanayama Y, Yonezawa T, Tarui S, Yamada T, Sakurai M, Kume H & Okudaira M (1986) *Aspergillus* vegetative endocarditis complicated with schizocytic hemolytic anemia in a patient with acute lymphocytic leukemia. *Acta Haematologica*, **76**, 60–62.

74. O'Brien H, Elliot PJ & Amess JAL (1981) Alcohol and relative polycythaemia. *Lancet*, **ii**, 987 (letter).

75. O'Brien H, Amess J & Mollin DL (1982) Recurrent thrombocytopenia, erythroid hypoplasia and sideroblastic anaemia associated with hypothermia. *British Journal of Haematology*, **51**, 451–456.

76. Paré PD, Chan-Yan C, Wass H, Hooper R & Hogy JC (1983) Portal and pulmonary hypertension with microangiopathic hemolytic anemia. *American Journal of Medicine*, **74**, 1093–1096.

77. Peto TEA, Pippard MJ & Weatherall DJ (1983) Iron overload in mild sideroblastic anaemia. *Lancet*, **1**, 375–378.

78. Pettit JE, Scott J & Hussein S (1976) EDTA-dependent red. cell neutrophil rosetting in autoimmune haemolytic anaemia. *Journal of Clinical Pathology*, **29**, 345–346.

79. Pickering D & Cuddigam B (1969) Infantile cortical hyperostosis associated with thrombocythaemia. *Lancet*, **ii**, 464–465.

80. Polliack A & Rachmilewitz EA (1973) Ultrastructural studies in β-thalassaemia major. *British Journal of Haematology*, **24**, 319–326.

81. Pryor DS & Pitney WR (1967) Hereditary elliptocytosis: a report of two families from New Guinea. *British Journal of Haematology*, **13**, 126–134.

82. Rauch AE, Tartaglia AP, Kaufman B & Kausel H (1984) RBC fragmentation and thymoma. *Archives of Internal Medicine*, **144**, 1280–1282.

83. Rieder RF & Bradley TB (1968) Hemoglobin Gun Hill: an unstable protein associated with chronic hemolysis. *Blood*, **32**, 355–369.

84. Ritchie JH, Fish MB, McMasters V & Grossman M (1968) Edema and hemolytic anemia in premature infants. A vitamin E deficiency syndrome. *New England Journal of Medicine*, **279**, 1185–1190.

85. Riggs SA, Wray NP, Waddell CC, Rossen RG & Gyorkey F (1982) Thrombotic thrombocytopenic purpura complicating Legionnaires' Disease. *Archives of Internal Medicine*, **142**, 2275–2280.

86. Rodin AE, Sloan JA & Nghiem QX (1972) Polysplenia with severe congenital heart disease and Howell–Jolly bodies. *American Journal of Clinical Pathology*, **58**, 127–134.

87. Rosa R, Prehu M-O, Beuzard Y & Rosa J (1978) The first case of a complete deficiency of diphosphoglycerate mutase in human erythrocytes. *Journal of Clinical Investigation*, **62**, 907–915.

88. Ryan FP, Smart RC, Holdsworth CD & Preston FE (1978) Hyposplenism in inflammatory bowel disease. *Gut*, **19**, 50–55.

89. Salyer WR, Salyer DC & Heptinstall RH (1973) Scleroderma and microangiopathic hemolytic anemia. *Annals of Internal Medicine*, **78**, 895–897.

90. Sansone G (1978) A new type of congenital dyserythropoietic anaemia. *British Journal of Haematology*, **39**, 537–543.

91. Schilling RF (1980) Platelet millionaires. *Lancet*, **ii**, 372–373 (letter).

92. Schulman I, Pierce M, Lukens A & Currmbhoy Z (1960) Studies on thrombopoiesis I. A factor in normal human plasma required for platelet production, chronic thrombocytopenia due to its deficiency. *Blood*, **16**, 943–957.

93. Seip M, Gjessing LR & Lie SO (1971) Congenital sideroblastic anaemia in a girl. *Scandinavian Journal of Haematology*, **8**, 505–512.

94. Serjeant GR & Serjeant BE (1972) A comparison of erythrocyte characteristics in sickle cell syndromes in Jamaica. *British Journal of Haematology*, **23**, 205–213.

95. Serjeant GR (1974) *The clinical features of sickle cell disease*. Amsterdam: North Holland Publishing Company.

96. Serjeant GR, Sommereux A, Stevenson M, Mason K & Serjeant BE (1979) Comparison of sickle cell-β⁰ thalassaemia with homozygous sickle cell disease. *British Journal of Haematology*, **41**, 83–93.

97. Serjeant GR, Grandison Y, Lowrie Y, Mason K, Phillips J, Serjeant BE & Vaidya S (1981) The development of haematological changes in homozygous sickle cell disease: a cohort study from birth to 6 years. *British Journal of Haematology*, **48**, 533–543.

98. Serjeant GR, Serjeant BE, Forbes M, Hayes RJ, Higgs DR & Lehmann H (1986) Haemoglobin gene frequencies in the Jamaican population: a study in 100,000 newborns. *British Journal of Haematology*, **64**, 253–262.

99. Sheehan RG & Frenkel EP (1983) Influence of hemoglobin phenotype on the mean erythrocyte volume. *Acta Haematologics*, **69**, 260–265.

100. Shilo S, Werner D & Hershko C (1985) Acute hemolytic anemia caused by severe hypophosphatemia in diabetic ketoacidosis. *Acta Haematologica*, **73**, 55–57.

101. Shine I & Lal S (1977) A strategy to detect β thalassaemia trait. *Lancet*, **i**, 692–694.

102. Srivastava PC (1973) Differentiation of thalassaemia minor from iron deficiency. *Lancet*, **i**, 154–155.

103. Steinberg MH, Gatling RR & Tavassoli M (1983) Evidence of hyposplenism, in the presence of splenomegaly. *Scandinavian Journal of Haematology*, **31**, 437–439.

104. Stewart GW, O'Brien H, Morris SA, Owen JS, Lloyd JK & Ames JAL (1987) Stomatocytosis, abnormal platelets and pseudohomozygous hypercholesterolaemia. *European Journal of Haematology*, **38**, 376–380.

105. Sugihara T, Miyashima K & Yawata Y (1984) Disappearance of microspherocytes in peripheral circulation and normalization of decreased lipids in plasma and in red cells in patients with hereditary spherocytosis after splenectomy. *American Journal of Hematology*, **17**, 129–139.

106. Tchernia G, Mohandas N & Shohet SB (1981) Deficiency of skeletal membrane protein band 4.1 in homozygous hereditary elliptocytosis. Implications for erythrocyte membrane stability. *Journal of Clinical Investigation*, **68**, 454–460.

107. Turnbull A & Almeyda J (1970) Idiopathic thrombocytopenic purpura in Kaposi's sarcoma. *Proceedings of the Royal Society of Medicine*, **63**, 603–605.

108. Turner RC, Chaplinski TJ & Adams HG (1986) Rocky Mountain Spotted Fever presenting as thrombotic thrombocytopenic purpura. *American Journal of Medicine*, **81**, 153–157.

109. Tzotzos S, Kanavakis E, Metaxotou-Mavromati A & Kattamis C (1986) The molecular basis of haemoglobin H disease in Greece. *British Journal of Haematology*, **63**, 263–271.

110. Upshaw JD (1978) Congenital deficiency of a factor in normal plasma that reverses microangiopathic hemolytic anemia. *New England Journal of Medicine*, **298**, 1350–1352.

111. Wardrop CAJ, Dagg JH, Lee FD, Sing H, Dyet JF & Moffatt A (1975) Immunological abnormalities in splenic atrophy. *Lancet*, **ii**, 4–7.

112. Weatherall DJ & Clegg JB (1981) *The thalassaemia syndromes*. Oxford: Blackwell Scientific Publications.

113. Willoughby MLN (1977) *Paediatric Haematology*. Edinburgh: Churchill Livingstone.

114. Wislöff F & Boman D (1979) Acquired stomatocytosis in liver disease. *Scandinavian Journal of Haematology*, **23**, 43–50.

115. Zarkowsky HS, Oski FA, Sha'afi R, Shohet SB & Nathan DG (1968) Congenital hemolytic anemia with high sodium, low potassium red cells. I Studies of membrane permeability. *New England Journal of Medicine*, **278**, 573–581.

116. Zarkowsky HS, Mohandas N, Speaker CB & Shohet SB (1975) A congenital haemolytic anaemia with thermal sensitivity of erythrocyte membranes *British Journal of Haematology*, **29,** 537–543.

117. Zauber NP & Echikson AB (1982) Giant cell arteritis and microangiopathic hemolytic anemia. *American Journal of Medicine*, **73,** 928–930.

Index